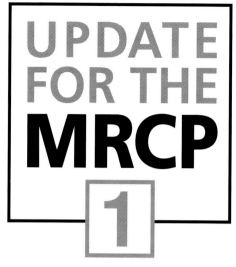

UPDATE FOR THE MRCP 1

SECOND EDITION

Edited by

Miles Witham BM BCh MRCP
Clinical Research Fellow, Section of Ageing and Health,
Ninewells Hospital and Medical School, Dundee

Timothy Gray MA MB BChir MRCP
Specialist Registrar in Cardiology,
Manchester Royal Infirmary, Manchester

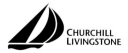

CHURCHILL
LIVINGSTONE

EDINBURGH   LONDON   NEW YORK   OXFORD   PHILADELPHIA   ST LOUIS   SYDNEY   TORONTO 2003

CHURCHILL LIVINGSTONE
An imprint of Elsevier Science Limited

First edition 1996
Second edition 2003

First edition by T. Andrews, P. Arlett, B. Brett and R. Jones

ISBN 0 443 07333 3

British Library Cataloguing in Publication Data
A catalogue record for this book is available from the British Library

Library of Congress Cataloging in Publication Data
A catalog record for this book is available from the Library of Congress

Notice
Medical knowledge is constantly changing. Standard safety precautions
must be followed, but as new research and clinical experience broaden
our knowledge, changes in treatment and drug therapy may become
necessary or appropriate. Readers are advised to check the most
current product information provided by the manufacturer of each drug to
be administered to verify the recommended dose, the method and
duration of administration, and contraindications. It is the responsibility of
the practitioner, relying on experience and knowledge of the patient, to
determine dosages and the best treatment for each individual patient.
Neither the Publisher nor the editors assumes any liability for any injury
and/or damage to persons or property arising from this publication.
The Publisher

The
publisher's
policy is to use
**paper manufactured
from sustainable forests**

Typeset by IMH(Cartrif), Loanhead, Scotland
Printed in China

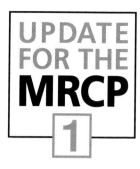

Commissioning Editor: Laurence Hunter
Project Development Manager: Hannah Kenner
Project Manager: Nancy Arnott
Designer: Erik Bigland

Preface

Revising for the MRCP examinations is never easy. Keeping up to date with key advances across the broad sweep of medicine while working in busy medical jobs is even harder. The previous editions of *Update for MRCP* successfully enabled many people to combine these two difficult tasks. Time and medical knowledge move on, and, in this new edition, we hope that we have succeeded in capturing a representative sample of the important advances that have occurred in medicine over the last few years.

The MRCP examination has itself undergone a metamorphosis in the last couple of years and the format of the book has changed in line with the changes in the examination. We have tried to balance the proportion of true/false and best-of-five-style questions in line with the part 1 MRCP exam; the proportion of questions asked in each field roughly parallels those asked in the examination as well. We have also reformatted the viva questions to bring them into line with the PACES examination format.

We hope that you find this book valuable, not only in keeping you one step ahead of the examiners, but we also hope that you find it useful in your everyday clinical practice – we wish you the best of luck.

Miles Witham
Timothy Gray

Contributors

Gavin Barlow MB ChB MRCP DTM&H
Specialist Registrar in Infectious Disease, Ninewells Hospital and Medical School, Dundee

Denise Braganza BSc MB ChB MRCP
Specialist Registrar in Cardiology, Addenbrooke's Hospital, Cambridgeshire

Ewen Cameron MA MB BChir MRCP
Specialist Registrar in Gastroenterology, Ipswich Hospital, Suffolk

Menna Clatworthy BSc MBBCh MRCP
Renal Registrar, Addenbrooke's Hospital, Cambridgeshire

Vicky Cleak MB ChB MRCPsych Dip
Specialist Registrar in Psychiatry, Royal South Hampshire Hospital, Southampton

Graeme Currie MB ChB MRCP DCH
Clinical Research Fellow, Asthma and Allergy Research Group, Ninewells Hospital and Medical School, Dundee

Justine Davies MB ChB MRCP
Clinical Lecturer in Clinical Pharmacology, Ninewells Hospital and Medical School, Dundee

Clare Galton MB BChir MRCP MD
Specialist Registrar in Neurology, Addenbrooke's Hospital, Cambridgeshire

Timothy Gray MA MB BChir MRCP
Specialist Registrar in Cardiology, Manchester Royal Infirmary, Manchester

Catherine Jury MB ChB MRCP
Specialist Registrar in Dermatology, Department of Dermatology, Monklands Hospital, Airdrie

Duncan McNab MB BS MPhil
Cardiology Research Fellow, Papworth Hospital, Cambridgeshire

Andrea Waring MB ChB MRCP
Clinical Lecturer in Medicine and Specialist Registrar in Rheumatology, Ninewells Hospital and Medical School, Dundee

Miles Witham BM BCh MRCP
Clinical Research Fellow, Section of Ageing and Health, Ninewells Hospital and Medical School, Dundee

Contents

Questions

ENDOCRINOLOGY
True/False questions

1. **Acromegaly**

   A 36-year-old woman presents with headache, thirst, polyuria and a gradual increase in her shoe size. MRI of the brain demonstrates a pituitary tumour 1.5 cm in diameter. Which of the following are true?

   A. IGF-1 can be used as a marker of her disease activity
   B. Pegvisomant could cause regression of her tumour
   C. Pegvisomant is an IGF-1 antagonist
   D. Cabergoline is now licensed for use in pregnancy
   E. She has a 6% chance of having multiple endocrine neoplasia type 1

2. **Thiazolidinediones in diabetes**

   A 45-year-old woman with type 2 diabetes is started on a thiazolidinedione by the diabetes clinic. Which of the following are true?

   A. Thiazolidinediones work by inhibition of the PPAR-γ receptor
   B. Thiazolidinediones act to reduce insulin resistance in muscle
   C. Thiazolidinediones are contraindicated in chronic heart failure
   D. Her liver function tests should be checked regularly
   E. Thiazolidinediones are indicated as add-on therapy to insulin

3. **Type 1 diabetes**

   A 16-year-old girl attends the diabetic clinic after recovering from diabetic ketoacidosis. Her parents accompany her with a list of statements that they have found on the internet. Which of them are true?

   A. Islet cell transplantation can obviate the need for exogenous insulin
   B. Continuous insulin pumps are proven to reduce the risk of myocardial infarction
   C. Insulin glargine is a short-acting insulin for use at mealtimes
   D. Brittle diabetes is due to sudden drops in the amount of insulin produced by the pancreas
   E. GAD antibodies are a good test to predict diabetes before it becomes clinically apparent

4.   **Thyroid function tests**

Regarding TSH:

A. High levels of β-hCG can stimulate the TSH receptor
B. Elevated TSH within the normal range is a marker of shortened life expectancy in older people
C. TSH testing is sufficient to detect secondary hypothyroidism
D. Low TSH levels can persist for months after successful treatment of thyrotoxicosis
E. TSH might be raised in the early stages of acute psychosis

5.   **Autoimmune polyendocrinopathy**

You see a young boy with hypoparathyroidism in the endocrinology clinic. His mother has been researching the condition and is concerned that he will develop autoimmune polyendocrinopathy syndrome type 1 (APS-1). Which of the following are true?

A. Hyperthyroidism is a common manifestation
B. You could test for the disease by probing for mutations in the APS gene on chromosome 16
C. Chronic mucocutaneous candidiasis is a characteristic part of the syndrome
D. Close monitoring for signs of Addison's disease is important
E. 5% of patients need pneumococcal vaccine

Best-of-5 questions

6.   **Obesity**

A 46-year-old woman with a history of hypertension attends your clinic. She is concerned about her weight as, despite having lost 4 kg over the last 2 months with help from her GP, she still weighs 86 kg. Her height is 1.55 m.
What is the best prescription for her?

A. Orlistat
B. Sibutramine
C. Orlistat plus exercise
D. Diet
E. Sibutramine plus diet

7.   **Diabetes therapy**

A 55-year-old man with type 2 diabetes has an HbA1c of 9.6%. His pre-meal glucostix readings are consistently below 7. He is currently taking 850 mg of metformin three times a day.
What would you add next to his existing therapy?

A. Glibenclamide
B. Repaglinide
C. A long-acting insulin
D. Insulin lispro
E. Rosiglitazone

8. **Hypertension in diabetes**

A 62-year-old woman has type 2 diabetes and a blood pressure of 165/83. This is the third occasion that her blood pressure has been elevated. Her creatinine is normal and she has no microalbuminuria. Which class of antihypertensive is most appropriate?

A. An ACE inhibitor
B. A thiazide
C. A dihydropyridine calcium channel blocker
D. A beta-blocker
E. Any of the above

9. **Hypercortisolaemia**

A 49-year-old woman presents with weight gain, hypertension, hirsutism and pigmented abdominal striae. She has a grossly elevated 24-h urinary cortisol. What would be your next test to ascertain the cause of the elevated cortisol?

A. CT of the adrenal glands
B. Adrenal scintigraphy
C. ACTH levels
D. Low-dose dexamethasone suppression test
E. High-dose dexamethasone suppression test

10. **The Barker hypothesis**

Which of the following statements best describes the Barker hypothesis?

A. Obesity in childhood is a risk factor for cardiovascular disease in adulthood
B. Exposure to multiple childhood infections is protective against autoimmune disease, including diabetes
C. Restricted growth in utero predisposes to impaired glucose tolerance and cardiovascular disease in adulthood
D. Exposure to high levels of glucose in utero changes the 'set point' for glycaemic control in adulthood, leading to impaired glucose tolerance and cardiovascular disease
E. Maternal hypertension predisposes the fetus to changes in vascular tone, leading to hypertension in adulthood

PACES questions

At the history-taking station you see a patient with a history of surgically treated acromegaly. The examiners ask 'What new medical treatments are available for acromegaly?' (*See* Answer 1)

At the history-taking station, you see a patient with diabetes who is taking glitazones. The examiners ask you 'What are the potential problems with glitazone therapy?' (*See* Answer 2)

You are taken to see a woman with signs of hypothyroidism. The examiners ask 'What do you think about using TSH as a sole screening test for hypothyroidism?' (*See* Answer 4)

At the ethics station, an obese woman demands one of the new 'fatbuster' drugs that she has read about in her weekly magazine. How do you go about counselling her? (*See* Answer 6)

At the history-taking station, you see a diabetic patient who is taking repaglinide. The examiners ask 'Tell us about postprandial hyperglycaemia and how you might go about treating it' (*See* Answer 7)

After the history-taking station, where you saw a diabetic patient with poorly controlled hypertension, the examiners ask 'If you were a diabetic patient with hypertension, which drug would you want as first-line therapy?' (*See* Answer 8)

You are taken to see a 46-year-old woman. She has moon facies, a buffalo hump, centripetal obesity, abdominal striae and a blood pressure of 165/100. The examiners ask 'How would you investigate this woman?' (*See* Answer 9)

RESPIRATORY

True/False questions

11.   Asthma

A 19-year-old student with asthma complains of nocturnal symptoms and peak flow variability while maintained on low-dose beclometasone. With regard to his current treatment and possible additional therapy:

A. Leukotriene receptor antagonists demonstrate both anti-inflammatory and bronchodilatory properties in vivo
B. Beclometasone dipropionate is a prodrug
C. Fluticasone propionate is more lipophilic than beclometasone dipropionate
D. Hydrofluoroalkane preparations of beclometasone dipropionate require to be given at twice the dose of chlorofluorocarbon formulations to ensure equivalent efficacy
E. Tolerance to the bronchoprotective properties of long-acting β_2-agonists is more marked than tolerance to their bronchodilatory properties

12.   Bronchial carcinoma

A 54-year-old smoker with cryptogenic pulmonary fibrosis of 10 years duration presents with haemoptysis and an abnormal chest X-ray. With respect to her likely diagnosis of bronchial carcinoma:

A. Finger clubbing is less common in small cell than squamous cell carcinoma
B. PET scanning has not been shown to increase the detection rate of local or distant metastasis
C. Cryptogenic fibrosing alveolitis is not an independent risk factor in its aetiology
D. Hypokalaemic alkalosis is associated with small cell bronchial carcinoma
E. Providing FEV_1 > 1.5 L, surgery should be performed in most patients presenting with small cell carcinoma

13.   Non-invasive ventilation

Non-invasive ventilation:

A. Should normally be avoided in patients with type II respiratory failure and GCS≤ 8
B. Is of no use in patients with cardiogenic pulmonary oedema
C. Is of benefit in weaning patients from mechanical ventilation
D. With bilevel support does not allow the recruitment of the underventilated lung
E. Is associated with a favourable outcome when the respiratory rate, but not acidosis, is reduced after 1 h

14.   Inflammation and asthma

In the pathogenesis, evaluation and management of asthma:

A. Type 1 helper T cells have a major role in the promotion of inflammation
B. Interleukin 5 is a proinflammatory cytokine
C. Normal spirometry precludes the diagnosis
D. Allergic rhinitis coexists in up to 40% of patients
E. Montelukast is useful as monotherapy in preventing exercise-induced bronchoconstriction

15.   Obstructive sleep apnoea

Regarding obstructive sleep apnoea syndrome:

A. The prevalence is high in patients with Marfan's syndrome
B. A body mass index < 25 virtually excludes the diagnosis
C. Nasal continuous positive pressure ventilation therapy improves cognitive function but does not reduce daytime somnolence
D. Individuals with Down syndrome are not predisposed to its development
E. The prevalence is approximately 16–20% of the middle-aged population

Best-of-5 questions

16.   **Chronic obstructive pulmonary disease**

A 60-year-old man who smokes 25 cigarettes a day complains of increasing breathlessness and wheeze. Spirometry reveals moderate airflow obstruction. His GP diagnoses chronic obstructive pulmonary disease. Which one of the following statements regarding his condition is true?

A. Most patients should undergo yearly pneumococcal and influenza immunisation
B. Up to 20% of patients demonstrate objective reversibility following a corticosteroid trial
C. Inhaled corticosteroids reduce the annual rate of decline in FEV_1 in most patients
D. Cigarette smoking increases the half-life of oral theophylline
E. In the provision of long-term oxygen therapy, oxygen should be used for up to 12 h per day to achieve maximum benefit

17.   **Primary pulmonary hypertension**

A 52-year-old woman, diagnosed as having primary pulmonary hypertension, demonstrates a positive response to acute vasodilator testing. Which one of these statements best describes her condition?

A. Familial cases tend to be transmitted in an autosomal dominant pattern of inheritance
B. The responsible gene has been localised to chromosome 7
C. Vasodilator testing should be reserved for patients with severe disease
D. Therapy with intravenous epoprostenol (prostacyclin) should now be instituted in view of the positive vasodilator response
E. Warfarin should be avoided unless pulmonary thromboembolism has been documented in the past

18.   **Community-acquired pneumonia**

A previously fit 50-year-old smoker is admitted to hospital with bilateral chest X-ray changes suggestive of community-acquired pneumonia. Which one of the following statements best describes his condition?

A. *Streptococcus pneumoniae* has been replaced by *Haemophilus influenzae* as the most frequent pathogen causing community-acquired pneumonia
B. Both a urea of < 4 mmol/L and systolic blood pressure < 90 mmHg are recognised adverse prognostic features
C. An associated parapneumonic effusion should normally be treated conservatively
D. Levofloxacin has good activity against *Streptococcus pneumoniae*
E. Cold agglutinin production occurs in approximately 5–10% of individuals with community-acquired pneumonia caused by *Mycoplasma pneumoniae*

19.   Tuberculosis

A 32-year-old man with HIV infection is diagnosed as having pulmonary tuberculosis. Which one of the following statements is true?

A. Visual acuity should be tested prior to commencement of pyrazinamide
B. Ethambutol is not necessary in conjunction with rifampicin, isoniazid and pyrazinamide
C. The clinical course of HIV is likely to be altered
D. Notification of pulmonary tuberculosis is no longer a statutory requirement
E. Care should be taken with isoniazid, as hepatic enzyme induction can reduce the efficacy of antiretroviral therapy

20.   Pulmonary embolism

A 28-year-old woman, using oral contraceptives, is admitted with suspected pulmonary thromboembolism. In the aetiology, diagnosis and management of thromboembolic disease, which one of these statements is true?

A. Third-generation oral contraceptives have a lower risk of venous thromboembolism than second-generation preparations
B. A negative D-dimer assay virtually excludes the diagnosis of pulmonary thromboembolism
C. Spiral CT angiography is not useful in detecting proximal pulmonary artery emboli
D. Unfractionated heparins demonstrate a superior safety and efficacy profile over low-molecular-weight heparins
E. Thrombolysis is contraindicated in pulmonary thromboembolism with systolic hypotension

PACES questions

At the history-taking station, you see a 30-year-old woman with chronic, difficult-to-control asthma. The examiners ask you 'How could you limit the amount of inhaled corticosteroid this woman has to take?' (*See* Answer 11)

At the history-taking station, you see a 57-year-old man with moderately severe COPD. The examiners ask 'What alternatives are there to intubation for patients with severe exacerbations of COPD?' (*See* Answer 13)

You see a 24-year-old man with asthma at the history-taking station. He is taking salbutamol, budesonide and montelukast. The examiners ask 'How does montelukast work?' (*See* Answer 14)

At the history-taking section, you see a very obese man with daytime somnolence, headaches, poor concentration and apnoeic attacks at night. The examiners ask 'What treatments are available for his condition?' (*See* Answer 15)

In the respiratory section, you examine a 60-year-old man with wheeze, a barrel chest, tar-staining of his fingers and reduced chest expansion. He breathes with pursed lips. The examiners ask 'Are steroids of any benefit in his condition? What other drugs besides bronchodilators are known to be useful in his condition?' (*See* Answer 16)

At the history-taking section, you see a woman with a diagnosis of primary pulmonary hypertension. The examiners ask 'What treatments are available for her condition?' (*See* Answer 17)

At the ethics station, you see a young man who is HIV positive. He presented with cough, fever and weight loss, and tubercle bacteria were found in his sputum. The examiners ask 'Explain to this man how you propose to treat him.' (*See* Answer 19)

DERMATOLOGY

True/False questions

21.   Psoriasis

Regarding psoriasis:

A. It arises due to an abnormality in the keratinocyte population
B. The Koebner phenomenon is pathognomonic of psoriasis
C. Type 2 T helper cells are important in the development of psoriasis
D. Antibodies to TNFα can be useful in the management of psoriasis
E. Ciclosporin has a direct effect on keratinocytes

Best-of-5 questions

22.   Pigmented lesions

A 36-year-old man attends with a lesion on his back. The lesion has been present since infancy and is 2 cm in diameter, darkly pigmented with a warty texture and coarse surface hair. He has recently noticed a prominent nodular portion in its centre. What is the most appropriate next step?

A. Thorough examination. If he has other similar lesions he can be reassured
B. Excise the entire lesion
C. Photograph the lesion and review in 4 months
D. Excise the nodular portion
E. Refer for laser resurfacing

23.   **Management of psoriasis**

A 34-year-old woman has been attending the dermatology clinic for many years. She has chronic plaque psoriasis unresponsive to topical treatment and has received high doses of UVB and UVA in the form of PUVA. Associated with her skin disease she has significant involvement of her wrists and distal interphalangeal joints. What is the most sensible next treatment?

A. Methotrexate
B. Ciclosporin
C. Acitretin (systemic retinoid)
D. Mycophenolate mofetil
E. Infliximab

24.   **Eczema**

Regarding the investigation and management of adult atopic eczema, which of the following statements is most appropriate?

A. Food allergy is a common exacerbating factor
B. Radioallergosorbent testing is helpful in identifying potential allergens
C. Sunlight can be an exacerbating factor
D. Strict housedust-mite avoidance should be encouraged
E. Topical steroid allergy is a common problem

25.   **Pruritus**

A 55-year-old woman presents with the following symptoms and signs – pruritus, recurrent oral candidiasis and a plaque of thin, yellow telangiectatic skin on the right shin. What investigation is most appropriate?

A. Full blood count
B. Serum glucose
C. Thyroid function test
D. Anti-nuclear factor
E. Urea and electrolytes

26.   **Chronic venous ulceration**

A 69-year-old woman attends your clinic with a chronic venous ulcer above her medial malleolus. Despite several months of compression bandaging, it has not healed. Her ankle brachial pressure indices are normal, as is her fasting glucose, and biopsy shows no evidence of malignancy or vasculitis.
    Which is the best additional treatment option?

A. Intermittent pneumatic compression
B. Pentoxifylline (oxpentifylline)
C. Zinc
D. Laser therapy
E. Hydrocolloid dressings

PACES questions

At the dermatology station, you are shown a woman with large psoriatic plaques over her extensor surfaces. The examiners ask 'What treatments are available for psoriasis that proves resistant to topical therapy and ultraviolet light therapy?' (*See* Answers 21 and 23)

At the dermatology station, you are shown a young woman with an excoriated eczematous rash. The examiners ask 'What factors are implicated in the development of adult eczema?' (*See* Answer 24)

CLINICAL PHARMACOLOGY

True/False questions

27. Angiotensin II receptor blockers

Regarding angiotensin II receptor blockers:

A. Losartan mediates its effects by inhibition of angiotensin at the AT_2 receptor
B. Angiotensin II receptor blockers are superior to ACE inhibitors in the treatment of diabetic nephropathy
C. The combination of an angiotensin II receptor blocker and an ACE inhibitor should not be used in diabetic patients with microalbuminuria
D. Losartan is as good as atenolol at reducing the incidence of myocardial infarction in patients with hypertension
E. Valsartan reduces mortality in patients with heart failure

28. Botulinum toxin

Regarding botulinum toxin:

A. Botulism is caused by the bacterium *Clostridium botulinum* and is an ascending paralysis that often affects the autonomic nervous system
B. *Clostridium botulinum* produces a neurotoxin that irreversibly blocks the release of acetylcholine
C. Botulinum toxin is a recognised treatment for strabismus
D. Botulinum toxin is injected around the affected muscles for clinical benefit
E. Botulinum toxin has no effect on overactive smooth muscles

29. Leptin

The following statements are correct concerning leptin in humans:

A. Serum leptin levels follow a diurnal pattern
B. Leptin inhibits OB-Rb receptors in the hypothalamus
C. Leptin is necessary for sexual maturation
D. Leptin levels fall out of proportion to fat mass during fasting and exercise programmes
E. Overfeeding decreases leptin concentrations

30.   Potassium

A patient with chronic heart failure is admitted in ventricular tachycardia and is found to have a potassium level of 2.8. Which of the following statements are true?

A. Hypokalaemia increases the risk of digoxin toxicity by suppressing renal digoxin excretion
B. A low potassium level improves endothelial function
C. Magnesium should not be given to this patient
D. In patients with heart failure on diuretic therapy, hypokalaemia is not related to mortality
E. This patient is at a lower risk of stroke than if his potassium was normal

31.   Cocaine use

Which of the following statements are true regarding cocaine use?

A. Cocaine increases noradrenaline (norepinephrine) reuptake in sympathetic nerve terminals
B. Cocaine use is not addictive
C. Cocaine users are at risk of myocardial infarction due to coronary artery vasospasm
D. Cocaine binds to dopamine and noradrenaline (norepinephrine) transport proteins, but not to serotonin transport proteins
E. The addictive effect of cocaine is mediated through the dopaminergic pathway

32.   Endothelial function

Regarding endothelial function:

A. Endothelial dysfunction is commonly associated with an increase in local nitric oxide production
B. The degree of endothelial dysfunction as assessed by arterial vasodilator response to acetylcholine is predictive of future cardiac events in hypertensive patients
C. Endothelial function in the peripheral arteries bears no relationship to that assessed in the coronary arteries
D. ACE inhibitor therapy does not improve endothelial function
E. Von Willebrand factor is elevated in states of endothelial dysfunction

33.   Endothelin

The following are true of endothelin:

A. Endothelin acts in an autocrine manner
B. Endothelin is an exclusive vasoconstrictor
C. Endothelin is released in response to adrenaline (epinephrine)
D. In pulmonary hypertension, treatment with the endothelin antagonist bosentan improves exercise capacity
E. Endothelin 1 triggers the release of nitric oxide

34. Complementary medicine

A patient with diabetes and hypertension presents to your clinic and asks your opinion regarding alternative therapies. Which of the following statements are correct?

A. Guar gum is useful in diabetes because it promotes the absorption of metformin
B. Yohimbine is a useful therapy for erectile dysfunction
C. Garlic is a useful therapy to prevent platelet-related bleeding
D. Yohimbine does not cause hypertension
E. Guar gum is able to chelate bile acids

35. Drugs and surgery

In patients undergoing surgery:

A. Ginkgo biloba increases the risk of bleeding
B. Cannabis is a useful treatment for nausea
C. Angiotensin converting enzyme inhibitors can be given by the intravenous route
D. β-blockers decrease the risk of death after vascular surgery
E. Withdrawal of cardiovascular medicines for up to 2 days postoperatively is associated with a negligible risk of cardiovascular complications

36. Drugs of abuse

Regarding drugs of abuse:

A. γ-hydroxybutyrate is a CNS depressant
B. Chronic usage of γ-hydroxybutyrate does not lead to dependency
C. Withdrawal of γ-hydroxybutyrate is associated with autonomic instability
D. Flunitrazepam is a slow- to medium-acting benzodiazepine
E. Disseminated intravascular coagulation is a recognised side-effect of amfetamine abuse

Best-of-5 questions

37. Bupropion (amfebutamone)

Which one of the following is true regarding smoking cessation using bupropion (amfebutamone)?

A. Smoking cessation using bupropion (amfebutamone) is commonly associated with weight gain
B. It should be started 2 days before the patient intends to quit
C. Serotonin reuptake inhibition is the main mechanism of action of bupropion (amfebutamone)
D. Treatment with bupropion (amfebutamone) is contraindicated in patients with epilepsy
E. 40% of bupropion (amfebutamone) is excreted unchanged in the urine

38.   Oxidative stress and antioxidants

Which one of the following statements is true?

A. Low-density lipoprotein particles that are small and dense are less prone to oxidation
B. Long-term treatment with antioxidant vitamins worsens endothelial function
C. High-dose vitamin E treatment is associated with a lower risk of cardiovascular disease in patients receiving haemodialysis
D. Vitamin E therapy is equivalent to fish oil in the secondary prevention of cardiovascular disease
E. In patients with a normal cholesterol, a combination of antioxidants is as good as simvastatin at reducing cardiovascular mortality

39.   COX II inhibitors

A 67-year-old man who is taking rofecoxib for osteoarthritis is admitted with 2 h of chest pain. His ECG shows 1 mm of ST depression in the inferior leads. Which of the following treatment combinations is most suitable for him?

A. Continue rofecoxib, start low-molecular-weight heparin
B. Stop rofecoxib, start aspirin and low-molecular-weight heparin
C. Continue rofecoxib, start aspirin, clopidogrel and low-molecular-weight heparin
D. Stop rofecoxib, start aspirin, clopidogrel and low-molecular-weight heparin
E. Stop rofecoxib, start clopidogrel and low-molecular-weight heparin

40.   Hypertension

Which one of the following statements is true regarding hypertension?

A. Carvedilol is not an appropriate antihypertensive for a patients with peripheral vascular disease
B. Cerebral oedema starts to develop at mean arterial pressures above 120 mmHg
C. Systolic blood pressure should be reduced gradually to below 130 mmHg in a patient with aortic dissection
D. ACE inhibitors are better than calcium channel blockers at preventing stroke
E. Hypertensive encepholopathy is associated with characteristic posterior leucoencephalopathy on MRI

41.   Acute mountain sickness

Which of the following are true regarding acute mountain sickness?

A. The risk of acute mountain sickness is directly proportional to altitude
B. The speed of ascent is of lesser importance than altitude in calculating the risk of acute mountain sickness
C. Furosemide (frusemide) is a worthwhile therapy for the prevention of acute mountain sickness

D. Dexamethasone 8–16 mg is beneficial for the prevention of acute mountain sickness

E. Signs of pulmonary oedema are necessary for the diagnosis of acute mountain sickness

PACES questions

At the history-taking station, you see a patient with a history of hypertension who has the criteria for left ventricular hypertrophy on his ECG. The examiners ask 'Would you start a beta-blocker or an angiotensin II receptor blocker?' (*See* Answer 27)

At the history-taking station, you see an obese, 45-year-old woman with type 2 diabetes. The examiners ask 'What role does leptin play in obesity?' (*See* Answer 29)

At the history-taking station, you see a 56-year-old man with a history of hypertension and type 2 diabetes. He sustained a myocardial infarction several months ago. The examiners ask 'What role does endothelial dysfunction play in this man's cardiovascular disease?' (*See* Answer 32)

At the history-taking station, you see a man with hypertension and peripheral vascular disease. He is due to have a femoral–popliteal bypass graft in a couple of weeks time. He currently takes aspirin, amlodipine and ginkgo biloba tablets. The examiners ask 'What changes to his medication regime would you suggest before he has surgery?' (*See* Answer 35)

At the ethics station, you see a man with angina who smokes 20 cigarettes per day. He is known to be a heavy drinker. He has read about the new wonder drug bupropion (amfebutamone), and wants you to prescribe this for him. How would you go about counselling him? (*See* Answers 37 and 46)

At the history-taking station, you see a woman with a history of cardiac failure, two previous myocardial infarctions and hypertension. The examiners ask 'Is there any evidence that vitamin supplements would be of benefit to this woman?' (*See* Answer 38)

PSYCHIATRY

True/False questions

42.   Alcohol dependency

Regarding alcohol dependency:

A. A history of withdrawal symptoms is required before a diagnosis of alcohol dependency can be made
B. Long-term exposure to alcohol is associated with an increase in GABA benzodiazepine receptor function
C. Depression in the context of alcohol dependency will often resolve with abstinence alone
D. Without treatment, the peak incidence of delirium tremens is at 72 h following abstinence
E. It is safe for patients to continue taking acamprosate even if they relapse with their drinking

43.   St John's wort

Regarding St John's wort (*Hypericum perforatum*):

A. It has tricyclic antidepressant properties
B. It has more side-effects than placebo
C. It is a potent inhibitor of hepatic enzymes
D. When used by patients with HIV who are taking indinavir, it may lead to drug resistance
E. It has been shown to be equally efficacious when compared with tricyclic antidepressants in moderate depression

44.   Chronic fatigue syndrome

Regarding chronic fatigue syndrome (myalgic encephalomyelitis):

A. The onset of chronic fatigue syndrome in childhood has a worse prognosis than onset in adulthood
B. Past psychiatric history is a risk factor
C. The number needed to treat for cognitive behavioural therapy in chronic fatigue syndrome is two
D. 'Pacing' of activities has been shown to be effective in clinical trials.
E. Antidepressants are a useful treatment for chronic fatigue syndrome

45.   Delirium

Which of the following are true in cases of delirium?

A. It is commonly misdiagnosed as depression on the general ward
B. Warfarin, digoxin and theophylline have sufficient anticholinergic activity to produce delirium in the elderly
C. Benzodiazepines are the treatment of choice in delirium that is not related to alcohol or substance abuse
D. The patient will have a relatively intact long-term memory but a poor short-term memory
E. Deafness decreases the risk of delirium

46.   Nicotine addiction

Regarding nicotine addiction:

A. Tolerance to nicotine occurs within a few days of starting to smoke
B. Buproprion (amfebutamone) is a less effective alternative treatment than nicotine patches
C. Part of the addictive quality of nicotine is because administration leads to the release of dopamine in the nucleus ambiguus
D. Flu-like symptoms are a recognised side-effect of nicotine patches
E. Simple advice given by doctors during routine care significantly increases the quit rate

Best-of-5 questions

47.   Psychosis

A 36-year-old man with a history of psychotic depression and cannabis misuse presents to the accident and emergency department with a 1-day history of generalised muscle stiffness, pyrexia and sweating. On examination, he is tachycardic with a blood pressure of 150/100 and rigidity in all four limbs. There is a lowered level of consciousness and he is unable to give much of a history, although his mother tells you that he takes lithium regularly and was started on risperidone by his GP a week ago as some psychotic symptoms had recurred. Which of the following tests is most important and would be diagnostic for his underlying condition?

A. White cell count
B. Lumbar puncture
C. Creatinine phosphokinase
D. Blood culture
E. Urinary drug screen

48.   Lithium toxicity

Which one of the following indicates lithium toxicity?

A. Coarse tremor
B. Polyuria
C. Vomiting
D. T-wave inversion on the ECG
E. Hypothyroidism

49.   Psychiatric drugs and weight gain

You are asked to see a 48-year-old obese Asian lady in the outpatient department. She has a recent diagnosis of type 2 diabetes as well as a long-standing diagnosis of schizoaffective disorder. Which one of the following medications is most likely to be significantly contributing to her weight gain?

A. Haloperidol
B. Olanzapine
C. Fluoxetine

D. Zopiclone
E. Carbamazepine

50.   Depression in older people

Which of the following is more likely to indicate depression in older people compared with a younger age group?

A. Suicidal thoughts
B. Hypochondriasis
C. Loss of interest or pleasure in things
D. Poor self care
E. Insomnia

51.   Dementia

Mr B is a 69-year-old male who is brought to accident and emergency in an ambulance. He has a 3-year history of dementia and has been cared for by his wife, who is having increasing difficulty coping with his behaviour. Mr B is troubled by visual hallucinations and examination reveals bruises from recurrent falls. His GP prescribed a low-dose neuroleptic to help with the hallucinations but this has led to severe parkinsonian features.

What is the most likely cause of his dementia?

A. Alzheimer's disease
B. Lewy body disease
C. Vascular disease
D. Alcohol
E. Frontotemporal dementia

PACES questions

You see a patient with signs of alcoholic liver disease at the abdominal station. The examiners ask 'What pharmacological therapy is available to help this man abstain from alcohol?' (*See* Answer 42)

At the ethics station, you see a 50-year-old mother whose daughter has been diagnosed with chronic fatigue syndrome. She wants to know what the treatment options are. Your task is to explain the treatment options to her. (*See* Answer 44)

At the history-taking station, you see an obese diabetic woman with a history of schizophrenia, for which she takes olanzapine. The examiners ask 'What medication could she be changed to in order to help her obesity?' (*See* Answer 49)

At the neurology station, you examine a man with tremor and rigidity in his upper limbs, worse on the right. You are told that his abbreviated Mental Test Score is 4/10. The examiners ask 'What is your differential diagnosis for his low mental test score?' (*See* Answer 51)

MISCELLANEOUS

True/False questions

52.   Visual impairment in older people

Which of the following statements are true?

A. Screening asymptomatic older people for early visual loss can lead to improvements in vision
B. The outcome of cataract surgery is as good in older people as it is in younger people
C. Latanoprost is a useful alternative to beta-blockers in older people with glaucoma
D. Macular degeneration is less common in patients who take statins
E. Vitamin E is not effective in retarding macular degeneration

53.   Thyroid eye disease

Which of the following statements are true regarding thyroid eye disease?

A. Radioiodine therapy for Graves' disease is associated with a lower incidence of thyroid eye disease than surgery
B. Steroids can reduce the incidence of thyroid eye disease seen after radioiodine therapy
C. Most thyroid eye disease does not require surgical intervention
D. Severe thyroid eye disease is more likely in younger patients and in women
E. Surgical intervention is required only if there are signs of optic nerve compromise

Best-of-5 questions

54.   Sexually transmitted diseases

A 26-year old male patient is admitted to an acute medical admissions unit with a febrile illness, a maculopapular rash, generalised lymphadenopathy and erosive oral lesions. There is a history of a painless penile ulcer, now healed, some weeks previously.
    What is the likely causative organism?

A. *Haemophilus ducreyi*
B. Herpes-simplex virus
C. *Treponema pertenue*
D. *Treponema pallidum*
E. *Calymmatobacterium granulomatis*

55.   Driving and the DVLA

In which of the following cases would a patient not be required to inform the Driving and Vehicle Licensing Agency (DVLA) of their medical condition?

A. Non-insulin dependent diabetes mellitus controlled by tablets
B. A diagnosis of Parkinson's disease without serious impairment
C. A diagnosis of Ménière's disease
D. A history of unstable angina
E. Following implantation of a pacemaker

PACES questions

At the ethics station, you see a patient who sustained a stroke a few months ago, leaving him with a left homonymous hemianopia. Despite this, he continues to drive and has not informed the DVLA of his condition, despite medical advice to do so. What do you do? (*See* Answer 55)

INFECTIOUS DISEASES

True/False questions

56.   Antibiotic resistance

Which of the following statements are true?

A. *Streptococcus pyogenes* is always sensitive to penicillin
B. Exposure to a third-generation cephalosporin is an important risk factor for colonisation with vancomycin-resistant enterococci
C. Ciprofloxacin resistance in salmonella is a recognised phenomenon
D. Common helminthic infections are often resistant to therapy
E. Uncomplicated urinary tract infections in females should be treated with short-course (3-day) antibiotic therapy

57.   Influenza

The following are true of influenza infection:

A. The duration of illness can be reduced by an inhaled haemagglutinin inhibitor
B. Vaccination should be avoided in HIV-positive patients
C. Bacteraemia is a common finding in patients admitted to the intensive care unit with influenza pneumonia
D. Amantadine has activity against influenza B virus
E. Patients admitted to an acute health care setting with suspected or confirmed infection should be isolated

58.   Lyme disease

A 45-year-old woman is admitted several days after receiving a tick bite whilst walking in the woods. She complains of a rash, arthritis and a low-grade fever. Serology for Lyme disease is positive.
    Which of the following are true:

A. Lyme disease is caused by the spirochaete *Borrelia recurrentis*
B. Acrodermatitis chronica atrophicans is the early dermatological hallmark
C. Rheumatological manifestations in Europe are less common than in the USA
D. Doxycycline for 14–21 days is an acceptable first-line regimen for early disease
E. A transient Jarisch–Herxheimer reaction can occur in some patients after commencing antibiotic therapy

59.   The systemic inflammatory response syndrome

The following parameters are consistent with one of the criteria used to assess the systemic inflammatory response syndrome:

A. Systolic BP < 90 mmHg and/or diastolic BP ≤ 60 mmHg
B. Urea > 7.0 mmol/L
C. Respiratory rate > 16/min
D. White cell count < 4.0×10^9/L or > 12×10^9/L
E. Temperature < 36°C or > 38°C

60.   Microbes, cancer and chronic diseases

Development of the following diseases has been associated with the stated microbe:

A. Kaposi's sarcoma and human herpesvirus 6
B. Nasopharyngeal carcinoma and cytomegalovirus
C. Hepatocellular carcinoma and hepatitis E virus
D. Adult T-cell leukaemia and human T-cell lymphotropic virus type 1
E. Anal carcinoma and human papillomavirus

61.   Severe sepsis and protein C

In severe sepsis:

A. Pro-inflammatory cytokines stimulate coagulation by the release of tissue factor from monocytes and vascular endothelium
B. Protein C levels are elevated in the majority of patients
C. Interleukin-6 levels are reduced in the majority of patients
D. Mortality can be reduced by administering an activated protein C infusion
E. Protein C promotes fibrinolysis and inhibits thrombosis

62.   Viral infections in pregnancy

The following viral infections occurring in pregnancy can have clinically significant fetal consequences:

A. Hand, foot and mouth disease
B. Parvovirus B19
C. Epstein–Barr virus
D. Cytomegalovirus
E. Varicella zoster virus

Best-of-5 questions

63. **Infection in the homeless and intravenous drug users**

A 23-year-old heroin user is admitted to hospital with severe sepsis associated with an area of pain, severe inflammation and oedema over the left thigh. A friend mentions that he had been 'popping' (injecting heroin into skin or muscle) at this site. A number of similar cases have been reported recently from other local hospitals. What is the most likely causal organism?

A. *Bacillus anthracis*
B. *Actinomyces israelii*
C. *Listeria monocytogenes*
D. *Clostridium novyi*
E. *Nocardia asteroides*

64. **Anthrax**

A traveller, recently returned from the USA, is admitted to hospital with influenza-like symptoms and signs of severe sepsis. The following morning the blood culture is found to contain 'anthrax-like organisms'. Which of the following intravenous antibiotics would be most appropriate?

A. Doxycycline
B. Benzylpenicillin
C. Ceftriaxone
D. Ciprofloxacin
E. Piperacillin and tazobactam

65. **Arboviruses**

A backpacker, recently returned from an overland trip through sub-Saharan Africa, presents with a febrile illness, jaundice and a significantly elevated aspartate aminotransferase. Which of the following is least likely to be the cause?

A. Leptospirosis
B. West Nile fever
C. Hepatitis E
D. Acute hepatitis B
E. Yellow fever

66. **Meningococcal disease**

A 21-year-old university student is admitted to hospital with a short history of an influenza-like illness, a progressive purpuric rash and a Glasgow Coma Score of 8. Which of the following investigations is it essential to perform for an early microbiological diagnosis?

A. Meningococcal serology
B. Bacterial throat swab
C. Blood culture
D. CSF analysis
E. Urinary meningococcal antigen

PACES questions

At the history-taking station, you are presented with a patient who has recently recovered from an episode of MRSA bacteraemia. The examiners ask 'What are the potential sources of this infection and are you are aware of any new treatments for MRSA?' (*See* Answer 56)

At the neurological station, you are presented with a 35-year-old female with unilateral facial nerve palsy thought to be due to Lyme disease. The examiners ask 'What treatment would you recommend?' (*See* Answer 58)

At the history-taking station, you are presented with a 54-year-old male who has recently recovered from Gram-negative sepsis. In the subsequent discussion, the examiners ask 'On admission to hospital, what objective criteria would you have used to assess the severity of this man's illness?' (*See* Answer 59)

At the dermatology station, you are presented with a 33-year-old male with several dark papules and plaques over his trunk. You make a correct diagnosis of Kaposi's sarcoma. As you walk to the next case the examiners ask 'What therapy might be available for that patient?' (*See* Answer 60)

At the history-taking station, you are presented with a 26-year-old homeless male who is currently being treated for tuberculosis. He has previously injected drugs. The examiners ask 'What other infections might this patient be at risk of and what preventative measures could be employed?' (*See* Answer 63)

At the history-taking station, you are presented with a traveller who has recently been admitted to the regional infection unit with malaria. The examiner asks 'When travelling, what precautions against malaria could this person have taken, other than chemoprophylaxis?' (*See* Answer 65)

At the history-taking station, you are presented with a 23-year-old female who has recently recovered from meningococcal disease. In the subsequent discussion, the examiner asks you 'What are the recommendations for meningococcal prophylaxis in healthcare staff?' (*See* Answer 66)

GASTROENTEROLOGY
True/False questions

67.   *Helicobacter pylori*

Regarding *Helicobacter pylori*:

A. Interleukin 1 beta is a potent inhibitor of gastric acid secretion
B. Duodenal ulceration is associated with pangastritis
C. Polymorphisms in the interleukin 1 beta gene are associated with gastric cancer
D. *Helicobacter pylori* infection occurs only within the stomach
E. *Helicobacter pylori* infection is associated with increased levels of somatostatin

68.   Pancreatic cancer

Regarding pancreatic cancer:

A. 75% of pancreatic cancers are caused by smoking
B. 40% of pancreatic cancers are operable at diagnosis
C. Patients with hereditary non-polyposis colorectal cancer are at increased risk of pancreatic cancer
D. Pancreatic cancer surveillance is effective in reducing mortality in individuals with a family history of pancreatic cancer
E. Pancreatic cancer is associated with germline mutations in *BRCA2*

69.   Microsatellite instability in colorectal cancer

Microsatellite instability:

A. Is more common in hereditary non-polyposis colorectal cancer than in sporadic colorectal cancer
B. Hereditary non-polyposis colorectal cancer is usually due to mutations in *hPMS1* and *hPMS2*
C. In sporadic colorectal cancer, microsatellite instability is usually due to mutations in mismatch repair genes
D. Can be caused by hypermethylation of the promoter regions of mismatch repair genes
E. Is found in 15% of sporadic colorectal cancers

70.   Non-alcoholic steatohepatitis

In non-alcoholic steatohepatitis:

A. Elevated ferritin and transferrin saturation in a patient with non-alcoholic steatohepatitis imply coexistent hereditary haemochromatosis
B. Biopsies from patients with cryptogenic cirrhosis frequently show signs of coexistent non-alcoholic steatohepatitis
C. Treatment of non-alcoholic steatohepatitis with statins often results in histological improvement
D. Liver biopsy is indistinguishable from alcoholic hepatitis
E. The prevalence of bacterial overgrowth is high

71.   **Genetics of inflammatory bowel disease**

Which of the following are true with regards to the genetics of Crohn's disease?

A. The genetic contribution to type I diabetes mellitus is greater than to Crohn's disease
B. Siblings of patients with Crohn's disease have a 5 times greater risk of developing the disease than individuals in the general population
C. Polymorphisms within the *NOD2* gene reduce an individual's risk of developing Crohn's disease.
D. Crohn's disease is not associated with the *IBD2* gene
E. Mutations in the *NOD2* gene are associated with an increased risk of ileal Crohn's disease

Best-of-5 questions

72.   **Screening for colorectal cancer**

A patient at normal risk of colorectal cancer attends clinic asking for advice regarding screening. Although not currently available in the UK, which of the following is proven to reduce colorectal cancer mortality?

A. Once-only barium enema aged 55
B. Once-only colonoscopy aged 55
C. Biennial faecal occult blood testing
D. Once-only flexible sigmoidoscopy aged 45
E. Annual digital rectal examination

73.   **Oesophageal cancer**

A 50-year-old man is diagnosed with oesophageal adenocarcinoma of the lower third of the oesophagus. Which investigation would be most useful to assess operability of this tumour?

A. Endoscopy
B. Endoscopic ultrasound
C. CT scan
D. PET scanning
E. Chest X-ray

74.   **Crohn's disease**

Which of the following is the most appropriate treatment for a patient with newly diagnosed severe active Crohn's disease?

A. Infliximab
B. Mesalazine
C. Prednisolone
D. Azathioprine
E. Methotrexate

75.   Familial adenomatous polyposis (FAP)

A 30-year-old patient presents to clinic having been told that his brother has been diagnosed with FAP at age 22. Which is the most straightforward test to establish whether this patient is also a gene carrier?

A. Colonoscopy
B. APC gene mutation analysis
C. Faecal occult blood testing
D. Flexible sigmoidoscopy
E. Fundoscopy

76.   Hepatitis C virus

A 35-year-old woman is seen in clinic with chronic hepatitis C infection. Which one test is most important in determining whether she should be offered combination therapy with interferon and ribavirin?

A. Viral genotype
B. Liver biopsy
C. Viral polymerase chain reaction
D. Level of transaminases
E. Mode of infection

PACES questions

At the history-taking section, you see an obese man with a history of liver disease. He tells you that his doctors are unsure of the diagnosis but think that there is a lot of fat in his liver. The examiners ask 'What is non-alcoholic steatohepatitis, and how can it be treated?' (*See* Answer 70)

At the history-taking section, you see a young woman recently diagnosed with Crohn's disease. She has a colostomy bag on with a fistula discharging into it. The examiners ask 'What contribution do genetics make to this disease, and what are the options for treating her?' (*See* Answers 71 and 74)

At the ethics station, you see a 40-year-old man who is very concerned about developing cancer of the colon. How would you go about counselling him? (*See* Answer 72)

At the history-taking station, you see a 23-year-old man who has recently undergone a total colectomy. He has FAP. The examiners ask 'What other features are associated with this condition, and how is FAP caused?' (*See* Answer 75)

At the history-taking section, you see a 25-year-old woman who has just been diagnosed as having hepatitis C. The examiners ask 'What factors could help to decide whether she is likely to respond to interferon and ribavirin?' (*See* Answer 76)

NEPHROLOGY

True/False questions

77.   Diabetic nephropathy

With regards to diabetic nephropathy:

A. Early microalbuminuria is usually associated with a raised glomerular filtration rate
B. In type II diabetes, microalbuminuria is associated with an increased risk of cardiovascular disease
C. Elevated HbA1c levels do not correlate with the development of diabetic nephropathy
D. The DD ACE gene polymorphism is associated with an increased risk of diabetic nephropathy
E. Raised plasma triglycerides have been correlated with the development of diabetic nephropathy

78.   Renal stones

Regarding renal stones:

A. Most renal calculi are composed of calcium urate
B. Once a renal stone has been passed or removed, recurrence is rare
C. High urine flow promotes stone formation
D. Loop diuretics can prevent calcium stone formation
E. In patients with idiopathic hypercalciuria and recurrent renal stones, a normocalcaemic, low animal protein, low salt diet can reduce the risk of recurrent episodes

79.   Anaemia in chronic renal failure

Which of the following are true?

A. The anaemia of chronic renal failure is usually hypochromic and macrocytic
B. The use of erythropoietin in patients with chronic renal failure can be associated with clinically significant hypertension
C. Resistance to erythropoietin therapy does not occur provided there are adequate iron stores
D. Anaemia in chronic renal failure often improves once patients are commenced on haemodialysis
E. Red cell aplasia can occur in association with erythropoietin treatment

80.   Autosomal dominant polycystic kidney disease

Which of the following are correct?

A. Extra-renal manifestations of autosomal dominant polycystic kidney disease include mitral valve prolapse, tricuspid regurgitation, aortic dissection and coronary artery aneurysms
B. Abnormalities of the *PKD1* gene are found in 85% of patients with autosomal dominant polycystic kidney disease

C. Patients with *PKD1* mutations tend to progress to end-stage renal failure at an earlier age than those with *PKD2* mutations

D. Polycystin-1 is a large integral membrane protein, which can bind polycystin-2 at its C terminal tail

E. Polycystin-2 can act as a calcium-ion-permeable cation channel

81. Renal vasculitis

Regarding renal vasculitis:

A. Microscopic polyangiitis is characterised by the presence of anti-GBM antibodies

B. Renal involvement occurs in 80% of patients with Wegener's granulomatosis

C. ANCA-associated vasculitides are associated with a pauci-immune crescentic glomerulonephritis

D. ANCA titres correlate tightly with disease activity

E. The addition of plasma exchange to cyclophosphamide and prednisolone can improve renal outcome in patients with severe acute renal impairment secondary to renal vasculitis

Best-of-5 questions

82.   Treatment of early diabetic nephropathy

Which of the following drug regimens (in addition to regular insulin) would you chose for a 25-year-old type 1 diabetic with hypertension, microalbuminuria and LDL cholesterol of 3.5 mmol/L?

A. Aspirin, β-blocker, statin

B. Aspirin, ACE inhibitor, statin

C. Angiotensin II receptor inhibitor, statin

D. ACE inhibitor, statin

E. Aspirin, calcium channel blocker

83.   Transplant failure

A 45-year-old man with a history of polycystic kidney disease is reviewed in the transplant clinic 6 years after renal transplantation and is found to be hypertensive with impaired renal function (serum creatinine 250 μmol/L, baseline 125 μmol/L) and to have trace proteinuria. The ciclosporin level is (and has always been) satisfactory. He initially had delayed graft function and has had two successfully treated episodes of acute rejection. He has been persistently hypercholesterolaemic despite treatment. The most likely diagnosis is:

A. Recurrent polycystic disease

B. Concurrent urinary tract infection

C. Chronic ciclosporin toxicity

D. Acute rejection

E. Chronic allograft nephropathy

84.   Transplant immunosuppression

A 48-year-old man with end-stage renal failure secondary to IgA nephropathy is admitted for a renal transplant. He is known to have diet-controlled diabetes mellitus. Which immunosuppressive agents would you use in combination with prednisolone?

A. Ciclosporin and azathioprine
B. Tacrolimus and azathioprine
C. Tacrolimus and rapamycin
D. Ciclosporin and mycophenolate mofetil
E. Tacrolimus and mycophenolate

85.   Membranous glomerulonephritis

A 25-year-old woman presents with nephrotic range proteinuria (3.5 g/24 h), normal renal function and an albumin of 27 g/L. A renal biopsy shows membranous glomerulonephritis. Secondary causes have been excluded. Which of the following would be the most appropriate plan of management?

A. Do nothing except monitor renal function on a monthly basis
B. Start an ACE inhibitor and monitor renal function
C. Start an ACE inhibitor, fully anticoagulate with warfarin and monitor renal function
D. Start an ACE inhibitor and treat with high dose oral prednisolone and chlorambucil alternate months
E. Start an ACE inhibitor and advise a high protein diet

86.   Renal cell carcinoma

A 55-year-old man presents with frank haematuria and fever and is found to have a renal cell carcinoma. Unfortunately, at presentation he also has pulmonary metastases bilaterally. Which of the following therapeutic regimens would be most appropriate?

A. Radical nephrectomy plus interferon α
B. Radical nephrectomy plus chemotherapy with 5-fluorouracil and cytarabine
C. Interferon α plus radiation therapy
D. Radical nephrectomy, interleukin-4 and radiation therapy
E. Interleukin-2 alone

PACES questions

At the history-taking station, you see a patient with type 2 diabetes and established diabetic nephropathy. The examiners ask 'What risk factors would you consider important to modify in order to limit the progression of diabetic nephropathy in a type 2 diabetic?' (*See* Answer 77)

At the abdominal station, you palpate two very large kidneys in a middle-aged man who has an AV fistula on his left forearm. You diagnose polycystic kidney disease. The examiners ask 'What is currently known about the genetics of polycystic kidney disease?' (*See* Answer 80)

At the history taking-station, you see a 64-year-old type 2 diabetic who has microalbuminuria on dipstick testing of urine. The examiners ask 'What tests would you like to perform and which drugs would you consider using?' (*See* Answer 82)

At the ethics station, the examiners ask 'The number of patients awaiting renal transplant in the UK continues to rise. Why might this be and how might this organ shortage be overcome?' (*See* Answer 83)

At the history-taking station, you see a man with a renal transplant. His immunosuppressive drugs include tacrolimus. The examiners ask 'What is tacrolimus and how does it work? (*See* Answer 84)

GENETICS
True/False questions

87.   Proteomics

Regarding proteomics:

A. The human genome project has identified over 100 000 genes
B. One gene ultimately results in one protein
C. Proteomics is the study of the qualitative and quantative information about the functional output of the genome, the proteome
D. Two-dimensional gel electophoresis separates proteins on the basis of size and weight
E. Two-dimensional gel electophoresis revealing the proteins p130 and p131 allows discrimination between Creutzfeldt–Jakob disease and other types of dementia

88.   DNA microarrays

Regarding DNA microarrays:

A. DNA microarrays are purely a research tool but might have implications for clinical practice in the future
B. DNA microarrays allow thousands of specific DNA or RNA sequences to be detected simultaneously
C. Oligonucleotide arrays allow the detection of proteins
D. Microarrays can yield information on whether a gene is present, and also its level of expression
E. Microarrays are often called DNA chips, as the technology for constructing the arrays was adapted from the semiconductor computing industry

89.   The cell cycle

Regarding the cell cycle:

A. DNA replication occurs during the mitotic phase of the cell cycle
B. The mitotic phase of the cell cycle is when DNA is distributed to opposite ends of the cell and division occurs to produce two daughter cells
C. The restriction point is the point at which the cell no longer requires mitogens to undergo cell division
D. Phophorylated retinoblastoma (rb) protein inhibits cell cycle progression
E. p53 mediates G1 cell-cycle arrest in response to DNA damage

IMMUNOLOGY

True/False questions

90.   Intravenous immunoglobulin

With regards to intravenous immunoglobulin:

A. The half-life in immunocompetent persons is 3 months
B. It is prepared from the pooled plasma of thousands of donors and contains IgG molecules with a distribution of IgG subclasses similar to that in normal human serum
C. Its action, in part, is due to the increased expression of inhibitory Fc receptors when used in autoimmune disorders
D. It contains antibodies which are unable to bind complement
E. Anti-idiotype antibodies account for its ability to neutralise autoantibody

91.   Monoclonal antibodies

With regards to monoclonal antibodies:

A. Humanised antibodies used therapeutically have only a human complementarity determining region, the remainder of the molecule being murine
B. The use of the anti-TNFα antibody infliximab in resistant Crohn's disease is not as yet supported by controlled trials
C. Etanercept is a recombinant IgG1 Fc fragment fused to two TNF receptors and is administered as a twice-weekly subcutaneous injection
D. Trastuzumab (Herceptin, humanised IgG1 antibody that targets HER2 growth receptor) has been recently licensed in the UK for treatment of patients with relapsed lung cancer
E. Abciximab is a chimeric monoclonal antibody that blocks the platelet membrane glycoprotein IIb/IIIa, thus preventing the binding of fibrinogen/vonWillebrand factor

92.   Pathogenesis of autoimmune disease

With regards to the pathogenesis of autoimmune disease:

A. Most autoimmune diseases are monogenic, with single gene defects leading to the development of clinical disease
B. Abnormalities in mechanisms of apoptosis can lead to autoimmunity
C. There might be an increase in the activation threshold of B cells
D. Complement deficiencies can lead to reduced clearance of immune complexes or potentially antigenic dead cells
E. Underexpression of TNFα can contribute to the development of SLE

93.   Immunotherapy for cancer

Which of the following statements are true?

A. Cancer cells can avoid elimination by the immune system by loss of expression of class I MHC molecules, thus avoiding recognition by cytotoxic T cells
B. The ideal target antigen for cancer immunotherapy should be strongly immunogenic and expressed on both tumour and normal cells
C. Whole irradiated tumour cells combined with BCG as an immunological adjuvant have been shown to be effective in increasing recurrence-free survival in some patients with Dukes B colorectal cancer
D. Neutrophils loaded with tumour antigen and infused into the patient can present tumour antigen to CD4 T cells and generate an antitumour immune response
E. Infusion of allogeneic lymphocytes can facilitate removal of leukaemic cells by a graft versus tumour effect

94.   Regulatory T cells

Which of the following are true?

A. Regulatory or suppressor T cells are characterised by the expression of CD8 and the interleukin-2 receptor alpha chain (CD25)
B. Cell-to-cell contact between suppressor T cells and responding cells is a prerequisite for suppression
C. Regulatory T cells do not produce interleukin-2
D. Depletion of CD25+ T cells in murine models precipitates the development of spontaneous autoimmune disease
E. In tumour immunotherapy, depletion of CD25+ T cells has been used to enhance the immune response to melanoma vaccine

95.   Vaccine development

Which of the following statements are correct?

A. Influenza vaccine can now be given intranasally
B. DNA vaccines always require a viral vector to produce an immune response
C. Transgenic plants are able to deliver antigens as an oral vaccine
D. Polysaccharide vaccines are particularly suitable for children below 1 year of age
E. Cutaneous application of anthrax toxin is effective in stimulating an immune response against anthrax infection

PACES questions

At the history-taking section, you see a woman who received intravenous immunoglobulin for Guillain–Barré syndrome. The examiners ask 'What is the rationale behind using intravenous immunoglobulin in autoimmune and inflammatory disorders?' (*See* Answer 90)

At the abdominal examination station, you see a woman with an enterocutaneous fistula. The examiners tell you that she has received infliximab and ask you to give some examples of other diseases where monoclonal antibodies are used therapeutically. (*See* Answer 91)

At the history-taking section, you see a woman with SLE. The examiners ask you 'The immune system normally functions to protect self from foreign invaders. What is currently known about why the body begins to react against self?' (*See* Answer 92)

At the dermatology station, you see a man with an irregular, pigmented lesion. You diagnose a malignant melanoma. The examiners ask 'How has the immune system been harnessed in therapeutic attempts to eliminate cancers?' (*See* Answer 93)

CARDIOLOGY

True/False questions

96. Aldosterone receptor blockade

Blockade of the aldosterone receptor:

A. Promotes loss of sodium by the kidneys
B. Is contraindicated in patients treated with digoxin
C. Is proven to provide symptomatic benefit in patients with NYHA class II heart failure
D. Reduces cardiac-related mortality in patients with symptoms of severe heart failure and poor ejection fraction
E. Reduces all cause mortality in patients with symptoms of severe heart failure and poor ejection fraction even if they are not on an ACE inhibitor

97. Cardiac resynchronisation therapy

A 30-year-old woman develops postpartum dilated cardiomyopathy. Although she gets some improvement in cardiac function, she still has poor ejection fraction 1 year later. ECG shows left bundle branch block. She is already being treated with diuretics and an ACE inhibitor. Cardiac resynchronisation with a biventricular pacemaker would:

A. Be indicated with NYHA class III heart failure for symptom relief
B. Reduce 12-month mortality
C. Probably reduce hospitalisation from heart failure over a 6-month period
D. Reduce the risk of sudden death from ventricular tachycardia
E. Not benefit patients not taking beta-blockers

98.   Statin therapy

A 50 year-old-woman attends your clinic. She is hypertensive on treatment with atenolol and she had a transient ischaemic attack 2 years ago. In addition to the atenolol, she takes aspirin. Her total cholesterol is 5.0 mmol/L. With regards to cholesterol lowering:

A. Simvastatin 40 mg once daily would significantly reduce the risk of death from a vascular cause
B. Simvastatin 40 mg once daily has been shown to rarely produce myopathy (total CK > 10 times the upper limit of normal)
C. Without statin therapy this patient is at significant risk of myocardial infarction
D. Statin therapy is known to increase the risk of cancer over a 5-year period
E. Statin therapy would not reduce the chance of this patient having further strokes if she also took an ACE inhibitor

99.   Clopidogrel

A 65-year-old man with hypertension is admitted with chest pain. He has a previous history of hypertension and hypercholesterolaemia, and has previously had an anterior myocardial infarction. ECG shows inferior T wave inversion. He is treated with aspirin and low molecular-weight heparin. He is already on a beta-blocker, a statin and an ACE inhibitor. Which of the following could be said for the use of clopidogrel in this situation?

A. Clopidogrel irreversibly inhibits the binding of ATP to platelets
B. Clopidogrel has been proven to reduce death from any cause in this situation
C. Clopidogrel has be shown to be more effective than aspirin in direct comparison
D. Clopidogrel should not be given for more than 28 days
E. Clopidogrel significantly increases the risk of bleeding when given with aspirin

100.   Asymptomatic aortic stenosis

A 50-year-old man who has been under regular cardiac follow-up for aortic stenosis comes to clinic. He is currently completely asymptomatic and has been researching his condition on the internet; he has come armed with a list of questions. Which of these are true?

A. The average increase in mean gradient is 7 mmHg per year
B. Surgery has not been proven to improve outcome in patients who have not yet developed symptoms

   C. Exercise testing in patients with asymptomatic aortic stenosis is contraindicated

   D. It is usually necessary to cross the aortic valve at the time of coronary angiography to confirm the echocardiographic estimate of valve gradient

   E. Event-free survival in asymptomatic patients with aortic stenosis is < 30% at 2 years

101. Exercise training in chronic heart failure

Which of the following are true?

A. Exercise training induces adverse remodelling of the heart in chronic heart failure

B. Weight training can improve peak oxygen uptake in chronic heart failure

C. Exercise training can improve quality of life and symptoms in chronic heart failure

D. Stamina training reverses the abnormalities seen in muscle metabolism in chronic heart failure

E. Exercise training can reduce fluid overload in chronic heart failure

Best-of-5 questions

102. Treatment of ventricular tachycardia

A 60-year-old man attends your department with an acute anterior myocardial infarction. He is treated with appropriate therapy including aspirin, thrombolysis, an ACE inhibitor and atenolol. Postdischarge he has a short run of non-sustained ventricular tachycardia on a 24-h monitor. Which strategy would best improve this man's prognosis?

A. Echocardiography shows ejection fraction of 45% and subsequent VT stimulation study is negative. The patient should have an implantable cardioverter defibrillator

B. Echocardiography shows an ejection fraction of 30% and subsequent VT stimulation study is negative. The patient should be treated with amiodarone

C. Echocardiography shows an ejection fraction of 45% and a subsequent VT stimulation study is negative. The patient should be treated with amiodarone

D. Echocardiography shows an ejection fraction of 30% and subsequent VT stimulation study is negative. The patient should have an implantable cardioverter defibrillator

E. Echocardiography shows an ejection fraction of 45% and a subsequent VT stimulation study is positive. The patient does not require additional therapy

103. Drug-eluting stents

A 50-year-old man presents to you with a classic history of angina pectoris. Exercise testing is strongly positive, so he is listed for diagnostic coronary angiography. This shows a discrete short stenosis in the proximal left anterior descending artery, with no other significant lesions seen. After discussion with the patient, he opts to proceed with coronary angioplasty. Which of the following best describes the current data for drug-eluting stents?

A. Drug-eluting stents have been shown to have lower revascularisation rates than coronary artery bypass surgery in two-vessel coronary artery disease
B. Drug-eluting stents show a reduction in restenosis at 6 months compared with standard stents in diabetic patients
C. Drug-eluting stents have been shown to reduce in-stent restenosis but slightly increase rates of acute thrombosis compared to standard stents
D. Drug-eluting stents reduce the rate of myocardial infarction over a 1-year period compared with standard stents
E. Drug-eluting stents reduce overall mortality over a 1-year period compared with standard stents

104. Driving following loss of consciousness

A 60-year-old man attends outpatients with two episodes of collapse with loss of consciousness in the last 3 months. These were both preceded by palpitations associated with feeling faint and sweating. His ECG shows left bundle branch block.

With regards to driving, which one of the following statements are correct?

A. He has a 'prospective disability'
B. He can legally drive after 6 months, presuming he is event free, without informing the DVLA
C. He can continue to drive so long as he informs the DVLA
D. He can drive after 6 months if he is found to have VT and has a defibrillator fitted, has no further events and has told the DVLA
E. He will never be allowed to hold a heavy goods vehicle licence

105. Vitamin E in arterial disease

With respect to the antioxidant vitamin E, which statement best describes its effect on coronary artery disease?

A. Vitamin E has not been shown to slow progression of atherosclerosis
B. Vitamin E has been demonstrated to reduce the composite endpoint of myocardial infarction, stroke and death from cardiovascular causes
C. Vitamin E has been shown to cause an increase in haemorrhagic stroke
D. Vitamin E taken in combination with vitamin C and beta carotene has not been shown to affect all-cause mortality
E. Vitamin E prevents oxidation of triglycerides so reducing accumulation in arterial walls

106.   Genetics of dilated cardiomyopathy

Which one of the following best describes the genetics of dilated cardiomyopathy?

A. The most common form of familial dilated cardiomyopathy is autosomal dominant
B. A mitochondrial familial condition has never been seen
C. The autosomal dominant form has 100% penetrance
D. Familial dilated cardiomyopathy makes up less than 10% of all cases
E. As yet, familial dilated cardiomyopathy has not been mapped at any specific gene loci

PACES questions

At the history-taking station, you see a man with a history of chronic heart failure who is taking furosemide (frusemide), lisinopril and spironolactone. The examiners ask 'Which patients with heart failure should receive spironolactone, and why does it improve survival in heart failure?' (*See* Answer 96)

At the history-taking station, you see a 67-year-old woman with dilated cardiomyopathy. She is severely symptomatic despite an ACE inhibitor and beta-blockers. Her ECG shows a left bundle branch block. The examiners ask 'What other therapies could you offer this woman?' (*See* Answers 96 and 97)

At the ethics station, you are asked 'Your Trust has run out of money, and has imposed restrictions on the indications for prescribing statins. What do you do?' (*See* Answer 98)

At the cardiovascular station, you examine a woman with signs of significant aortic stenosis. The examiners ask 'Given that this woman is asymptomatic, how would you follow her up, and when would you refer her for valve surgery?' (*See* Answer 100)

At the cardiovascular station, you examine a man with obvious signs of congestive cardiac failure. The examiners ask 'What role does exercise have in the management of this man's condition?' (*See* Answer 101)

At the history-taking station, you see a man with an implanted cardioverter–defibrillator. The examiners ask 'What are the indications for fitting this device?' (*See* Answer 102)

At the communications station, you see a woman who is under investigation for episodes of collapse. She is keen to resume driving as soon as possible. What do you tell her? (*See* Answer 104)

RHEUMATOLOGY

True/False questions

107.   Rheumatoid arthritis

Which of the following are true?

A. Rheumatoid factor is an IgG antibody against the antigenic determinants on the Fc fragment of IgM
B. Lymphocytes are the predominant cell in rheumatoid synovial fluid
C. Agents that inhibit TNFα might be associated with CNS demyelination
D. The pharmacological activity of infliximab is inhibited by methotrexate
E. The risk of myocardial infarction is substantially increased

108.   Systemic lupus erythematosus (SLE)

Which of the following statements are true?

A. Antinuclear antibody is always positive
B. After 10 years of disease, the most common cause of death is active disease
C. Hydroxychloroquine increases serum cholesterol
D. Discoid lupus almost always progresses to SLE
E. SLE is uncommon in black Africans

109.   Myositis

A 60-year-old man presents with mild proximal muscle weakness. He has found it increasingly difficult to climb stairs. He has also noticed a rash on his face and scalp. He feels slightly short of breath but is otherwise well. His weight is steady. Examination does indeed confirm the presence of some thigh muscle weakness and tenderness. He has an erythematous facial rash and a flaky rash on his scalp. His chest is clear. Blood tests reveal an ESR of 60 mm/h and a creatinine kinase of 1000.

Which of the following statements are correct?

A. He has a greater than 90% chance of having a malignancy
B. His symptoms are likely to respond to penicillamine
C. He should have a barium enema
D. After 3 years of follow-up, he is unlikely to develop a malignancy
E. Hydroxychloroquine is a useful therapy for his skin problems

110.   Non-steroidal anti-inflammatory drugs (NSAIDs)

An 87-year-old man is referred to the clinic. He has osteoarthritis. His past medical history includes a myocardial infarction 5 years ago. He also has a history of dyspepsia; gastroscopy in the past showed a superficial gastritis. Co-codamol is no longer helping his pain. His GP asks you for advice on the use of a COX II inhibitor.

Which of the following statements are correct regarding NSAIDs and their use?

A. More than 20% of patients suffer side-effects when taking NSAIDs
B. COX II selective NSAIDs have no effect on the gastric mucosa
C. He is more likely to develop renal toxicity than with a standard NSAID
D. The use of COX II selective NSAIDs with low-dose aspirin is thought to be safe
E. The co-prescription of a proton pump inhibitor with a COX II selective NSAID has been shown to further reduce the incidence of gastrointestinal bleeding

Best-of-5 questions

111. Glucosamine

A 64-year-old female with joint pains attends the rheumatology outpatients. She has read about glucosamine in an arthritis magazine. She asks you for some information on the preparation.
Only one of the following pieces of information is correct; which one?

A. Glucosamine has disease-modifying effects in the treatment of osteoarthritis
B. Glucosamine can safely be used in diabetics
C. Glucosamine cannot be prescribed by a registered medical practitioner
D. Glucosamine is a component of synovium
E. Glucosamine has disease-modifying effects in the treatment of rheumatoid arthritis

112. Ankylosing spondylitis

A 23-year-old man attends your clinic complaining of a 6-month history of lower back pain and stiffness first thing in the morning. He also has some pain in his right heel. On examination he has a reduced range of movement in his back and some tenderness over the right Achilles tendon. His ESR is 50.
Which one of the following statements is incorrect?

A. HLA-B27 is likely to be positive
B. Physiotherapy alone is likely to provide prognostic benefit
C. Local steroid injection of the Achilles tendon should be considered
D. Sulfasalazine is unlikely to help his symptoms
E. X-ray of the sacroiliac joints is likely to be abnormal

113. Gout

A 45-year-old male presents with a 3-day history of a hot painful left knee. He has been previously well. He smokes 20 cigarettes per day and drinks 40 pints of beer per week. He suffers from dyspepsia. His body mass index is 32. His serum urate is normal.
Which one of the following statements is correct?

A. A normal serum urate excludes the diagnosis of gout
B. The absence of crystals excludes the diagnosis of gout

C. Gout is associated with negative birefringent crystals under polarised light
D. Septic arthritis can usually be excluded clinically, therefore joint aspiration is unnecessary
E. A high C-reactive protein means he has septic arthritis

114.   Temporal arteritis

A 75-year-old woman complains of a new onset of left-sided headache associated with pain in the jaw region when eating. She also complains of some pain in her groin. She has a history of mild angina. Her ESR is 30. On examination she has thickening and tenderness over the left temporal artery.

In view of the normal ESR, which course of action would you take?

A. Observe – she is very unlikely to have temporal arteritis in view of the normal ESR
B. Carry out temporal artery biopsy; then start 15–20 mg of prednisolone
C. Arrange urgent temporal artery biopsy and start treatment only if the result is positive
D. Start 40–60 mg of prednisolone, arrange temporal artery biopsy and continue steroids even if result is negative
E. Start 40–60 mg of prednisolone, arrange temporal artery biopsy and discontinue steroids if result is negative

115.   Pseudogout

A 70-year-old woman, who has a history of mild osteoarthritis, presents with acute confusion. She has a temperature of 37.5°C. Her chest is clear and urinalysis is normal. She is commenced on oral co-amoxiclav. She fails to improve by the next day. The senior house officer on the ward notices that she has a swollen right knee.

Which one of the following statements is incorrect?

A. She is likely to have acute pseudogout
B. Her symptoms might well respond to colchicine
C. She should have the joint aspirated immediately to exclude infection
D. The absence of positive birefringent crystals excludes the diagnosis of pseudogout
E. Plain X-ray of the knee may help with diagnosis

116.   Reactive arthritis

A 27-year-old man presents to the medical admissions ward. He has a 1-week history of dysuria and a 6-day history of urethral discharge. He also tells you that for the past 2 days he has had a very painful swollen right knee. On examination his temperature is 37.2°C and he does indeed have a synovitic right knee. His CRP is 55.

Which one of the following would not be useful?

A. Knee aspiration
B. HLA typing
C. Course of doxycycline
D. Penile swab
E. Rheumatoid factor assay

PACES questions

You are taken to see a patient with rheumatoid changes in her hands and evidence of active synovitis. The examiners ask 'What new treatments are available for rheumatoid arthritis that is resistant to standard therapies, and what are their side-effects?' (*See* Answer 107)

At the history-taking station, you see a woman with SLE. The examiners ask 'What is the survival rate for patients with SLE, and from what do they die?' (*See* Answer 108)

At the dermatology station, you see a man with a violaceous rash. On being told that he has proximal muscle weakness you make a diagnosis of dermatomyositis. The examiners ask 'What investigations would be appropriate to search for underlying disease?' (*See* Answer 109)

At the history-taking station, you see a 78-year-old woman with severe osteoarthritis. She has a previous history of myocardial infarction and peptic ulcer disease. The examiners ask 'What would a COX II selective non-steroidal anti-inflammatory drug have to offer this woman?' (*See* Answer 110)

At the history-taking station, you see a woman with osteoarthritis. She states that her life has been transformed by her glucosamine supplements. The examiners ask 'What is the evidence that glucosamine actually works?' (*See* Answer 111)

At the history-taking station, you see a young man with recently diagnosed ankylosing spondylitis. The examiners ask 'What therapies are effective in this disease?' (Answer 112)

At the history-taking station, you see an 85-year-old woman with headaches, morning shoulder stiffness and scalp tenderness. You make a provisional diagnosis of temporal arteritis. The examiners ask 'How would you investigate and treat this woman?' (*See* Answer 114)

EPIDEMIOLOGY

True/False questions

117.   Confounding

The following methods can be used to prevent or control for the potential effects of confounding factors in epidemiological studies:

A. Matching
B. Blinding
C. Randomisation
D. Restriction
E. Regression

118.   Observational studies

The following statements regarding issues of the design of observational studies are correct:

A. The results of a correlational study are typically expressed as an odds ratio
B. Case-control studies are well suited to study diseases with a long latency period
C. Subjects in case-control studies are selected on the basis of their exposure history
D. Cohort studies are designed to facilitate the examination of multiple exposures of a single disease
E. Case-control studies are particularly susceptible to bias, as both exposure and disease have already occurred at the time subjects are selected for the study

Best-of-5 questions

119.   Homocysteine and ischaemic heart disease

A 68-year-old man with ischaemic heart disease is reviewed in outpatients. He has recently read in a newspaper that homocysteine is an important risk factor for ischaemic heart disease and that taking vitamins like folate will lower his risk of a heart attack in the future. He now seeks your advice on whether folate supplementation is indicated for his condition. Which of the following is the most appropriate advice on the basis of the best, current epidemiological evidence?

A. There is no convincing evidence that homocysteine is a risk factor for ischaemic heart disease
B. There is convincing evidence that homocysteine is not a risk factor for ischaemic heart disease
C. The contribution of homocysteine to the development of ischaemic heart disease remains unclear but it is unlikely to be a major determinant
D. Homocysteine is likely to be a strong contributor to the development of ischaemic heart disease but folate supplementation does not modify homocysteine level
E. Homocysteine is likely to be a strong contributor to the development of ischaemic heart disease but folate supplementation does not alter ischaemic heart disease outcomes

NEUROLOGY

True/False questions

120. Paraneoplastic syndromes

Which of the following statements are correct?

A. Anti-Yo antibodies are associated with sensory neuropathy
B. Lambert–Eaton myasthenic syndrome can be treated with plasma exchange
C. Small cell lung carcinoma can be associated with encephalomyelitis
D. 50% of patients with myasthenia gravis have a thymoma
E. Retinal degeneration is associated with anti-Ri antibodies

121. Inflammatory neuropathies

Which of the following statements are correct?

A. Guillain–Barré syndrome is associated with anti-GM1 antibodies in 25% of cases
B. The treatment of choice for Guillain–Barré syndrome is high-dose steroids
C. Neuropathies associated with a monoclonal gammopathy do not respond to immunotherapy
D. Chronic inflammatory demyelinating neuropathies can be treated with steroids or intravenous immunoglobulin.
E. Chronic inflammatory demyelinating neuropathies are associated with antibodies against GQ1b ganglioside

122. Subarachnoid haemmorhage

In the diagnosis of subarachnoid haemorrhage:

A. A normal CT scan 24 h after presentation excludes a significant subarachnoid haemorrhage
B. A lumbar puncture is only positive if there are over 100×10^6 red blood cells per mL present
C. Once the diagnosis is established, nimodipine 60 mg 4-hourly should be started to prevent rebleeding
D. If the patient deteriorates clinically then an urgent CT scan is indicated
E. A ruptured aneurysm is the cause in 85% of cases

123. Epileptic seizures

A 24-year-old female presents with an episode of loss of consciousness. The event was unwitnessed but she had a feeling of déjà vu and an odd feeling in her stomach prior to the event. Afterwards she was drowsy for 30 min and noticed she had been incontinent and had bitten her tongue:

A. The diagnosis is most likely to be a generalised tonic–clonic seizure
B. An anticonvulsant should be started immediately

C. She should be counselled regarding the risk of fetal abnormalities for all anticonvulsant medication
D. An interictal EEG may be normal
E. MRI imaging of her head should be undertaken

124. Genetics of neurological disease

Which of the following statements are true?

A. Charcot–Marie–Tooth disease (hereditary motor sensory neuropathy 1) is a triplet repeat disorder
B. Heteroplasmy accounts for the variation in tissue susceptibility to mitochondrial disorders
C. Mutations in the dystrophin gene cause myotonic dystrophy
D. Patients with trisomy 21 have an increased risk of Alzheimer's disease
E. von Hippel–Lindau syndrome is an autosomal dominant disorder

Best-of-5 questions

125. Multiple sclerosis

Patients with which one of the following types of multiple sclerosis should be offered beta-interferon treatment?

A. Relapsing remitting disease with over two relapses a year
B. Primary progressive
C. Relapsing remitting disease, unable to walk 100 yards
D. Secondary progressive disease, unable to walk unaided
E. Relapsing remitting disease with less than one relapse per year

126. Emergency neurology

Which one of the following scenarios requires urgent neurological investigation?

A. Internuclear ophthalmoplegia
B. Sudden onset foot drop
C. Seventh nerve palsy with onset over several days
D. Sudden onset cerebellar syndrome
E. Painless incomplete third nerve palsy

127. Variant Creutzfeldt–Jakob disease

Which one of the following statements best describes this condition?

A. Neurological features tend to be seen earlier than psychiatric features
B. Variant Creutzfeldt–Jakob disease has been seen only in patients who are homozygous for methionine at codon 129 of the prion protein gene
C. Insomnia tends to occur late in the course of the disease
D. Median survival of the disease is less than 9 months
E. Cerebellar signs tend to occur early in the course of the disease

128. Parkinson's disease

A 61-year-old man presents with a 6-month history of progressive unilateral stiffness and bradykinesia together with a resting tremor. Which treatment option is most appropriate?

A. Levodopa treatment alone
B. Levodopa and dopamine agonist combined
C. Dopamine agonist alone
D. Selegiline alone
E. No treatment should be given until the patient is functionally disabled

129. Reversible causes of dementia

A 78-year-old man presents with increasing falls and reduced mobility over the last year. He has had difficulty reaching the toilet and has had episodes of urinary incontinence for 8 months. His wife reports that he has become increasingly forgetful over the last few months. He has no vascular risk factors and no head injuries but had viral meningitis 11 years ago. The most likely diagnosis is:

A. Normal pressure hydrocephalus
B. Alzheimer's disease
C. Brain tumour
D. Chronic bilateral subdural haematomas
E. Depression

PACES questions

At the history-taking station, you see a man with myasthenia gravis. The examiners ask 'What other neurological diseases are caused by autoantibodies?' (*See* Answer 120)

At the communication station, you see a 29-year-old woman who has had a second fit within a year. MRI of the brain shows no abnormality. How would you discuss treatment options with her? (*See* Answer 123)

At the neurology station, you see a 32-year-old woman with cerebellar signs and internuclear ophthalmoplegia. The examiners ask 'Which patients with multiple sclerosis should be offered interferon therapy?' (*See* Answer 125)

At the neurology station, you see a woman with unilateral resting tremor, rigidity and bradykinesia. Her gait is markedly slow. You make a diagnosis of Parkinson's disease. The examiners ask 'What are the treatment options for her disease?' (*See* Answer 128)

At the history-taking station, you see a 71-year-old man with a 3-month history of intellectual impairment. The examiners ask 'What treatable causes for his condition would you like to exclude?' (*See* Answer 129)

HAEMATOLOGY

True/False questions

130. Blood transfusion

Which of the following statements are true?

A. All blood in the UK is currently screened for the Creutzfeldt–Jakob disease prion
B. Leucodepletion is used to reduced the transmission of Creutzfeldt–Jakob disease and cytomegalovirus infections
C. The chance of contracting hepatitis C from a unit of transfused blood is 1 in 100 000
D. Blood transfusion can lead to a worse outcome in colorectal cancer
E. Aprotinin reduces the amount of blood transfusion needed during liver transplantation

131. Haemolytic–uraemic syndrome/thrombotic thrombocytopenic purpura

Which of the following statements are true?

A. Clopidogrel has been associated with thrombotic thrombocytopenic purpura
B. Deficiency of complement factor B is responsible for some familial cases of haemolytic–uraemic syndrome
C. Haemolytic–uraemic syndrome in children is associated with a poor prognosis
D. Early antibiotic therapy in haemolytic–uraemic syndrome improves outcome
E. Excess von Willebrand factor binds platelets into clumps, causing the microthrombi seen in thrombotic thrombocytopenic purpura

132. Deep venous thrombosis

Which of the following statements are true?

A. Antipsychotic use is associated with idiopathic deep venous thrombosis
B. Third-generation oral contraceptive pills are associated with an increased risk of deep venous thrombosis
C. Extended duration deep venous thrombosis prophylaxis does not reduce the incidence of thromboembolic disease after hip or knee surgery when compared to standard duration prophylaxis
D. D-dimers are a highly specific test for deep venous thrombosis
E. Asymptomatic deep venous thromboses on long-haul flights can be prevented by wearing elastic compression stockings

Best-of-5 questions

133. Thalassaemias

Which one of the following statements is true?

A. Bone marrow transplantation is not an effective treatment for β-thalassaemia
B. β-thalassaemia is usually undetectable until after birth
C. Deferiprone is an oral chelating agent that can cause thrombocytopenia
D. *Yersinia* infection is a recognised complication of desferrioxamine therapy
E. Splenectomy is no longer indicated in β-thalassaemia

134. Stem cell transplantation

A 42-year-old man with acute myeloid leukaemia is being worked up for myeloablation and transplantation. Which one of the following statements regarding stem cell transplantation is incorrect?

A. Autologous peripheral blood stem cell transplantation leads to faster repopulation than autologous bone marrow stem cell transplantation
B. HLA-A2 positive recipients of cytomegalovirus positive allogenic stem cell donations have an improved survival compared to HLA-A2 negative recipients of cytomegalovirus positive donations
C. Immunocompetent cells in allogeneic stem cell donations can produce a graft versus tumour effect
D. Umbilical cord blood donations are an important source of donor cells for adult transplantation
E. Allogeneic transplants from siblings have a lower morbidity and mortality than those from unrelated donors

PACES questions

At the ethics station, you see a 50-year-old woman who is due to undergo major surgery soon. She is very concerned at the fact that she might receive a blood transfusion, as she has heard about the infections that one can get from blood. How would you counsel her? (Answer 130)

At the history-taking station, you see a woman who has recently sustained a deep venous thrombosis. The examiners ask 'What are the risk factors for deep venous thrombosis?' (Answer 132)

MOLECULAR BIOLOGY
True/False questions

135.   Biofilms

Which of the following statements are true regarding biofilms?

A. Biofilms usually consist of one type of bacterium
B. Bacteria in biofilms are highly resistant to antibiotics
C. Bacteria in biofilms divide rapidly
D. Some bacteria in biofilms can enter a spore-like state
E. Prolonged courses of multiple antibiotics will usually eradicate biofilms

136.   Apoptosis

Regarding apoptosis:

A. The final common effectors in apoptosis are membrane-bound tyrosine kinases
B. Some cancers show an increased rate of apoptosis
C. Cancer cells can defend themselves against cytotoxic lymphocytes by inducing apoptosis
D. HIV infection causes an increased rate of apoptosis
E. TRAIL receptors can induce apoptosis

137.   Oxidative phosphorylation

Which of the following diseases has been associated with defects in the oxidative phosphorylation pathway?

A. Huntington's chorea
B. MELAS syndrome
C. MERRF syndrome
D. Friedreich's ataxia
E. Chronic progressive external ophthalmoplegia (CPEO)

138.   Selenium

Which of the following statements are true regarding selenium?

A. Selenium binds to aspartate to form a reaction centre in enzymes
B. Selenium-containing enzymes play a role in converting thyroxine to triiodothyronine
C. Selenium supplementation enhances cell-mediated immune activity
D. Lack of selenium can cause viruses to mutate into more virulent forms
E. Selenium supplementation can retard the progression of atherosclerotic lesions

139. Angiogenesis

Which of the following substances are known to promote angiogenesis?

A. Thyroxine
B. Fibroblast growth factor
C. Interferon alpha
D. Leptin
E. Endothelin

140. Mechanisms of bone turnover

Which of the following statements are correct?

A. Osteoclast formation is driven primarily by the RANK ligand
B. Osteoclast formation is inhibited by osteoprotegerin
C. Oestrogen levels are an important determinant of bone mineral density loss in older men
D. Genetic influences dominate in determining peak bone mineral density in young adults
E. Osteoblast lifespan is decreased in the postmenopausal state

141. Biology of the senses

Which of the following statements are true?

A. Menthol receptors are present on trigeminal neurons
B. The sensation of cold is mediated by excitatory ion channels
C. Heat receptors can be activated by capsaicin
D. Pheromone receptors have not been detected in the human nose to date
E. A glutamate receptor is responsible for mediating the bitter taste sensation

142. Channelopathies

Regarding channelopathies:

A. Long QT syndrome can be caused by mutations of the KCNQ1 potassium channel
B. Brugada syndrome is caused by mutations in the CHP4 calcium channel
C. Heart failure produces an acquired potassium channelopathy
D. Familial hypokalemic periodic paralysis is caused by a mutation in a skeletal muscle potassium channel
E. Channelopathy affecting neuronal sodium channels is the primary cause of disordered nerve function in multiple sclerosis

143.   Antimicrobial peptides

Which of the following statements are true regarding antimicrobial polypeptides?

A. Defensins are large hydrophobic polypeptides
B. The activity of antimicrobial peptides in human lung is reduced in cystic fibrosis
C. Secreted histone proteins in the gut are the precursors for antimicrobial peptides
D. Many antimicrobial peptides also act as chemotactic agents
E. Many antimicrobial peptides bind to and inactivate bacterial ribosomes

144.   Molecular biology of hypoxia

Which of the following statements are true?

A. Increased erythropoietin levels directly induce tissue tolerance to hypoxia
B. Hypoxia-inducible factor promotes glucose transport and glycolysis
C. Tissue hypoxia is sensed via high intracellular ADP/ATP ratios
D. The von Hippel–Lindau tumour suppressor gene plays a key role in hypoxic sensing
E. Hypoxia-inducible factor is inhibited by angiogenic growth factors

145.   Hypocretin/orexin

Which of the following are true of the hypocretin/orexin system?

A. It plays an important part in the pathogenesis of adrenoleucodystrophy
B. Hypocretin acts as an inhibitory neurotransmitter
C. Hypocretin could play an important role in regulating sleep
D. Hypocretin-producing neurons are concentrated in the dorsolateral hypothalamus
E. Hypocretin supplementation reduces appetite in humans

ONCOLOGY

True/False questions

146.   Therapy for malignant gliomas

Regarding therapy for malignant gliomas:

A. Temozolomide therapy is associated with a 30% 5-year survival rate
B. Chemotherapy demonstrates a small survival benefit when added to radiotherapy
C. Temozolomide therapy worsens quality of life
D. Radiotherapy can be associated with a decline in cognitive function
E. Biopsy using a gamma knife is less likely to cause seeding of the tumour

147. Estrogen and breast cancer

Which of the following are true regarding estrogen and breast cancer?

A. Hormone replacement therapy including progesterones does not increase the risk of breast cancer
B. Serum estradiol levels correlate with the development of breast cancer
C. Anastrozole can reduce the incidence of first-presentation breast cancer in high-risk patients
D. Soya confers an increased risk of developing breast cancer
E. Low catechol-O-methyl transferase activity protects against breast cancer

148. Hypercalcaemia of malignancy

A 67-year-old woman with known metastatic breast cancer presents with tiredness, nausea and vomiting. Routine bloods show a urea of 16.4, creatinine 237, calcium 3.57. Which of the following are true?

A. Bisphosphonate therapy has an antitumour effect on her disease
B. Elevated PTHrP levels are an important part of the mechanism of her hypercalcaemia
C. Renal calcium excretion is likely to be elevated
D. Osteoprotegerin is an alternative therapy to bisphosphonates to lower her calcium levels
E. Endothelin receptor antagonists can reduce the metabolic activity of bony metastases in her disease

Best-of-5 questions

149. Non-small cell lung cancer

A 54-year-old man presents with a persistent cough and weight loss. Chest radiography reveals a 2 cm mass in the right lung field. He undergoes lobectomy and histology confirms a squamous cell carcinoma of the lung. Which one of the following statements is correct?

A. Neoadjuvant chemotherapy would have improved his chance of survival
B. Adjuvant chemotherapy can reduce his risk of local recurrence
C. Palliative chemotherapy is inappropriate if he relapses
D. CT screening for lung cancer may reduce mortality from the disease
E. Chest X-ray screening can reduce mortality from lung cancer when combined with sputum cytology

150.   **Second malignancy after chemotherapy and radiotherapy**

Which of the following is not a risk factor for increased incidence of second malignancy after therapy for Hodgkin's disease?

A. Combined chemotherapy and radiotherapy
B. Duration of follow-up
C. Size of radiation field
D. Young age at first presentation
E. Male sex

PACES questions

At the communication station, you see a 58-year-old woman who is taking hormone replacement therapy. She is worried by recent reports in the press of a new trial that showed an increased risk of cancer, and is considering stopping her hormone replacement therapy. How do you counsel her? (*See* Answer 147)

At the history-taking station, you see a woman with breast cancer who is receiving a pamidronate infusion for her high calcium level. The examiners ask 'How does malignancy produce hypercalcaemia?' (*See* Answer 148)

At the communication station, you see a 42-year-old man who wants to be screened for lung cancer. He smokes, finds it difficult to give up, but wants the reassurance of a chest X-ray. What do you tell him? (*See* Answer 149)

Answers

ENDOCRINOLOGY

True/False answers

1. **Acromegaly**

   A. **T**   B. **F**   C. **F**   D. **F**   E. **T**

   Acromegaly is an uncommon endocrine disorder characterised by excess growth hormone secretion, usually from a pituitary macroadenoma. Symptoms can be due to mass effects from the tumour (headache, visual field defects) or metabolic, due to excess growth hormone. Features include sweating, joint pains, head, jaw and limb enlargement, deepening of the voice, carpal tunnel syndrome, hypertension and glucose intolerance. Organomegaly can occur and the condition predisposes to cardiovascular disease, including cardiomyopathy. Six per cent of patients diagnosed with acromegaly do have the MEN-1 syndrome (multiple endocrine neoplasia type 1).

   Pegvisomant is a genetically engineered growth hormone analogue that acts as a highly selective growth hormone receptor antagonist. The recombinant protein is attached to a polyethylene glycol backbone, giving a long half-life and thus allowing once-daily subcutaneous dosing. It has been shown to improve the signs and symptoms of acromegaly, including soft tissue swelling, sweating and fatigue, and might also reduce fasting insulin and glucose levels in patients with acromegaly. It causes significant falls in circulating levels of insulin-like growth factor-1 (IGF-1); 90% of patients treated with pegvisomant in fact achieve normal levels of IGF-1. Growth hormone levels, on the other hand, tend to rise slightly on therapy.

   Pegvisomant produces no statistically significant reduction in adenoma volume; surgery is therefore required if symptoms indicate a mass effect from the tumour. Regular follow-up with serial MRI scans is advocated because there is some theoretical concern that growth hormone blockade could remove a source of inhibition of adenoma growth, thus leading to accelerated tumour growth.

   IGF-1 is a commonly used marker of disease activity in acromegaly; it is the hormone that mediates the biological effects of growth hormone. Plasma levels reflect the average growth hormone level and do not vary greatly throughout the day. Single measurements of growth hormone convey little information; growth hormone release is pulsatile and rises as a result of stress in normal individuals. A dynamic suppression test (e.g. the glucose tolerance test) is needed to diagnose acromegaly using levels of growth hormone. Although IGF-1 levels can easily be measured as a static test, they might be less reliable after pituitary surgery and, whereas normalisation of growth hormone levels is thought to support an improved long-term outcome, there is less evidence regarding long-term outcome with normalisation of IGF-1 levels. Patients undergoing growth hormone receptor blockade should have IGF-1 measured in preference to growth hormone, as the above example shows. In practice, both dynamic testing of growth hormone, together with IGF-1 measurements, could be performed.

Although pituitary surgery holds out the best chance of a cure, drug therapy is useful as a holding measure, or as an option where surgery or radiotherapy have failed. The somatostatin analogues octreotide and the longer-acting lanreotide are both effective. The dopamine agonists bromocriptine or cabergoline can also be used. Cabergoline is not licensed for use during pregnancy; the manufacturer recommends discontinuing the drug 1 month prior to conception. However, there is no evidence of teratogenicity and there are a number of anecdotal reports of healthy babies being born despite conception occurring while on cabergoline therapy.

References

Duncan E, Wass J A H 1999 Investigation protocol: Acromegaly and its investigation. Clinical Endocrinology 50:285–293

Trainer P J, Drake W M, Katznelson L et al 2000 Treatment of acromegaly with the growth hormone-receptor antagonist pegvisomant. New England Journal of Medicine 342:1171–1177

Van der Lely A J, Hutson R K, Trainer P J et al 2001 Long-term treatment of acromegaly with pegvisomant, a growth hormone receptor antagonist. Lancet 358:1754–1759

2.   Thiazolidinediones

A. **F**   B. **F**   C. **T**   D. **T**   E. **F**

The thiazolidinediones (glitazones) are a novel class of oral hypoglycaemic agents. They work by binding to and activating peroxisome proliferator-activated receptor gamma (PPAR-γ). This receptor is a nuclear transcription factor, found predominantly in adipocytes. Activation of PPAR-γ leads to an increase in adipose tissue mass and increased uptake of fatty acids, with a consequent reduction in circulating glucose concentrations via the Randle cycle. Insulin resistance is also decreased.

Glitazone therapy reduces blood glucose, glycosylated haemoglobin (HbA1c) and circulating insulin levels. Insulin resistance as measured by glucose clamp techniques is reduced. Glitazones are able to reduce serum glucose in patients already taking metformin, a sulphonylurea, insulin, or all three. However, 25% of patients are resistant to the effects of glitazones; no appreciable improvement in glycaemic control is seen in this subgroup.

Glitazones are currently licensed as add-on therapy for patients with type 2 diabetes who have inadequate glycaemic control on metformin plus a sulphonylurea. Metformin plus a glitazone is the preferred combination, especially in obese individuals, as it causes less weight gain than sulphonylurea plus glitazone. There is no evidence to support using triple therapy and glitazones are not currently licensed for use with insulin. Glitazones are not licensed as monotherapy in the UK, although they are in the USA.

As with many new drugs, long-term evidence of efficacy is lacking. In particular, there are no data as to whether glitazones can reduce the incidence of microvascular or macrovascular endpoints.

Troglitazone, the first licensed glitazone, was withdrawn soon after its introduction because of serious hepatotoxic reactions, but two newer analogues – rosiglitazone and pioglitazone – have not as yet been associated with serious liver toxicity. Despite this, increases in transaminases do occur and regular liver function monitoring is advised.

All of the glitazones can cause fluid retention; their use in cardiac failure is thus contraindicated. The gain in adipocyte mass translates into a total body weight gain; there is some concern that this gain in weight could eventually lead to increasing insulin resistance over a long period of time. Other concerns include the effect of glitazones on lipid profile; both HDL and LDL levels increase and it is unclear how this will translate into overall cardiovascular risk.

Evidence is accumulating that the PPAR-γ receptor is involved in the regulation of many genes in a number of metabolic pathways. This has the potential to lead to therapy in a number of other disease processes; a direct effect on vascular remodelling has been suggested but such wide-ranging actions also carry the possibility that glitazones could have long-term mutagenic effects, perhaps in combination with other carcinogenic events.

References

NICE 2000 Full guidance on rosiglitazone for type 2 diabetes mellitus. Technology appraisal guidance No 9. Online. Available: www.nice.org.uk/article.asp?a=1189

NICE 2001 Full guidance on the use of pioglitazone for type 2 diabetes mellitus Technology appraisal guidance No 21. Online. Available: www.nice.org.uk/article.asp?a=1189

Schoonjans K, Auwerx J 2000 Thiazolidinediones: an update. Lancet 355:1008–1010

3. Type 1 diabetes

A. **T**   B. **F**   C. **F**   D. **T**   E. **F**

The autoimmune basis of type 1 diabetes has been appreciated for many years but recent insights have helped to paint a clearer picture of the natural history of the disease. A variety of anti-islet-cell antibodies can be detected before the disease becomes clinically apparent, and dysregulation of cellular immunity is also apparent long before the disease becomes overt. In infants, islet-associated antigen

(IAA) antibodies usually precede the occurrence of glutamic acid decarboxylase (GAD) antibody. In adults developing type 1 diabetes, GAD antibodies are much more common than IAA. Other antibodies commonly found include ICA512A and IA2A. These antibodies can be detected prior to the onset of clinically overt disease and often become detectable sequentially. Although detection of GAD antibodies increases the likelihood that type 1 diabetes will occur in the future, it is insensitive for predicting the occurrence of overt disease that will occur several years hence. Detection of multiple autoantibodies greatly increases the likelihood of developing the disease but this can occur close to the time of overt disease, leaving no time for any future preventive agent to exert an effect.

Several attempts have been made to transplant islet cells as a therapy for diabetes; the success rate was very low until a group from Edmonton, Canada, reported seven consecutive patients being successfully transplanted. All seven patients became independent of exogenous insulin, with normal HbA1c values. At least two donor pancreases per patient were required; more in one case. Islets were isolated from donor pancreases before embolisation into the liver via a catheter placed in the portal vein. The immunosuppressive regimen avoided steroids, using instead tacrolimus, sirolimus and daclizumab (an interleukin-2 receptor antibody). Patients remained independent of exogenous insulin during follow-up of several months. Several centres around the world are now collaborating to trial this protocol in a much larger number of type 1 diabetic patients.

Subcutaneous insulin infusion is a relatively new way of administering insulin. A subcutaneous cannula is connected to a belt-worn pump, which administers a constant basal supply of rapid-acting insulin. The user can administer boluses at mealtimes by pressing a button. The advantage of such a system is that tight glycaemic control is maintained, possibly with fewer episodes of hypoglycaemia. It might lead to improved nocturnal glycaemic control in some patients and can avoid the 'dawn' phenomenon of rising glucose levels before breakfast. There is no evidence that insulin pumps reduce the risk of microvascular or macrovascular events compared with a standard basal-bolus injection regime. HbA1c might be slightly better with pump therapy (0.2% in one study). Brittle diabetics might not benefit. Not all patients can be educated to use the pump system and cannula dislodgement and infection can be problems. Very frequent blood glucose monitoring is also required with pump systems.

Insulin glargine is a very long-acting modified insulin; the order of the amino acids within the insulin has been changed. Insulin lispro is another modified insulin that acts very rapidly. It does not dimerise, unlike natural insulin, and is thus absorbed rapidly. It is used at mealtimes to ensure a rapid peak of insulin action that coincides with peak glucose absorption. Insulin aspart is another modified insulin with rapid onset of action.

The cause of 'brittle' diabetes; i.e. type 1 diabetes characterised by recurrent episodes of diabetic ketoacidosis, is unclear but does not appear to be related to sudden drops in the amount of insulin produced by the pancreas; in type 1 diabetes, little or no insulin is produced by the pancreas. Poor adherence to therapy certainly plays a role in brittle diabetes, however; patients with insulin use that is less than predicted from their prescriptions are much more likely to present with diabetic ketoacidosis.

References

Atkinson M A, Eisenbarth G S 2001 Type 1 diabetes: new perspectives on disease pathogenesis and treatment. Lancet 358:221–229

Morris A D, Boyle D I R, McMahon A D et al 1997 Adherence to insulin treatment, glycaemic control, and ketoacidosis in insulin-dependent diabetes mellitus. Lancet 350:1505–1510

Pickup J, Keen H 2002 Continuous subcutaneous insulin infusion at 25 years. Diabetes Care 25(3):593–598

Shapiro A M J, Lakey J R T, Ryan E A et al 2000 Islet transplantation in seven patients with type 1 diabetes mellitus using a glucocorticoid-free immunosuppressive regimen. New England Journal of Medicine 343:230–238

4.   Thyroid function tests

A. **T**   B. **F**   C. **F**   D. **T**   E. **T**

Thyroid stimulating hormone (TSH) is produced by the anterior pituitary gland and is the major factor governing release of the hormone thyroxine by the thyroid gland. Thyroxine and triiodothyronine both exert negative feedback on the release of TSH. The TSH receptor can also be activated by very high levels of beta human chorionic gonadotrophin (β-hCG), e.g. during molar pregnancy. Rare mutations of the TSH receptor can also make the receptor much more sensitive to β-hCG. In such patients, pregnancy-associated thyrotoxicosis can occur as a result of high levels of β-hCG.

Considerable controversy continues regarding the best combination of thyroid function tests. Although TSH alone as a first-line test is undoubtedly the most cost-efficient strategy, cases of secondary hypothyroidism, usually as a result of hypopituitarism, will be missed when this strategy is used. Such cases often present with a normal TSH (often in the lower half of the normal range) and a low thyroxine level.

Low TSH levels can persist for months after successful treatment of thyrotoxicosis. Such levels do not necessarily indicate inadequate treatment; indeed patients can become profoundly hypothyroid, e.g. after radioiodine treatment, yet still have a low TSH.

A number of systemic disease processes can cause derangement of thyroid function tests. The sick euthyroid syndrome is well recognised; the most common pattern is low or normal TSH, normal thyroxine and low triiodothyronine. Such derangements usually resolve once the intercurrent illness resolves. Similarly, TSH might indeed be elevated in the first 2 weeks of an acute psychotic illness;

levels usually return to normal. The significance of such changes is unclear.

Recent work suggests that TSH levels at the lower end of normal are a predictor of increased mortality in older people. Most of the excess risk appears to be due to death from cardiovascular disease. Such individuals have been postulated to have 'subclinical hyperthyroidism', that is, low–normal TSH but normal triiodothyronine and thyroxine levels and no overt signs or symptoms of thyrotoxicosis. Whether such biochemical disturbances cause excess cardiovascular disease or are an epiphenomenon is not clear, but thyroxine has been shown to have potentially adverse effects on pulse rate, blood pressure and left ventricular mass – an important prognostic marker for cardiovascular disease.

References

Dayan C M 2001 Interpretation of thyroid function tests. Lancet 357:619–624

Parle J V, Masionneuve P, Sheppard M C et al 2001 Preduction of all-cause and cardiovascular mortality in elderly people from one low serum thyrotropin result: a 10-year cohort study. Lancet 358:861–865

Wardle C A, Fraser W D, Squire C R 2001 Pitfalls in the use of thyrotropin concentration as a first-line thyroid-function test. Lancet 357:1013–1014

5.   Autoimmune polyendocrinopathy

A. **F**   B. **F**   C. **T**   D. **T**   E. **F**

Autoimmune polyendocrinopathy syndrome type 1 (APS-1) is an autosomal recessive disease caused by mutation of the *AIRE1* gene on chromosome 21; over 30 mutations of this gene have now been reported. It is a rare disease; a recent Norwegian study found a prevalence of 1 in 80 000, and reported prevalence varies from 1 in 14 000 in Sardinia to 2–3 per million in northern England. The disease causes a wide spectrum of ectodermal dystrophic changes, as well as organ-specific autoimmune disease. The diagnosis is made on the presence of two out of three of Addison's disease, chronic mucocutaneous candidiasis and primary hypoparathyroidism.

Chronic mucocutaneous candidiasis typically presents at age around 5 years, with hypoparathyroidism becoming apparent at age 8 and Addison's disease presenting later, at around age 12. Careful and frequent review is thus necessary to detect the onset of Addison's disease before an Addisonian crisis occurs. Survival in the past was poor; nowadays however, survival is probably better than 90% at 20 years. Deaths do occur from sepsis as well as from the complications of organ specific autoimmune disease such as diabetic ketoacidosis and Addisonian crisis; the candidiasis seen in the disease is thought to be due to a defect of T lymphocyte function (B cells and therefore antibody production are unaffected).

Other organ-specific features include gonadal failure, hypopituitarism, pernicious anaemia, hepatitis, vitiligo and type 1 diabetes. Organ-specific autoantibodies are often found that accompany these clinical manifestations. Hypothyroidism is uncommon (5–10%) and hyperthyroidism is rare. Hyperparathyroidism is not a recognised association with APS-1. Ectodermal changes include nail dystrophy, keratopathy, enamel hypoplasia and alopecia. Malabsorption affects 25–30% of sufferers and hyposplenism occurs in up to 40% of cases.

APS-2 has a polygenic inheritance, with linkage to human leucocyte antigen (HLA) DR3 and DR4. Mutations of the *AIRE* gene do not appear to play a part in the development of APS-2. It is diagnosed by the presence of Addison's disease plus either autoimmune thyroid disease or type 1 diabetes. Vitiligo, pituitary failure, gonadal failure, pernicious anaemia and alopecia do occur, but are relatively uncommon (each < 5%). Candidiasis and hypoparathyroidism are not associated with the syndrome. APS-2 is not uncommon; 40–50% of patients with Addison's disease have another APS-2-associated endocrinopathy.

References

Betterele C, Greggio N A, Volpato M 1998 Clinical review 93. Autoimmune polyglandular syndrome type 1. Journal of Clinical Endocrinology and Metabolism 83:1049–1055

Myhre A G, Halonen M, Eskelin P et al 2001 Autoimmune polyendocrinopathy syndrome type 1 (APS 1) in Norway. Clinical Endocrinology 54:211–217

Obermayer-Straub P, Manns M P 1998 Autoimmune polyglandular syndromes. Ballière's Clinical Gastroenterology 12:293–315

Pearce S H S, Cheetham T D 2001 Autoimmune polyendocrinopathy syndrome type 1: treat with kid gloves. Clinical Endocrinology 54:433–435

Best-of-5 answers

6.   Obesity

Answer: **C**

The Western world is in the grip of a pandemic of obesity. The prevalence of obesity (which is defined as having a body mass index (BMI) > 30 kg/m^2) is well over 20% and rising in the UK; the prevalence is over 30% in the USA. Obesity is a risk factor for atherosclerotic disease, a major risk factor for developing type 2 diabetes and hypertension, and contributes to osteoarthritis, back pain and other musculoskeletal complaints. Obesity also carries a burden of psychological morbidity and is a risk factor for the development of some cancers.

Orlistat is a pancreatic lipase inhibitor that reduces the absorption of fat from dietary intake. It is not absorbed systemically but can cause side-effects of steatorrhoea, flatulence and abdominal discomfort if significant quantities of dietary fat are ingested when taking the drug. It is contraindicated in patients with known malabsorption or cholestasis. NICE guidelines on the use of orlistat suggest that it should be prescribed only for those patients who have already lost 2.5 kg in the month prior to prescription as a result of diet and exercise and who have either: (1) a BMI of $\geq$ 28 kg/m^2 plus significant comorbidities (e.g. hypertension, diabetes, hypercholesterolaemia); or (2) a BMI of $\geq$ 30 kg/m^2 with no associated comorbidities. It is further suggested that prescription of orlistat be accompanied by further advice on diet and exercise strategies.

The woman in this example has a body mass index of 35.8; she thus qualifies for orlistat therapy, which should be accompanied by exercise and continuing diet therapy. Therapy should normally not be prescribed for longer than a year, and is not licensed for use beyond 24 months. The NICE guidelines suggest that weight loss of 5% at 3 months and 10% at 6 months should be documented to justify continuing with the therapy.

Sibutramine is a noradrenaline (norepinephrine) and serotonin reuptake inhibitor. It induces a feeling of having eaten enough and might also help to prevent the decline in energy expenditure often seen during weight-loss programmes based on dieting. It is contraindicated in patients with established coronary artery disease, heart failure, peripheral vascular disease, stroke or arrhythmias. NICE guidelines suggest that sibutramine be used in patients with a BMI of $\geq$ 30, or $\geq$ 27 kg/m^2 where other comorbid disease (see above) is present. It should not be used for longer than 1 year and should be accompanied by ongoing dietary and exercise therapy and counselling. Weight loss of 2 kg in the first 4 weeks and 5 kg at 3 months should be achieved if therapy is to continue.

Sibutramine can increase blood pressure and so is not recommended for use in hypertensive patients. It can also cause nausea and vomiting, dry mouth, insomnia, constipation, headache and palpitations. There is some evidence that sibutramine can slow the rate of weight reaccumulation over a longer period. Small and often non-significant improvements in lipid profile and, in diabetics, glycaemic control, have been noted.

Neither of the above therapies has yet been subjected to trials involving hard endpoints such as death or cardiovascular events. There is no evidence to support combining the therapies.

References

James W P T, Astrup A, Finer N et al 2000 Effect of sibutramine on weight maintenance after weight loss: a randomised trial. Lancet 356:2119–2125

NICE 2001 Full guidance on the use of orlistat for the treatment of obesity in adults Technology appraisal guidance No 22. Online. Available: www.nice.org.uk/article.asp?a=1189

NICE 2001 Full guidance on the use of sibutramine for the treatment of obesity in adults. Technology appraisal guidance No 31. Online. Available: www.nice.org.uk/article.asp?a=1189

7.   Diabetes therapy

Answer: **B**

Given the fact that this man's glucostix readings are below 7 before each meal, his poor diabetic control is likely to be due to postprandial hyperglycaemia. Normally, the pancreas secretes a low basal level of insulin and responds to a glucose load (such as that provided by a meal) with a rapid release of insulin. Type 2 diabetes is characterised not only by insulin resistance but also by inadequate beta-cell function. Thus the ability of the pancreas to respond to a glucose load is compromised, leading to postprandial hyperglycaemia.

Postprandial hyperglycaemia is correlated with HbA1c at least as tightly as fasting glucose levels are. Postprandial hyperglycaemia is associated with both microvascular and macrovascular events and some studies suggest that therapy targeted at postprandial hyperglycaemia is more effective at lowering HbA1c than therapy targeted at fasting glucose levels.

Traditional sulphonylurea drugs are typically slow acting and are thus unable to stimulate insulin secretion rapidly when a meal is taken. Furthermore, their duration of action means that insulin levels can stay high long after a glucose load has been absorbed, leading to the risk of hyporglycaemia. Awareness of this risk has knock-on effects for the diabetic patients in terms of dietary behaviour and consequent weight gain; patients who experience hypoglycaemia tend to eat between meals and eat when not hungry so as to minimise the risk of a 'hypo'.

This man is not on insulin therapy and is unlikely to benefit much from a long-acting insulin, as his fasting glucose levels are well controlled. Insulin lispro is a rapidly acting insulin that could be used to control postprandial hyperglycaemia but it might be possible to avoid the use of exogenous insulin in this man, at least for the moment.

Repaglinide is a meglitinide analogue, meglitinide being the non-sulphonylurea moiety of glibenclamide, which was noted to have insulin-releasing properties independent of the sulphonylurea moiety. Repaglinide binds to a separate site on the sulphonylurea receptor, a potassium channel present on pancreatic beta cells. The drug has a rapid onset of action, with peak insulin levels occurring 1–2 h after ingestion. It has a short half-life – insulin returns to fasting levels within 6 h of ingestion – thus reducing the risk of hypoglycaemia. Furthermore, the ability of the drug to release insulin from beta cells is dependent on the glucose concentration; at low glucose levels, little insulin is released. This also contributes to the low incidence of hypoglycaemia seen with meglitinide analogue therapy.

Repaglinide can be used in mild to moderate renal impairment. It is contraindicated in pregnancy and in severe liver impairment. Side-effects are nausea and vomiting, diarrhoea and constipation. Although hypoglycaemia is a recognised side-effect, the incidence is lower than with sulphonylureas.

There is some evidence that meglitinide analogues can reduce HbA1c levels and they also appear to have an effect on eating patterns; fewer people report eating when not hungry to reduce the chance of a hypo. The effect of meglitinide analogues on hard outcomes such as microvascular and macrovascular disease is unknown at present. Exactly how these agents will fit into the therapeutic armamentarium is also unclear but their use in cases of predominantly postprandial hypoglycaemia seems logical.

References

Dornholst A 2001 Insulinotropic meglitinide analogues. Lancet 358:1709–1716

Inzucchi S E 2002 Oral antihyperglycemic therapy for type 2 diabetes. Journal of the Americal Medical Association 287:360–372

8. Hypertension in diabetes

Answer: **E**

Several trials give good long-term data using hard endpoints such as death, myocardial infarction, stroke or other vascular events, involving a number of classes of antihypertensives. Head-to-head comparisons between classes of antihypertensive are scarce, however. All of the above choices of antihypertensive have now been shown to reduce the incidence of cardiovascular events in diabetic patients.

Angiotensin converting enzyme (ACE) inhibitors are a good first-line choice for diabetic patients with raised blood pressure. The UK prospective diabetes study (UKPDS) showed that patients treated with ACE inhibitors showed a 25% reduction in microvascular endpoints and a reduction in combined macrovascular endpoints. Several trials have now shown that in diabetic patients with microalbuminuria or established diabetic nephropathy, ACE inhibitors can retard the progression of nephropathy and delay the time to end stage renal failure. The recent RENAAL and CALM studies have demonstrated similar effects of angiotensin II receptor blockers in patients with microalbuminuria or established diabetic nephropathy.

The HOPE trial showed that in patients with diabetes, the ACE inhibitor ramipril reduced the combined endpoint of death, myocardial infarction or other vascular event; the reduction in events was out of proportion to the small reduction in blood pressure seen in this trial. Some, but not all, studies suggest that ACE inhibitors might improve insulin sensitivity.

Both beta-blockers and thiazides can have adverse effects on the lipid profile; they can also worsen insulin resistance, with consequent adverse effects on glycaemic control. Beta-blockade can exacerbate problems with impotence in diabetes. However, UKPDS showed that beta-blockers were as effective as ACE inhibitors at reducing macrovascular and microvascular endpoints, and the SHEP and INSIGHT trials showed that thiazides could also reduce the rate of cardiovascular events.

Both the SYST-EUR and HOT trials showed that calcium-antagonist-based therapy can also reduce the incidence of cardiovascular events in hypertensive diabetic patients, and the

INSIGHT trial showed equivalence of efficacy between co-amilozide (hydrochlorothiazide plus amiloride) and a long-acting nifedipine formulation.

Recently, the LIFE study compared the effect of losartan versus atenolol on cardiovascular events in hypertensive patients with left ventricular hypertrophy (LVH) diagnosed on ECG criteria. In diabetic patients, there was a 25% reduction in the combined endpoint of cardiovascular death, stroke and myocardial infarction with losartan. This was despite the blood pressure reduction being slightly less in the losartan group.

References

Feher MD 2002 Diabetes and hypertension. Medicine 30:30–32

Heart Outcome Prevention Evaluation (HOPE) study investigators 2000 Effects of ramipril on cardiovascular and microvascular outcomes in people with diabetes mellitus. Results of the HOPE study and MICRO-HOPE substudy. Lancet 355:246–259

Julius S, Majahalme S, Palatini P 2001 Antihypertensive treatment of patients with diabetes and hypertension. American Journal of Hypertension 14:310S–316S

Lindholm L, Ibsen H, Dahlof B et al 2002 Cardiovascular morbidity and mortality in patients with diabetes in the Losartan Intervention for Endpoint reduction in hypertension study (LIFE): a randomised trial against atenolol. Lancet 359:1004–1010

9.   Hypercortisolaemia

Answer: **C**

Cushing's syndrome is caused by an excess of circulating cortisol. This leads to a wide range of signs and symptoms, including truncal obesity, weight gain, hypertension, mood disorders, thinning of skin, striae, easy bruising, impaired glucose tolerance, hirsutism, acne, muscle weakness and amenorrhoea. Cushing's syndrome can be caused by a pituitary adenoma (Cushing's disease), by ectopic adrenocorticotrophic hormone (ACTH) secretion (as a result of small cell lung carcinoma or carcinoid tumours), or by adrenal tumours or hyperplasia. Pseudo-Cushing's syndrome can occur in people with severe depression or alcoholism.

Elevated 24-h urinary free cortisol levels, preferably collected on three occasions, have a sensitivity and specificity of > 95%. This investigation alone is usually adequate to make a diagnosis of Cushing's syndrome. Only in borderline cases is a low-dose dexamethasone suppression test required; this can be useful for distinguishing pseudo-Cushing's syndrome.

Once the diagnosis is established, the focus shifts to finding out the cause of the hypercortisolaemia. ACTH levels are useful because they can distinguish between pituitary (normal or high ACTH), ectopic (very high ACTH) and adrenal (low ACTH) sources of disease. Once this distinction has been made, the appropriate imaging can be carried out: MRI of the pituitary, chest X-ray and perhaps CT of the chest for high ACTH; CT or MRI of the adrenals for low ACTH.

Between 1 and 8% of people have adrenal adenomas on CT or MRI of the adrenals. The vast majority of these are non-functioning ('incidentalomas'), thus indiscriminate imaging of the adrenals without testing ACTH can lead to erroneous conclusions as to the site of pathology. Adrenal scintigraphy can be helpful in assessing whether adrenal masses are functional adenomas.

Up to 50% of pituitary microadenomas are invisible on MRI of the pituitary and not all adenomas of the pituitary seen on MRI are functional; some are 'incidentalomas'. Thus, in cases with elevated ACTH, the high-dose dexamethasone test should be used – pituitary adenomas are usually suppressed by this test, whereas ectopic sources of ACTH are not. In difficult cases, inferior petrosal sinus sampling of ACTH will confirm or refute a pituitary origin of the hormone excess.

Reference

Bertagna X 2001 Cushing's syndrome. Medicine 29:16–19

Boscaro M, Barzon L, Fallo F et al 2001 Cushing's syndrome. Lancet 357:783–791

10.   The Barker hypothesis

Answer: **C**

Barker's hypothesis states that low birth weight, as caused by poor growth in utero, is a risk factor for adverse cardiovascular outcomes in adulthood. It is postulated that relative malnutrition in utero leads to a long-term resetting of several metabolic and endocrine homeostatic mechanisms, such that risk factors for atherogenesis, e.g. impaired glucose tolerance, dyslipidaemia, hypertension and raised fibrinogen levels, become more likely in adulthood.

More recently, this hypothesis has been extended to form the 'thrifty phenotype' hypothesis; changes in utero as described above help to prepare the newborn child for life in a nutritionally poor environment, but if this 'thrifty phenotype' is then exposed to a plentiful supply of food (as is the case nowadays in the Western world), weight gain, hypertension and impaired glucose tolerance result. This could help to explain the massive increase in cardiovascular disease seen in the Western world over the last century, as fetal and childhood malnourishment have given way to the current dietary overabundance enjoyed by most adults. It further helps to explain the rapid rise in cardiovascular disease being seen amongst South Asian immigrants to Western countries, and indeed within the more affluent in South Asia itself. Similarly high levels of diabetes, hypertension and cardiovascular disease are seen amongst Australian aboriginal populations. The risk posed by low fetal growth and that posed by environmental events appear to be additive; the group of patients at highest risk of cardiovascular events are those with low birth weight who become obese adults; those who have higher birth weights and do not become obese in adulthood have the lowest risk.

Work is underway to elucidate the mechanisms behind these findings; there is evidence that the response of the hypothalamic–pituitary–adrenal axis is different in individuals who were small at birth, and low birth weight babies display a higher degree of insulin resistance even in childhood. There is also evidence that slow growth in the first year of life has similar effects, independent of birth weight, and that those with a low birth weight are more susceptible to environmental risk factors for cardiovascular disease (e.g. smoking). It appears to be low birth weight, not prematurity, that determines adult cardiovascular risk.

References

Barker D J P, Forsen T, Uutela A et al 2001 Size at birth and resilience to effects of poor living conditions in adult life: longitudinal study. British Medical Journal 323:1273–1276

Barker D J P 1997 Intrauterine programming of coronary heart disease and stroke. Acta Paediatrica (suppl):178–182

Eriksson J, Forsen T, Tuomilehto J et al 2001 Early growth and coronary heart disease in later life: longitudinal study. British Medical Journal 322:949–953

Robinson R 2001 The fetal origins of adult disease. British Medical Journal 322:375–376

RESPIRATORY

True/False answers

11.   Asthma

A. **T**   B. **T**   C. **T**   D. **F**   E. **T**

Asthma is characterised by reversible airflow obstruction, bronchial hyperresponsiveness and inflammation. Inflammation (mediated by histamine, prostaglandins and leukotrienes) is found from large airways to alveoli, indicating that treatment targeted at the entire bronchial tree is necessary. Metered-dose inhalers are the most common means of facilitating topical delivery of drugs to the airway, and oral antiasthma treatments provide a more systemic approach. In addition to the higher mortality rate found among uncontrolled asthmatics, untreated inflammation can lead to development of relatively fixed airways, which become less responsive to conventional therapy.

Corticosteroids are the most effective anti-inflammatory therapy available in the treatment of asthma, but have a limited impact on leukotriene levels. The cysteinyl leukotrienes (consisting of leukotrienes C_4, D_4 and E_4) are important pro-inflammatory mediators implicated in the pathogenesis of asthma and resulting in bronchoconstriction, inflammatory cell recruitment, mucous hypersecretion and smooth muscle proliferation. Arachidonic acid is the precursor molecule from which cysteinyl leukotrienes are produced after activation of the 5-lipoxygenase pathway. Further down the cascade, leukotriene C_4 synthase is an integral enzyme involved in their biosynthesis converting leukotriene A_4 to C_4.

Pharmacologically, antagonism of the leukotriene pathway can be achieved with blockade of the leukotriene receptor (using a leukotriene receptor antagonist such as montelukast or zafirlukast) or with use of a 5-lipoxygenase inhibitor (e.g. zileuton). Because they are orally active and permit once- or twice-daily dosing, leukotriene receptor antagonists can be advantageous in patients who find coordination with inhalers a problem. Studies indicate that they demonstrate both anti-inflammatory and bronchodilatory properties and exhibit additive effects when given with inhaled corticosteroids.

Inhaled corticosteroids are the gold-standard therapy in asthma and bind to glucocorticoid receptors found throughout the entire bronchial tree. Fluticasone propionate was introduced as an alternative for patients requiring high doses of beclometasone dipropionate; it is more lipophilic and has a longer duration of action than the latter. Beclometasone dipropionate undergoes first-pass metabolism (in the lung and liver) and is subsequently converted to beclometasone-17-monopropionate (the active component) and beclometasone-21-monopropionate (the inactive component). In patients prescribed inhaled corticosteroids, doses up to 800 µg/day results in a fairly steep dose–response curve for antiasthma beneficial effects, whereas at doses above this the curve flattens off. The dose–response curve for systemic adverse effects is initially flat but becomes steep at doses above 800 µg/day. Maximising the distance between these two curves results in a favourable therapeutic ratio.

Because of their deleterious effects upon the ozone layer, inhalers using chlorofluorocarbon as the propellant are being phased out and replaced by inhalers using hydrofluoroalkane as the propellant. Beclometasone is one of the most commonly prescribed inhaled corticosteroids in asthma and its hydrofluoroalkane preparation, when given at half the dose, results in comparable efficacy. The particles in these new formulations are also of a smaller size and are in solution, allowing easier passage to the smaller airways and thus facilitating more widespread anti-inflammatory activity.

Long-acting β_2-agonists act directly upon bronchial smooth-muscle β_2-adrenoceptors and suppress the release of inflammatory mediators from primed mast cells in the airway. As a consequence, they exert their beneficial effects by means of bronchodilation and protection against bronchoconstrictor stimuli. Tolerance to both these properties has been demonstrated, but far more consistently with the latter. When used on a regular basis, tolerance to their bronchoprotective effects occurs more readily in patients possessing a polymorphism of the β_2-adrenoceptor, which occurs in about 40% of the UK population. Despite these concerns, however, a recent meta-analysis has demonstrated the superiority of salmeterol over doubling the dose of inhaled corticosteroid in terms of improved lung function and symptom-free days. Moreover, the recent OPTIMA study investigated the management of mild asthma in patients already receiving low-dose inhaled corticosteroids. It demonstrated that the addition of formoterol had a superior effect, in terms of increasing the time to first exacerbation, than doubling the dose of inhaled corticosteroid.

References

Gross G, Thompson P J, Chervinsky P, Van den Burgt J 1999 Hydrofluoroalkane-134a beclomethasone dipropionate, 400 μg, is as effective as chlorofluorocarbon beclomethasone dipropionate, 800 μg, for the treatment of moderate asthma. Chest 115:343–351

O'Byrne P M, Barnes P J, Rodriguez-Roisin R et al 2001 Low dose inhaled budesonide and formoterol in mild persistent asthma: the OPTIMA randomized trial. American Journal of Respiration and Critical Care Medicine 164:1392–1397

Shrewsbury S, Pyke S, Britton M 2000 Meta-analysis of increased dose of inhaled steroid or addition of salmeterol in symptomatic asthma (MIASMA). British Medical Journal 320:1368–1373

12. Bronchial carcinoma

A. **T**   B. **F**   C. **F**   D. **T**   E. **F**

Bronchial carcinoma is the most common malignancy in the developed world. Despite many advances in diagnosis and treatment, the 5-year survival rate is still < 20%, although patients who present early with stage I disease can have a significantly improved 5-year survival. Whether mass screening will be beneficial in the detection of early disease in asymptomatic individuals remains to be established.

Bronchial carcinoma is generally divided into two main categories according to cell type. Non-small cell bronchial carcinoma (squamous cell, adenocarcinoma, and large cell) accounts for 70–80% of all new cases; the remainder are of small cell histology. One of the most common cell types in the UK is squamous cell carcinoma, although the incidence of adenocarcinoma is increasing. Squamous carcinomas tend to be central in origin, present with haemoptysis, arise in previous tuberculous cavities and metastasise late. Finger clubbing is strongly associated with squamous but not small cell bronchial carcinoma, and can disappear after successful tumour resection. Small cell carcinoma tends to present after local, haematogenous or lymphatic spread has already occurred. It is this cell type that is associated with production of hormones such as antidiuretic hormone (ADH) or ACTH. Ectopic ACTH production causes bilateral adrenal hyperplasia and subsequent secretion of cortisol. This leads to high levels of cortisol, which are not suppressed with dexamethasone, loss of diurnal variation in cortisol levels and a hypokalaemic alkalosis. Hypercalcaemia is more commonly due to bone metastasis but squamous carcinoma can produce parathyroid hormone (PTH)-related peptide, which can cause confusion, polyuria with thirst, constipation, nausea and vomiting. Despite small cell lung cancer being sensitive to chemotherapy, it still has a dismal long-term prognosis in view of early metastasis. Four to six cycles of chemotherapy using combinations of cisplatin, etoposide, cyclophosphamide, doxorubicin and vincristine-based chemotherapy are usually administered.

Most cases of bronchial carcinoma are caused by cigarette smoking, which is quantitated by pack years (the product of the number of packs smoked per day and the number of years spent smoking). Smoking cessation therefore plays an important step in the prevention of bronchial carcinoma. Bupropion (amfebutamone), an antidepressant, has been shown to help people stop smoking. In a recent randomised, placebo-controlled trial, patients were given bupropion (amfebutamone), nicotine patch or placebo. Treatment with bupropion (amfebutamone) in combination with a nicotine patch was significantly more effective than placebo or nicotine patch alone. Smokers who have not quit after 2 months of therapy should be advised to stop taking bupropion (amfebutamone). Previous contact with asbestosis is the most common occupational association for bronchial carcinoma, and radon, nickel, chromate and aromatic hydrocarbon exposure is also implicated in its pathogenesis. Cryptogenic fibrosing alveolitis is an independent risk factor.

Once diagnosed, accurate clinical staging is important in determining those patients who will benefit most in terms of surgery, chemotherapy and radiotherapy. Positron emission tomography (PET) using 18-fluorodeoxyglucose, which is preferentially taken up by neoplastic tissue, has been developed. This has shown to improve diagnostic sensitivity of both local and distant metastasis in non-small cell bronchial carcinoma. This might subsequently improve the preoperative staging of patients and tailoring of appropriate treatment to patients. Interest has grown in potential new therapies for lung cancer including inhibition of angiogenesis, immunotherapy and gene therapy. Mutations in the p53 tumour suppressor gene are associated in the development of malignancy. Whether correction of genetic abnormalities will prove effective remains to be seen.

References

British Thoracic Society and Society of Cardiothoracic Surgeons of Great Britain and Ireland Working Party 2001 Guidelines on the selection of patients with lung cancer for surgery. Thorax 56:89–108

Hoffman P C, Mauer A M, Vokes E E 2000 Lung cancer. Lancet 355:479–485

Jorenby D E, Leischow S J, Nides M A et al 1999 A controlled trial of sustained-release bupropion, a nicotine patch, or both for smoking cessation. New England Journal of Medicine 340:685–691

Pieterman R M, van Putten J W, Meuzelaar J J et al 2000 Preoperative staging of non-small-cell lung cancer with positron-emission tomography. New England Journal of Medicine 343:254–261

13.   Non-invasive ventilation

A. **T**   B. **F**   C. **T**   D. **F**   E. **F**

Non-invasive ventilation is a useful therapeutic adjunct in the management of patients with hypercapnic respiratory failure. An adjustable facemask provides an interface between patient and portable ventilator, allowing assisted ventilation to take place without problems such as nosocomial pneumonia, sinusitis and upper airway injury associated with intubation and mechanical ventilation, and occupation of an intensive care bed. Patients are thus able to eat, drink, communicate and receive nebulised medication while receiving non-invasive ventilation in various settings. Providing appropriate expertise and experience is available from medical and nursing staff, it can be used in general medical and respiratory wards in addition to high dependency units. It can also be used successfully on a domiciliary basis in patients with chronic hypercapnic respiratory failure, such as those with chronic neuromuscular disorders, chest wall deformity or spinal cord and brainstem lesions.

Non-invasive ventilation is particularly beneficial in patients with exacerbations of chronic obstructive pulmonary disease (COPD) and especially in those with a respiratory acidosis of between pH 7.25 and 7.35. When used in this situation, it has been shown to reduce the requirement for intubation and reduce the mortality rate compared to standard therapy. It also causes a more rapid improvement in physiological parameters such as pH and respiratory rate. The efficacy of non-invasive ventilation has been demonstrated in a number of other clinical settings, including hypercapnic pulmonary oedema, as an aid to wean patients from mechanical ventilation and in patients with pneumonia. Its use can also be considered as a 'ceiling of treatment' when mechanical ventilation is considered inappropriate.

Non-invasive ventilation is not suitable for all patients with respiratory failure. It should generally be avoided in those with orofacial burns or trauma, vomiting and intestinal obstruction, haemodynamic instability, untreated pneumothorax and obtunded patients unable to protect their airway. Non-invasive ventilation should also be used with caution in patients who have copious respiratory secretions, such as in cystic fibrosis or bronchiectasis, although a break can allow time for adequate physiotherapy and postural drainage. Doxapram, a respiratory stimulant, is sometimes used in patients unable to tolerate non-invasive ventilation who have hypercapnic respiratory failure. However, doxapram is often poorly tolerated because of confusion, agitation, tachycardia and nausea.

Analysis of arterial blood gases is imperative when non-invasive ventilation is used in patients with acute hypercapnic respiratory failure. In those patients with a deteriorating pH despite non-invasive ventilation in conjunction with routine medical therapy, mechanical ventilation should be considered. Physiological variables associated with a favourable outcome are an improvement in pH, $p\text{CO}_2$ and respiratory rate 1 h after its commencement.

Most non-invasive ventilation machines have the ability to provide bilevel support allowing both inspiratory and expiratory positive airway pressure support. The expiratory positive airway pressure support allows recruitment of underventilated alveoli and helps splint open the distal airways allowing improved gas exchange. Machines also permit the provision of oxygen through a port, which is vital for most patients.

References

British Thoracic Society Standards of Care Committee 2002 Non-invasive ventilation in acute respiratory failure. Thorax 57:192–211

Plant P K, Owen J L, Elliott M W 2000 Early use of non-invasive ventilation for acute exacerbations of chronic obstructive pulmonary disease on general respiratory wards: a multicentre randomised controlled trial. Lancet 355:1931–1935

14. Inflammation and asthma

A. **F**   B. **T**   C. **F**   D. **T**   E. **T**

Inflammation is one of the classic features of asthma in which type 2 helper T cells (Th2 cells) are thought to play a critical role. Th2 cells secrete a variety of cytokines, which cause production of IgE by B lymphocytes and initiate and promote airway inflammation. By contrast, type 1 helper T cells (Th1 cells) have a role in the protection against various organisms, secrete interferon gamma and have an inhibitory effect on Th2 cell production. An imbalance between these two CD4 T cell types is considered to be central to the underlying allergic inflammatory process in asthma. Cytokines such as interleukin-3 and interleukin-5 are involved in the activation and survival of eosinophils, and recent work has been carried out investigating the anti-inflammatory effects of administration of anti-interleukin-5 antibodies. Interest has also arisen involving treatment with subcutaneous injections of anti-IgE antibodies. This monoclonal antibody is known to prevent the binding of IgE molecules to receptors on mast cells, thereby preventing the release of proinflammatory mediators.

Allergic rhinitis, which can be perennial, seasonal or a combination of both, is an inflammatory condition of the nasal mucosa causing itch, sneeze, watery nose and excess mucous production. Because the upper and lower respiratory tracts are in direct continuation with one another, they often share similar responses to inhaled stimuli and treatments options. Allergic rhinitis, which commonly coexists with asthma and occurs in approximately 40% of asthmatics, is associated with bronchial hyperresponsiveness and is a risk factor for the subsequent development of asthma. Some studies have reported that treatment of allergic rhinitis is associated with a commensurate improvement in asthma symptoms and reduction of exacerbations.

Montelukast, a leukotriene receptor antagonist, is useful in patients with exercise-induced asthma, as add-on therapy in patients not controlled on inhaled corticosteroids and in concomitant allergic rhinitis. It is also of value in patients with aspirin-sensitive asthma who overproduce cysteinyl leukotrienes. Leukotriene receptor antagonists possess less anti-inflammatory activity than inhaled corticosteroids and are less effective bronchodilators than long-acting β_2-agonsits. Recent concerns have been raised regarding the use of leukotriene receptor antagonists and development of Churg–Strauss syndrome (characterised by peripheral blood eosinophilia, vasculitis and asthma). Following the introduction of a leukotriene receptor antagonist, some patients have been able to reduce their inhaled corticosteroid dose with consequent unmasking of features suggestive of Churg–Strauss syndrome. It remains uncertain whether this has been due to masking effects of the inhaled corticosteroid or due to the leukotriene receptor antagonist itself.

By definition, asthma is associated with reversible airflow obstruction, thereby allowing the diagnosis to be made in patients with normal spirometry. In asthmatic patients with abnormal spirometry, the FEV_1 is reduced, often with a maintained FVC, whereas the FVC can also be reduced in patients who have had airway remodelling as a result of untreated inflammation. Reduction in the mid-expiratory flow during expiration is considered to be suggestive of obstruction of the smaller airways. People with asthma often demonstrate hyperresponsiveness to inhaled bronchoconstrictor stimuli, such as methacholine or histamine, and a positive response (a fall in FEV_1 often of 20% from initial baseline) following either of these agents can aid confirmation of a diagnosis.

References

Drazen J M, Israel E, O'Byrne P M 1999 Treatment of asthma with drugs modifying the leukotriene pathway. New England Journal of Medicine 340:197–206

Frew A J, Plummeridge M J 2001 Alternative agents in asthma. Journal of Allergy and Clinical Immunology 108:3–10

Leff J A, Busse W W, Pearlman D et al 1998 Montelukast, a leukotriene-receptor antagonist, for the treatment of mild asthma and exercise-induced bronchoconstriction. New England Journal of Medicine 339:147–152

Lipworth B J, White P S 2000 Allergic inflammation in the unified airway: start with the nose. Thorax 55:878–881

15.   Obstructive sleep apnoea

A. **T**   B. **F**   C. **F**   D. **F**   E. **F**

The prevalence of obstructive sleep apnoea syndrome is in the order of 1–4% of the middle-aged population and is increasingly being recognised as an important clinical entity. During normal sleep, pharyngeal muscles relax causing a reduction in the airway diameter. In patients with sleep apnoea, complete or partial pharyngeal obstruction can result in snoring, apnoea, hypoxia and increased respiratory effort and arousal. Once increased arousal has occurred with resolution of hypoxia, the process is repeated throughout the night. The recurrent hypoxia that accompanies these changes can in severe cases result in pulmonary hypertension and cor pulmonale.

The association between sleep apnoea and hypertension has been extensively investigated. Various comorbid conditions such as obesity have made analysis difficult, but it is thought likely that sleep apnoea is a risk factor for subsequent development of daytime hypertension.

Despite being strongly associated with obesity, obstructive sleep apnoea commonly occurs in patients with a normal BMI. Individuals with orofacial anatomical abnormalities such as macroglossia (acromegaly, hypothyroidism, amyloidosis), Down syndrome, Marfan syndrome, adenoid and tonsillar hypertrophy, and retro- or micrognathia (Pierre–Robin syndrome) are also predisposed. Drugs that cause relaxation of the pharyngeal muscles such as alcohol, benzodiazepines and opiates can lead to prolonged periods of apnoea and blunting of arousal responses resulting in symptoms.

Often the patient's partner describes witnessed apnoeas and complains of excessive and loud snoring, which is audible despite sleeping in different rooms. Subjective complaints include unrefreshing sleep, daytime somnolence especially in potentially disastrous circumstances such as when driving, impotence, lack of concentration and energy, and morning headache. A subjective questionnaire employed in the evaluation of sleep apnoea is the Epworth sleepiness scale in which individuals comment on how easily they could fall asleep in a particular situation.

Patients are often referred for overnight sleep studies (polysomnography) in which different physiological variables are measured to help confirm or refute the diagnosis. In particular, overnight oxygen saturation, EEG analysis and frequency of apnoeas are assessed along with other parameters.

Conservative measures such as weight reduction and avoidance of alcohol and sedatives underlie the management strategies in many patients. However, nasal continuous positive airway pressure (nasal CPAP) is often required in the treatment of patients. Application of a nasal mask with an entrained oxygen supply splints the airway open, thereby maintaining airway patency. Nasal CPAP reduces daytime somnolence and improves quality of life, mood and cognitive function. Since the introduction of nasal CPAP, surgical measures such as uvulopalatopharyngoplasty and fashioning of a tracheostomy are far less commonly performed, although adenotonsillectomy can be of benefit, particularly in children.

References

Jenkinson C, Davies R J, Mullins R, Stradling J R 1999 Comparison of therapeutic and subtherapeutic nasal continuous positive airway pressure for obstructive sleep apnoea: a randomised prospective parallel trial. Lancet 353:2100–2105

Stradling J R, Pepperell J C, Davies R J 2001 Sleep apnoea and hypertension: proof at last? Thorax 56(suppl 2):ii45–ii49

Best-of-5 answers

16. Chronic obstructive pulmonary disease

Answer: **B**

Chronic obstructive pulmonary disease (COPD) is a chronic progressive irreversible condition characterised by airflow obstruction ($FEV_1/FVC < 70$) and $FEV_1 < 80\%$ predicted. The term COPD has largely replaced diseases formerly known as chronic bronchitis and emphysema. Recent British Thoracic Society guidelines have categorised patients into having mild (60–80%), moderate (40–59%) and severe (< 40%) disease, according to the percentage FEV_1 predicted. Unlike asthma, in which eosinophils, mast cells and lymphocytes predominate, the associated inflammatory airway response is associated with neutrophils. Cigarette smoking causes the vast majority of cases, although deficiency of the alpha-1 antitrypsin enzyme, an antiprotease enzyme synthesised in the liver, is associated with airflow obstruction. Individuals with the ZZ genotype often develop emphysema in their third or fourth decade, which progresses rapidly in cigarette smokers. Irrespective of its aetiology, COPD causes progressive hypoxaemia (a potent vasoconstrictor of the pulmonary vasculature) and development of pulmonary hypertension and right ventricular strain. The subsequent appearance of clinical signs and symptoms of right ventricular failure signifies a poor prognosis.

In all but the mildest of disease, a corticosteroid trial is probably indicated to determine those who will gain benefit from long-term use. Following an oral or high-dose inhaled corticosteroid trial, less than 20% of patients demonstrate objective reversibility, that is, an absolute 200 mL and 15% improvement in baseline FEV_1. On the whole, whether patients gain long-term benefit from inhaled corticosteroids remains a contentious issue. In the recent multicentre placebo controlled ISOLDE trial, patients with COPD with a mean FEV_1 of 50% predicted were given fluticasone propionate 500 μg twice daily from a metered-dose inhaler. In agreement with other studies, this trial demonstrated that fluticasone did not alter the rate of decline in FEV_1 but did produce a small increase in FEV_1 in association with fewer exacerbations. However, the propensity of inhaled corticosteroids to cause dose-related adverse effects has to be weighed against their modest efficacy.

Theophylline, a non-selective phosphodiesterase inhibitor, is an orally active bronchodilator that also possesses some anti-inflammatory activity. One of its main drawbacks is its narrow therapeutic window between toxic and therapeutic doses. Monitoring patients blood concentration and starting patients on a low dose of theophylline is therefore required to minimise the risk of cardiac and gastrointestinal adverse effects. The half-life is increased in patients with heart failure, cirrhosis and in those taking ciprofloxacin and erythromycin, whereas it is decreased in current cigarette smokers and patients taking rifampicin, phenytoin and carbamazepine. A recent study was carried out using a new selective phosphodiesterase inhibitor, cilomilast, in patients with COPD. When given twice daily, FEV_1 was significantly improved, however quality of life evaluation was no different from placebo. Mucolytics such as carbocisteine encourage expectoration by reducing the viscosity of sputum. A recent systematic review examined the effects of prolonged treatment with oral mucolytics and confirmed that their use was associated with a reduction in number of exacerbations. Yearly vaccination against influenza is recommended and a one-off pneumococcal vaccination should also be given but is specifically contraindicated within 3 years of previous administration.

Hypoxic patients with COPD benefit from supplemental oxygen, which has been shown to improve survival when used for at least 15 h a day. Current guidelines suggest that long-term oxygen therapy should be prescribed (providing there are no contraindications) when the pO_2 is < 7.3 kPa on two successive occasions 3 weeks apart in the stable patient. It can also be prescribed to hypoxic patients who have peripheral oedema, pulmonary hypertension or secondary polycythaemia. Prior to its prescription by concentrator or cylinder, smoking cessation should be strongly encouraged.

Despite other beneficial manoeuvres, such as pulmonary rehabilitation and the use of non-invasive ventilation in acidotic patients, COPD remains an enormous problem in both primary and secondary care. Smoking cessation remains the only effective measure in altering the progressive decline in FEV_1 and altering the actual diseases process. This emphasises the importance of encouraging all patients to quit smoking.

References

The COPD Guidelines Group of the Standards of Care Committee of the BTS 1997 BTS guidelines for the management of chronic obstructive pulmonary disease. Thorax 52(suppl 5):S1–S28

Burge P S, Calverley P M, Jones P W et al 2000 Randomised, double blind, placebo controlled study of fluticasone propionate in patients with moderate to severe chronic obstructive pulmonary disease: the ISOLDE trial. British Medical Journal 320:1297–1303

Compton C H, Gubb J, Nieman R et al 2001 Cilomilast, a selective phosphodiesterase-4 inhibitor for treatment of patients with chronic obstructive pulmonary disease: a randomised, dose-ranging study. Lancet 358:265–270

Poole P J, Black P N 2001 Oral mucolytic drugs for exacerbations of chronic obstructive pulmonary disease: systematic review. British Medical Journal 322:1271–1274

17.   Primary pulmonary hypertension

Answer: **A**

Pulmonary hypertension is present when the mean resting pulmonary arterial pressure is > 25 mmHg at rest and > 30 mmHg on exercise; primary pulmonary hypertension is diagnosed when no aetiological agent is identified. Pulmonary hypertension can also be caused by chronic thromboembolic disease, COPD, HIV infection, use of anorectic agents (such as fenfluramine), sarcoidosis and congenital heart disease (because of increased pulmonary blood flow through cardiac shunts). It can also occur in association with connective tissue disease (e.g. rheumatoid arthritis, systemic sclerosis and SLE).

Primary pulmonary hypertension has an annual incidence of 1–2 per million and occurs more commonly in females than males, with a ratio of 2:1. It often presents between the ages of 20 and 40 years. Untreated, it leads to a progressive decrease in lung function and worsening of symptoms. Most cases of primary pulmonary hypertension occur sporadically but about 6% of cases are familial, demonstrating an autosomal dominant pattern of inheritance with incomplete penetrance. The responsible gene has been localised to chromosome 2 and recently mapped to an abnormality in the *BMPR2* gene.

Symptoms tend to be non-specific with dyspnoea, fatigue, chest pain and syncope typical initial presentations. As the disease progresses, clinical signs of right heart failure develops. All patients in whom the diagnosis is suspected should have a chest X ray, ECG, pulmonary function tests with gas transfer and transthoracic echocardiography. Further investigations should be carried out if a secondary cause, such as rheumatoid factor, is considered and imaging should be performed to exclude pulmonary thromboembolism. The diagnosis of primary pulmonary hypertension is normally confirmed during right heart catheterisation, which should be performed in most patients irrespective of stage. This also allows the opportunity to perform vasodilator testing. Following the administration of a vasodilator such as nitric oxide, a positive response is confirmed by a 20% reduction in pulmonary artery pressure without a fall in cardiac output. It is these patients who should be given long-term therapy with oral vasodilators such as diltiazem or nifedipine, which have demonstrated improved mortality and reduction of symptoms. Amlodipine can be considered, as an alternative, when right ventricular dysfunction is present.

Pulmonary hypertension *per se* is associated with an increased risk of thromboembolism. Subsequent treatment with warfarin is indicated in patients with pulmonary hypertension secondary to thromboembolic disease and is of benefit in those with primary pulmonary hypertension.

Irrespective of vasodilator response, patients with primary pulmonary hypertension should be considered for long-term treatment with intravenous prostaglandins. Prostaglandins have an antiplatelet effect in addition to bronchodilatory properties. Long-term treatment has demonstrated improved survival and results in fewer symptoms in patients with primary pulmonary hypertension. Due to associated risks and impracticalities associated with permanent intravenous access, there has been recent interest in aerosolised formulations of prostaglandins.

Vasoconstriction of the pulmonary arterial bed is one of the hallmark features of primary pulmonary hypertension and has prompted the investigation of an endothelin-1 (a potent pulmonary vasoconstrictor) receptor antagonist. A recent study has evaluated the effects of bosentan, an orally active endothelin receptor antagonist, in patients with primary pulmonary hypertension or pulmonary hypertension secondary to connective tissue disease. This demonstrated that twice-daily dosing improved 6-min walking distance compared to placebo in conjunction with less symptoms of breathlessness. A heart–lung transplant remains the only option for prolonging survival in resistant cases despite adequate medical treatment.

References

Hoeper M M, Schwarze M, Ehlerding S et al 2000 Long-term treatment of primary pulmonary hypertension with aerosolized iloprost, a prostacyclin analogue. New England Journal of Medicine 342:1866–1870

Recommendations on the management of pulmonary hypertension in clinical practice. Heart 2001; 86(suppl 1):I1–13

Rubin L J, Badesch D B, Barst R J et al 2002 Bosentan therapy for pulmonary arterial hypertension. New England Journal of Medicine 346:896–903

18.   Community-acquired pneumonia

Answer: **D**

Community-acquired pneumonia is a common cause of hospitalisation in the UK. *Streptococcus pneumoniae*, a Gram-positive diplococcus, remains the most common aetiological pathogen, indicating that antibiotics effective against this organism are usually required. Inadequate treatment of streptococcal pneumonia can result in local and haematogenous spread leading to pericarditis, meningitis, septic arthritis, lung or brain abscess, empyema, peritonitis and septicaemia. Infection with *Haemophilus influenzae* or *Moraxella catarrhalis* can be more common in patients with COPD. Infection due by *Mycoplasma pneumoniae* occurs in 4-yearly epidemics and often infects young adults. Pneumonia due to *M. pneumoniae* is associated with extrapulmonary features such as pericarditis, Stevens–Johnson syndrome, haemolytic anaemia, arthralgia, hepatitis and meningoencephalitis. Cold agglutinin production can be detected in 50% of cases. In the elderly, community-acquired pneumonia often results in symptoms not localised to the chest such as confusion, diarrhoea or vomiting. In all age groups, clinical improvement precedes radiological improvement. Many reasons account for patients failing to improve. Relatively common causes for treatment failure include inadequate dose, poorly absorbed antibiotic, resistant organism, viral infection or overwhelming infection. Additional or alternative diagnoses should also be considered, including bronchial carcinoma, pulmonary embolism, left ventricular failure, pulmonary eosinophilia, fibrosing alveolitis and allergic alveolitis.

Patients requiring hospital admission with severe community acquired pneumonia often require a β-lactamase-stable antibiotic (e.g. co-amoxiclav) in conjunction with a macrolide (erythromycin or clarithromycin) to cover potential atypical pathogens. In those patients intolerant of penicillins or macrolides, levofloxacin, a newer fluoroquinolone, demonstrates efficacy against *S. pneumoniae.* Additional supportive treatment such as oxygen to maintain saturation above 92%, deep vein thrombosis prophylaxis, analgesia and adequate nutritional supplementation are required for a satisfactory outcome.

In community-acquired pneumonia, features associated with an adverse outcome include the presence of comorbid illness, a respiratory rate ≥ 30 bpm, confusion, systolic blood pressure < 90 mmHg and/or diastolic blood pressure ≤ 60 mmHg, bilateral chest X-ray changes, leucopenia (WCC < 4) or leucocytosis (WCC > 20), hypoxaemia and a urea > 7 mmol/L. Inadequate treatment or delayed presentation of pneumonia can result in its extension into the pleural cavity, causing the development of a parapneumonic effusion or empyema. Frank pus is found in the pleural space with an empyema, often with absence of bacterial growth due to prior treatment with antibiotics. Clinically an empyema can manifest as persisting pyrexia, raised inflammatory markers, failure to improve and can cause drainage through the chest wall or formation of a bronchopleural fistula. If parapneumonic effusion or empyema is considered to be a possible complication, thoracocentesis is generally required. Those individuals discovered to have an empyema or complicated parapneumonic effusion (pH < 7.2, low glucose and raised LDH) should proceed to have tube thoracostomy often accompanied by instillation of intrapleural streptokinase. Treatment with intrapleural streptokinase or urokinase have been shown to be associated with an improved clinical and radiological outcome, without significant risk of systemic or local bleeding complications.

References

BTS Guidelines for the management of community acquired pneumonia in adults. Thorax 2001; 56(suppl 4):IV1–64

Sahn S A 1998 Use of fibrinolytic agents in the management of complicated parapneumonic effusions and empyemas. Thorax 53(suppl 2):S65–S72

19.   Tuberculosis

Answer: **C**

Mycobacteria are aerobic Gram-positive rods that do not lose their colouring following staining with acid or alcohol, hence the term 'acid–alcohol fast'. Infection with the human tubercle bacillus can cause both respiratory and non-respiratory tuberculosis. Tuberculosis has been a notifiable disease in the UK since the early twentieth century and any physician making the diagnosis is required to report it to the relevant statutory body.

Pulmonary tuberculosis is generally treated for a period of 6 months. In uncomplicated cases in which resistance is unlikely, the initial period should consist of a 2-month treatment block with rifampicin, isoniazid and pyrazinamide followed by a 4-month treatment block with rifampicin and isoniazid. If sensitivities are not available after 2 months of initial treatment, all three drugs should be continued until they are known. Once 2 weeks of effective treatment has elapsed in smear-positive patients, they are considered non-infectious. The addition of ethambutol is considered appropriate in patients who have a higher chance of isoniazid resistance, for example those who have been previously treated for tuberculosis, immigrants and the immunosuppressed such as those infected with HIV. Ethambutol can cause ocular toxicity manifesting as visual-field disturbance and impaired acuity, and should therefore be used with caution in young children or the elderly, who might be unable to report deterioration in eyesight. Treatment with isoniazid can cause peripheral neuropathy, which is more commonly seen in patients with HIV infection, alcoholics, the malnourished and diabetics. In such cases pyridoxine should be given once daily on a prophylactic basis.

In patients who fail to improve, poor adherence to therapy is the most likely explanation, however, the presence of single- or multidrug-resistant tuberculosis should be considered in all cases. Poor adherence can sometimes be improved by the use of combination tablets and by formal supervision/directly observed therapy.

HIV infection is an important risk factor in the development of tuberculosis, which can be from either reactivation of tubercle bacilli or newly acquired infection. Pulmonary tuberculosis often presents in a similar fashion to the non-HIV infected individual when the CD4 count is normal. In patients with a low CD4 count the clinical course can be varied and the traditional predilection of the organism to demonstrate upper zone changes in chest X-rays is less common. Due to altered cell-mediated immunity, the tuberculin test tends to be negative. The standard four-drug treatment should normally be instituted unless drug resistance is considered likely, in which case alternative combinations should be considered. Physicians should be aware that the chance of having multidrug-resistant disease is greater and adverse drug reactions are also more common in HIV-infected individuals. Care has to be taken because rifampicin can cause induction of hepatic enzymes, rendering protease inhibitor drugs used to treat HIV inactive. A possible compromise is to continue with standard antituberculous treatment and use an alternative antiretroviral. Alternatively, rifampicin can be omitted from the usual drug regime and the patients continue with their usual antiretrovirals but with an extension to the antituberculous treatment period. It is thought that the clinical course of HIV is accelerated in the presence of pulmonary tuberculosis. Moreover, the mortality rate is greater in HIV-positive subjects with tuberculosis, and can be twice that of HIV negative individuals.

References

Joint Tuberculosis Committee of the British Thoracic Society 1998 Chemotherapy and management of tuberculosis in the United Kingdom: recommendations 1998. Thorax 53:536–548

Joint Tuberculosis Committee of the British Thoracic Society 2000 Control and prevention of tuberculosis in the United Kingdom: code of practice 2000. Thorax 55:887–901

Subcommittee of the Joint Tuberculosis Committee of the British Thoracic Society 2000 Management of opportunist mycobacterial infections: Joint Tuberculosis Committee Guidelines 1999. Thorax 55:210–218

20.   Pulmonary embolism

Answer: **B**

Pulmonary thromboembolism is a relatively common life-threatening disorder in which mortality is high in the initial hour. Diagnosis on clinical grounds can be unreliable and, because of risk of haemorrhage, unnecessary treatment with anticoagulants should be avoided. As a result, weight is increasingly put upon diagnostic strategies. Pulmonary angiography is the gold standard investigation but is invasive and not readily available in many centres. D-dimer is a breakdown product of cross-linked fibrin and is raised in patients with thromboembolism. D-dimer assays demonstrate a very low false-negative rate, suggesting that if a negative result is obtained, the risk of pulmonary embolism is very low. Ventilation perfusion isotope scans (VQ scans) are available in many hospitals. They should be carried out within 24 h of the diagnosis, if possible, as the development of pleural effusions or pulmonary haemorrhage can make the interpretation of scans less reliable. Perfusion defects in the presence of adequate ventilation are the hallmark of pulmonary embolism. According to the criteria used in the PIOPED trial, VQ scans should be interpreted as being normal, or have low, intermediate or high probability. The diagnostic accuracy is increased when the chest X-ray is normal or practically normal. Conditions that can therefore cause diagnostic uncertainty include COPD, pulmonary fibrosis, left ventricular failure or previous pulmonary embolism. Spiral CT angiography is a useful method of diagnosis even when the chest X-ray is abnormal. Following injection of contrast medium, pulmonary emboli are demonstrated as filling defects in the pulmonary vasculature. This method of diagnosis is perhaps less useful in detecting patients with subsegmental emboli, although it tends to be useful in patients with intermediate VQ scans. Transthoracic echocardiography can also be useful in diagnosing large pulmonary emboli and identifying other conditions such as aortic dissection, myocardial infarction and pericardial and valvular heart disease, which can at times present similarly.

Concern has been raised regarding the risks of venous thromboembolism with third-generation oral contraceptives. A recent meta-analysis has demonstrated that individuals using third-generation oral contraceptives, such as those containing desogestrel and gestodene, have an almost twofold greater chance of venous thromboembolism. This is compared with second-generation contraceptives, such as those containing levonorgestrel or norethisterone. It should be noted, however, that pregnancy has at least a two- to threefold greater risk of venous thromboembolism when compared to most oral contraceptive preparations.

Discovery or clinical suspicion of pulmonary embolism requires prompt treatment with anticoagulants. In this respect, unfractionated heparins are increasingly being replaced by low molecular-weight heparins in the treatment of pulmonary embolism. They have a superior efficacy and adverse effect profile (less haemorrhage, thrombocytopenia and osteoporosis) and their prolonged duration of action allows once-daily subcutaneous dosing.

In patients with massive pulmonary embolism causing haemodynamic instability, heparin is often inadequate and mechanical (embolectomy) or pharmacological (thrombolysis) removal is warranted. Often, patients with smaller emboli, but who have comorbid cardiopulmonary disease, present with severe haemodynamic compromise. In patients with pulmonary embolism that results in right ventricular dysfunction, the outcome is generally worse than in those without. Thrombolysis is particularly indicated in patients with systemic hypotension, and successful outcomes can be achieved with streptokinase or with rtPA, which has a lower risk of systemic hypotension. As in myocardial infarction, the former should be given only once because of the risks of antibody development. Embolectomy is not commonly performed and is reserved for patients with contraindications to thrombolysis or in those failing to respond to thrombolysis. Inferior vena cava filters can be inserted under local anaesthetic in patients who experience recurrent pulmonary emboli despite adequate anticoagulation or in those with contraindications to long-term prescription of warfarin administration.

References

Kemmeren J M, Algra A, Grobbee D E 2001 Third generation oral contraceptives and risk of venous thrombosis: meta-analysis. British Medical Journal 323:131–134

Lorut C, Ghossains M, Horellou M H et al 2000 A noninvasive diagnostic strategy including spiral computed tomography in patients with suspected pulmonary embolism. American Journal of Respiration and Critical Care Medicine 162:1413–1418

British Thoracic Society (BTS) Standards of Care Committee 1997 Suspected acute pulmonary embolism: a practical approach. Thorax 52(suppl 4):S1–S24

Wood K E 2002 Major pulmonary embolism: review of a pathophysiologic approach to the golden hour of hemodynamically significant pulmonary embolism. Chest 121:877–905

DERMATOLOGY

True/False answers

21.   Psoriasis

A. **F**   B. **F**   C. **F**   D. **T**   E. **T**

Psoriasis is a common disease affecting approximately 2% of the UK population. It broadly fits into two categories. Type 1 psoriasis presents before the age of 40 and is associated with a positive family history and HLA-CW6. Type 2 (sporadic) psoriasis presents after the age of 50 with no familial association.

The areas of the body classically affected are the scalp, extensor surfaces of the elbows and knees and the sacrum. Nails can be involved with pitting and onycholysis. Flexures are another common site of disease involvement. The groin and inframammary, areas are particularly affected, and the appearance can be mistaken for candidal intertrigo.

The Koebner phenomenon refers to the appearance of a skin disease at the site of trauma such as an operation scar. It is a common feature of psoriasis but is also seen in a number of other conditions, such as lichen planus and vitiligo. Interestingly, psoriasis can also demonstrate the 'reverse Koebner' phenomenon where plaques spare areas of trauma.

For many years it was assumed that an abnormality in the keratinocyte population was the primary cause of psoriasis. It is now understood that psoriasis is an immune mediated disease with abnormal T cells stimulating keratinocyte proliferation and differentiation. The pathway involved is the type 1 T helper cell immune response. The T cells infiltrating the skin are activated CD4+ T helper cells and CD8+ cytotoxic cells. These in turn produce proinflammatory cytokines such as IFN-γ, TNF-α and interleukin-2.

TNF-α antibodies have been an important development in the management of severe psoriasis. Initially used in rheumatoid arthritis and Crohn's disease, trials have shown that plaque psoriasis responds rapidly to infusions of the monoclonal antibody infliximab. The most widely known of these trials is a placebo-controlled trial of infliximab in 33 patients with moderate to severe psoriasis. Patients receiving the active treatment responded rapidly, the median time to response being 4 weeks as measured by the physician's global assessment.

Ciclosporin is commonly used in the management of psoriasis. It blocks the production of helper T cells inhibiting the production of proinflammatory lymphokines notably interleukin-2. It also has a direct action on DNA synthesis and keratinocyte proliferation. In effect, ciclosporin modifies both the immune stimulus and the end-organ response in psoriatic patients. It has been show to be effective in double-blind, placebo-controlled trials. One 4-month cross-over trial in 85 patients showed that 72% of those treated had cleared or nearly cleared their psoriasis by 4 months. The optimal dose for treatment in this group was 4.2 mg/kg; it is recommended that the dose does not exceed 5 mg/kg because of the risk of renal side effects and hypertension.

References

Chaudhari U, Romano P, Mulcahy, LD et al 2001 Efficacy and safety of Infliximab monotherapy for plaque-type psoriasis: a randomised trial. Lancet 357:1842–1847

Ellis C N 1991 Cyclosporine for plaque type psoriasis; results of a multidose double blind trial. New England Journal of Medicine 324:277–284

Best-of-5 answers

22.   Pigmented lesions

Answer: **B**

Congenital melanocytic naevi affect 1% of newborns. They are usually pale, macular lesions, easily missed at birth, which gradually thicken and darken over time. The most dramatic changes often occur at puberty when the naevi can become very thickened and warty with dark terminal hairs across their surface.

Congenital naevi have been divided into three size categories. Small lesions are less than 1.5 cm in diameter, medium lesions range from 1.5 to 20 cm and giant lesions are those over 20 cm in diameter. The malignant potential of these lesions is largely dependent on their size. In giant naevi the lifetime incidence of malignancy is reported as 4–6%. The risk associated with small and medium sized naevi remains unclear.

The concern in the patient presented above is that the new nodular portion of a long-standing naevus might represent a malignant melanoma. The sensible next step is therefore to proceed to complete excision. Removal of the nodular portion alone would be appropriate only if removal of the whole lesion was impossible, for example in a giant congenital naevus.

Thorough examination is important to rule out the presence of another primary tumour and to assess how many and what type of naevi the patient has. Many people with congenital naevi have more than one naevus, but this further increases their risk of, rather than protecting them from, the development of melanoma. Clinical photography does have a role in the follow-up of patients with multiple atypical naevi but does not replace thorough history taking and examination. In this case, the history of change should be regarded as highly suspicious and should prompt definitive action.

Laser resurfacing is a technique that can be used in the management of epidermal naevi, which often have a warty or scaly surface. Resurfacing is of limited benefit in pigmented naevi as the naevus cells extend into the dermis. To remove them all would result in significant scarring whereas leaving them in place leads to recurrence. Lasers that remove pigment are not recommended in the management of melanocytic naevi because they target the melanin within the naevi rather than the melanocytes. Removing the pigment in this way therefore makes no difference to the risk of developing melanoma but makes any malignancy that develops harder to detect because the lesion is amelanotic.

Reference

Lanigan S W 2000 Lasers in dermatology. Medicine 28:16–18

Owen C M, Telfer N R 2000 Skin cancer. Medicine 28:39–43

---

23.   Management of psoriasis

Answer: **A**

Decisions regarding second-line therapy for the treatment of psoriasis are complex. Each option has benefits and risks that need to be carefully considered. In some instances, the side-effects of treatment might be associated with a higher mortality than the disease itself. As in all chronic disease, decisions regarding second-line therapy are made in partnership with the patient following discussion of all the pros and cons.

In this patient, methotrexate would appear to be the most sensible choice as it would help her skin and joint disease. It can be continued long term if effective, usually up to a maximum of 3 g cumulative dose. It is also not a bar to pregnancy. Should she wish to become pregnant it is simply advised that she waits 6 months after stopping the drug.

Ciclosporin is relatively contraindicated here due to the previous high dose phototherapy. The combination of ciclosporin on a background of previous PUVA greatly increases the incidence of cutaneous squamous cell carcinoma to approximately seven times that of PUVA alone. Although this might be considered a risk worth taking in an elderly patient, it is not recommended in younger people.

Systemic retinoids can often be useful in palmoplantar psoriasis or in combination with phototherapy. When combined with light they both reduce the amount of light required (because of their photosensitising effect) and also protect against the development of non-melanoma skin cancer through their antiproliferative effect on keratinocytes. Unfortunately, they have no beneficial action on joints and are profoundly teratogenic, an effect that persists for up to 2 years after their withdrawal, making them essentially unsuitable for women of childbearing age.

Mycophenolate mofetil has recently been re-introduced in the management of psoriasis; it was abandoned in the 1980s following fears about carcinogenicity. It works by blocking the synthesis of purines, which are important in the production of T cells. In clinical trials it has been effective at reducing the psoriasis area severity score but the doses required for efficacy tend to be associated with gastrointestinal side-effects. To date there have been no trials comparing its efficacy with other systemic agents for psoriasis but current clinical opinion is that it is less effective at clearing psoriatic plaques than ciclosporin or methotrexate. Currently it is reserved largely for people not responsive to more mainstream treatment.

Infliximab is a newly available TNF-α antibody. It is highly effective in the management of psoriatic arthropathy and plaque psoriasis, however, its cost at this stage (approximately £3000 per course) makes it a treatment reserved for patients who have failed on all other available therapies or those with life-threatening disease.

References

Lebwohl M 2001 Treatment of psoriasis. Part 2. Systemic therapies. Journal of the American Academy of Dermatology 45:649–661

Marcil I, Stern R S 2001 Squamous-cell cancer of the skin in patients given PUVA and ciclosporin: nested cohort crossover study. Lancet 358:1042–1045

Roenigk H H 1998 Methotrexate in psoriasis: consensus conference. Journal of the American Academy of Dermatology 38(3):478–485

24.   Eczema

Answer: **C**

Adult atopic eczema presents a challenge to most dermatologists because it tends to be more severe, more difficult to manage and associated with a wider range of complications than childhood disease. Whereas atopic eczema is common in children, affecting 10–15% of those under 10 years old, only 5–10% of these children continue to have disease in adulthood. These adults tend to have more severe atopic eczema with extensive skin involvement and frequent acute flares often associated with infection. Photosensitivity is also relatively common in adults with atopic eczema, with patients reporting that their skin is more active during the summer. Phototesting to identify the exact wavelength of light triggering the eczema is often unhelpful because it is the combination of infrared and ultraviolet radiation found in natural sunlight that causes the flare. This means that rather than a true allergy to a specific wavelength of light, these patients are deemed to be aggravated by the combination of radiation wavelengths in sunlight.

Food allergy remains a contentious subject in the management of atopic eczema. It is thought that approximately 10% of children with atopic eczema have a food allergy, with symptoms ranging from delayed exacerbation of eczema to anaphylaxis. Some clinicians are sceptical about the ability of foods to flare eczema in the absence of a type 1 (immediate hypersensitivity) response whereas others will investigate children for the possibility that foods can induce a delayed hypersensitivity reaction (type 4), resulting in a flare of eczema. In adults, it is very uncommon for food to play an important role in disease activity. Unless patients present with a history of a type 1 reaction to food, lip or tongue swelling, wheeze or dysphagia further investigation is not usually undertaken.

The role of IgE in atopy also remains unclear. About 80% of patients with atopic eczema will have increased levels of IgE on radioallergosorbent testing to a mixture of inhaled and ingested antigens. Mixed high levels of IgE are difficult to interpret because there is often no history of the substance triggering a flare in eczema and strict avoidance of allergens, such as housedust mite, rarely leads to a dramatic improvement in disease. In addition, approximately 50% of UK adults have increased levels of IgE to a variety of substances with no evidence of atopic eczema. Radioallergosorbent testing is therefore not routinely performed in adults with atopic eczema, as the results tend not to be helpful in their management.

Contact dermatitis is thought to be more common in this group of patients because the increased permeability of the skin allows greater movement of allergens across the skin. As in the general population, nickel and fragrances account for most cases of allergic contact dermatitis in atopic eczema. Contact sensitivity to topical steroids remains uncommon but should be considered in any patient complying with treatment who fails to improve. Patch testing is the investigation of choice but can only be performed when the skin is settled.

References

Bindslev-Jensen C 1998 ABC of allergies: food allergy. British Medical Journal 316:1299–1302

Gutgesell C, Heise S, Seubert S et al. 2001 Double blind placebo controlled trial of house dust avoidance measures in adult patients with atopic dermatitis. British Journal of Dermatology 145:70–74

25.   Pruritus

Answer: **B**

The most common cause for this combination of signs and symptoms is diabetes mellitus. Pruritus is considered to be a classic symptom of diabetes, although its exact incidence and mechanism is unknown. Random blood glucose should form part of the basic screen in any patient who presents with itch in the absence of obvious cutaneous disease. In general, a pruritus screen should include a thorough history, general examination (especially for lymphadenopathy), full blood count, urea and electrolytes, liver function tests, serum glucose, thyroid function tests and plasma protein electrophoresis. In the absence of an obvious underlying cause for pruritus, treatment is with simple emollients, topical steroids, antihistamines and avoidance of irritants such as fragrance, which can exacerbate the problem. If simple measures are not effective, a variety of modalities can be used, although the evidence for efficacy of each is limited. These include UVB phototherapy, naltrexone, thalidomide and topical or systemic doxepin.

Candida albicans infections of the oral and genital mucosae, nail folds and intertriginous areas are all more common in diabetics and might be the initial presenting feature. High glucose levels in the saliva, urine and sweat are thought to increase susceptibility, acting as a good food source. In addition, the maceration and increased moisture levels seen in the skin folds of overweight type 2 diabetics further encourage yeast growth. Oral disease can be especially difficult to eradicate in the presence of false teeth. These should be removed and soaked in an anticandidal agent to avoid recurrence. Genital disease in men is referred to as candidal balanitis and can result in phimosis if not treated.

Necrobiosis lipoidica is a degenerative disease of collagen, which presents as well-defined plaques of shiny, atrophic, yellow skin with surface telangectasia commonly on the shins. It is reported to occur in 0.3% of diabetics, whereas 60–75% of patients with necrobiosis lipoidica have diabetes. It can occur in the absence of diabetes and can predate the development of diabetes by several years. The natural history of these lesions is unrelated to diabetic control; improvement of blood sugar levels will not increase their chance of healing. Management of these lesions is difficult as little has been shown to make any impact. Potent topical or intralesional steroids can improve the appearance. Ulcerated lesions can be treated with excision and grafting, although recurrence in the treated site can occur. In general, these lesions are a cosmetic problem and no specific treatment is offered.

References

Braun M, Lowitt M H 2001 Pruritus. Advances in Dermatology 17:1–27

Ferranger T, Miller F 2002 Cutaneous manifestations of diabetes mellitus. Dermatology Clinics 20:483–492

Schmelz M 2002 Itch: mediators and mechanism. Journal of Dermatological Science 28:91–96

26. Chronic venous ulceration

Answer: **B**

The best available treatment for chronic venous leg ulcers is compression bandaging, usually delivered as a four-layer system. It has been shown to improve ulcer healing rates and results in complete healing of a higher percentage of ulcers. It is contraindicated in patients with arterial disease; care is required in patients with diabetes or rheumatoid arthritis. Most other treatments for venous ulceration have little evidence to recommend them. Simple dressings appear to be as effective as more complex dressings (e.g. hydrocolloid) when used in combination with compression bandaging. A number of dressings incorporating growth factors, as well as topical agents such as cultured skin and mesoglycan, have been trialled; there is little evidence of benefit. Injection of the growth factor

GM-CSF into the area around the ulcer did lead to an increase in the number of ulcers that were completely healed. However, the trial was small and requires corroborating.

Physical therapies, including electromagnetic therapy, ultrasound and laser therapy, also lack strong evidence in their favour. Ultrasound has improved ulcer healing rates in several small studies but in most studies the effect did not reach statistical significance.

Intermittent pneumatic compression, although a theoretically attractive way of reducing venous stasis, does not appear to lead to improved healing when added to compression bandaging. Oral agents including aspirin, zinc and thromboxane antagonists appear similarly ineffective at promoting ulcer healing. There is weak evidence that flavonoids can improve ulcer healing rates but the strongest evidence is for the effectiveness of pentoxifylline (oxpentifylline). Pentoxifylline (oxpentifylline) has a number of effects that might explain its beneficial effect on ulcer healing: it improves red cell deformability and improves blood flow; it also inhibits production of cytokines, including IFN-γ, interleukin-12 and TNF. A systematic review of eight randomised trials concluded that pentoxifylline (oxpentifylline) leads to an increase in the number of completely healed and substantially improved venous leg ulcers when compared with placebo; this remained true for patients with and without compression bandaging.

References

Nelson E A, Cullum N, Jones J 2001 Clinical evidence, 5th edn. BMJ Publishing, London, p 1366–1375

Jull A, Waters J, Arroll B 2002 Pentoxifylline for treatment of venous leg ulcers: a systematic review. Lancet 359:1550–1554

CLINICAL PHARMACOLOGY

True/False answers

27.   Angiotensin II receptor blockers

A. **F**   B. **F**   C. **F**   D. **T**   E. **F**

Angiotensin II receptor blockers such as irbesartan, valsartan and losartan, block the effects of angiotensin II at the AT_1 receptor. In patients treated with an ACE inhibitor there is still production of angiotensin II and aldosterone from local and systemic sites. Angiotensin II receptor blockers further reduce levels of angiotensin II and aldosterone.

It is now well established that ACE inhibitors slow the progression of diabetic nephropathy, and trials have recently been carried out looking at the effects of angiotensin II blockers on renal disease in type 2 diabetic, hypertensive patients. Losartan has been shown to reduce the progression of renal disease in patients with proteinuria, and irbesartan reduces the progression to proteinuria in patients with microalbuminuria. These studies did not allow concurrent ACE inhibitor therapy, although the CALM study found that lisinopril and candesartan were equally good at reducing blood pressure and microalbuminuria, and that the combination gave the best results. Although this study did not include patients with established renal failure, the combination certainly seems to be beneficial in preventing progression to nephropathy. There is no evidence that angiotensin II receptor blockers are superior in efficacy to ACE inhibitors when used alone.

The LIFE study enrolled hypertensive patients with left ventricular hypertrophy (on ECG criteria) and compared losartan to atenolol. Losartan was superior to atenolol in the reduction of cardiovascular events, but this was mainly due to a reduction in stroke as the incidence of myocardial infarction was the same in each group. This suggests that losartan has beneficial cerebrovascular effects that are not shared by atenolol. Subgroup analysis of the LIFE trial showed that in diabetic patients losartan was better than atenolol at improving cardiovascular outcomes, in contrast to some previous studies.

The Val-HeFT trial compared valsartan with placebo added to standard heart failure treatment, including an ACE inhibitor. Although valsartan reduced morbidity and hospital admissions, there was no effect on overall mortality, and the addition of valsartan to patients receiving a β-blocker and an ACE inhibitor was associated with an increased mortality rate.

References

Brenner B M, Cooper M E, de Zeeuw D et al 2001 Effects of losartan on renal and cardiovascular outcomes in patients with type 2 diabetes and nephropathy. New England Journal of Medicine 345:861–969

Dahlof B, Devereux R B, Kjeldsen S E et al 2002 Cardiovascular morbidity and mortality in the Losartan Intervention For Endpoint reduction in hypertension study (LIFE): a randomised trial against atenolol. Lancet 359:995–1003

Mogensen C E, Neldam S, Tikkanen I et al 2000 Randomised controlled trial of dual blockade of renin–angiotensin system in patients with hypertension, microalbuminuria, and non-insulin dependent diabetes: the candesartan and lisinopril microalbuminuria (CALM) study. British Medical Journal 321:1440–1444

Parving H H, Lehnert H, Brochner-Mortensen J et al 2001 The effect of irbesartan on the development of diabetic nephropathy in patients with type 2 diabetes. New England Journal of Medicine 345:870–878.

28. Botulinum toxin

A. **F**   B. **T**   C. **T**   D. **F**   E. **F**

Botulism is a descending paralysis that often affects the bulbar muscles and commonly involves the autonomic nervous system. It is caused by *Clostridium botulinum*, an anaerobic spore-forming organism that is often found in soil. Botulism usually results from eating contaminated food; the spore can survive brief heating at 100°C. It can also occur as a result of a wound infection, e.g. in neonates with umbilical stump infection.

C. botulinum produces botulinum toxin, a heat-labile neurotoxin of which there are seven different serotypes (A–G). They all interfere with neurotransmission by blocking the release of acetylcholine; binding is irreversible, thus botulism cannot be reversed with antitoxin. Nerve function takes 2–3 months to recover and is due to the formation of new synapses.

Botulinum toxin also has therapeutic benefits as a result of its long-lasting effects on nerve terminals. It affects parasympathetic and cholinergic postganglionic sympathetic neurons, as well as α motor neurons in striated muscle. The potential uses are thus great and include treating spasticity, various dystonias (e.g. torticollis, blepharospasm, laryngeal dystonia and writer's cramp), strabismus, dysphagia due to achalasia, and hyperhidrosis. Botulinum toxin is also widely used for cosmetic purposes.

Serotype A is the serotype that is commercially available for use. Two preparations exist: Botox and Dysport. The preparations have to be injected into the affected muscle. Side-effects of botulinum toxin are mostly due to weakness of the muscles; both those injected and those adjacent to the injection site can be affected, for example, if used for the treatment of torticollis, a dysphagia might develop. Inappropriate muscle injection can be minimised by the use of electromyographic guidance. Generalised muscle weakness is very rare. The systemic side-effect that is most commonly seen is an influenza-like illness. Tolerance to the injections can occur due to the development of neutralising antibodies; this is more likely with more frequent or higher-dose injections.

References

Ghoshal U C, Chaudhuri S, Pal B B et al 2001 Randomized controlled trial of intrasphincteric botulinum toxin A injection versus balloon dilatation in treatment of achalasia cardia. Diseases of the Esophagus 14:227–231

Munchau A, Bhatia K P 2000 Uses of botulinum toxin injection in medicine today. British Medical Journal 320:161–165

Wollina U, Karamfilov T, Konrad H 2002 High-dose botulinum toxin type A therapy for axillary hyperhidrosis markedly prolongs the relapse-free interval. Journal of the Americal Academy of Dermatology 46:536–540

29. Leptin

A. **T**   B. **F**   C. **T**   D. **T**   E. **F**

Leptin is a 167-amino-acid protein that is synthesised and released by white adipose tissue. It is produced in greater quantities by subcutaneous fat than by visceral fat. It circulates in plasma in free and bound forms. Plasma levels follow a diurnal pattern with superimposed pulsatile release. The mechanisms underlying the control of this diurnal pattern are not known but it is interesting that the pattern shifts with a shift in meal times, and that cortisol levels have little correlation with leptin, suggesting a lack of true circadian control.

Insulin increases serum leptin concentrations in both the short and long term, however leptin mRNA levels are increased only after long-term exposure to insulin. Leptin levels do not increase immediately after food; increases usually occur 4–7 h after a meal. Glucocorticoids also increase both leptin concentrations and leptin mRNA. In addition, the sympathetic system is a key regulator of leptin production. Sympathomimetic amines and cold exposure decrease leptin production and gene expression. These are only a few of the pathways that are likely to be involved in leptin regulation.

Although it has peripheral sites of action, the principal site of action is thought to be on the hypothalamus. Leptin crosses the blood–brain barrier and binds to the long form OB-Rb receptors in the hypothalamus, which it stimulates. The result is to decrease food intake and increase energy expenditure.

Although initially thought to be a satiety hormone, leptin is now thought of as a hormone to prevent starvation. In an environment where food is scarce one of the main roles of leptin would be to conserve energy by decreasing thyroid-hormone-induced thermogenesis. It would also mobilise energy stores by increasing the secretion of stress glucocorticoids while at the same time suppressing gonadal function – all achieved by a decrease in leptin levels. Leptin levels are increased in conditions of overeating and are decreased in conditions of fasting, although leptin levels are decreased out of proportion to the amount of fat tissue lost. It is known that leptin is needed for sexual development; people who are genetically deficient in leptin present with early morbid obesity, no pubertal development and dysfunction of the growth hormone and thyroid hormone axes.

Leptin levels are proportional to body fat, probably because there is more adipose mass to synthesise leptin in obese people. However, acute changes in leptin levels are thought not to reflect actual fat stores or adipocyte numbers, but more likely the state of the adipocyte mass, that is, whether there is triglyceride synthesis or hydrolysis.

Most obese people have high levels of leptin, although the link between obesity and leptin levels is not yet clear. It could be that they are resistant to leptin as a primary mechanism of their obesity, or it might be that the leptin receptors become desensitised because of the high levels of leptin in obese people. Leptin as a treatment for obesity is being trialled at the moment; the method of administration is subcutaneous. Early results show that weight loss can be achieved, although the results are no better than with current obesity therapies. It might be that to overcome leptin resistance very high doses need to be used.

References

Fried S K, Ricci M R, Russell C D, Laferrere B 2000 Regulation of leptin production in humans. Journal of Nutrition 130:3127S–3131S

Hickey M S, Calsbeek D J 2001 Plasma leptin and exercise: recent findings. Sports Medicine 31:583–589

Mantzoros C S 1999 The role of leptin in human obesity and disease: a review of current evidence. Annals of Internal Medicine 130:671–680

30.   Potassium

A. **T**   B. **F**   C. **F**   D. **F**   E. **F**

Interest in the beneficial effects of potassium has been stimulated by the observation that treatments that increase serum potassium (e.g. ACE inhibitors and spironolactone) are associated with a beneficial effect on survival. Hypokalaemia is arrhythmogenic, as it makes the resting potential of myocytes more negative, hastens depolarisation and lengthens the action potential. It also increases QT interval dispersion, a known risk factor for cardiovascular death. Hypokalaemia also exacerbates the arrhythmogenic effects of digoxin, the major mechanism being via promotion of myocardial digoxin binding to the Na/K ATPase pump. Hypokalaemia also decreases the renal excretion of digoxin. In patients with hypertension, those treated with diuretics such that the potassium falls below 3.5 mmol/L have been shown to lose the protective effect of blood pressure lowering. In the Multiple Risk Factor Intervention trial, patients on higher doses of diuretics had an increased risk of sudden death. Hypertensive patients treated with thiazide diuretics who are hypokalaemic have an increased occurrence of ventricular ectopics, which disappear when the hypokalaemia is corrected. Conversely, a higher potassium intake (as assessed by 24-h urine potassium excretion) is associated with a lower blood pressure, although it is not known if the beneficial effect of a high potassium on blood pressure is maintained once the sodium intake is reduced. One possible mechanism is that a higher potassium level appears to improve endothelial function in hypertensive patients; potassium also reduces the vascular response to angiotensin II.

Magnesium and potassium loss often go hand in hand, especially if the patient is on diuretics. Therefore, if a patient is hypokalaemic it is always worth checking the magnesium level. Hypomagnesaemia also contributes to digoxin toxicity and magnesium is a recognised adjunctive treatment for arrhythmias associated with digoxin use.

Whether due to the beneficial effects on the blood pressure on the endothelium or the fact that many studies commenting on the effect of potassium on stroke have used fruit and vegetables to increase potassium (which might have other beneficial effects) it appears that a high dietary intake of potassium can reduce the risk of suffering a stroke. Avoidance of low potassium is also probably beneficial in patients with heart failure. Heart failure causes neurohormonal activation, increasing the levels of aldosterone leading to sodium retention and hypokalaemia. The diuretics used to treat heart failure worsen the hypokalaemia, the hyponatraemia that results leads to greater aldosterone release thus exacerbating the hypokalaemia. Hypokalaemia is a strong independent predictor of mortality in heart failure; the increase in mortality in trials involving heart failure patients taking potassium-wasting diuretics is probably due to an increase in ventricular arrhythmias in these patients.

As well as its beneficial cardiovascular effects, potassium also reduces calcium excretion, might reduce hypercalcuria in patients with renal calculi and improves bone mass in postmenopausal women.

References

Heart Outcomes Prevention Evaluation Study Investigators 2000 Effects of ramipril on cardiovascular and microvascular outcomes in people with diabetes mellitus: results of the HOPE study and MICRO-HOPE substudy. Lancet 355:253–259

He F J, MacGregor G A 2001 Fortnightly review: beneficial effects of potassium. British Medical Journal 323:497–501

Pitt B, Zannad F, Remme W J et al 1999 The effect of spironolactone on morbidity and mortality in patients with severe heart failure. Randomized Aldactone Evaluation Study Investigators. New England Journal of Medicine 341:709–717

31. Cocaine use

A. **F**   B. **F**   C. **T**   D. **F**   E. **T**

Cocaine is found in the leaves of the South American coca shrub. Other than having local anaesthetic properties, cocaine is a stimulant; it has central and peripheral actions. It stimulates central sympathetic outflow and binds directly to the dopamine, serotonin and noradrenaline (norepinephrine) transport proteins, preventing the reuptake of dopamine, serotonin and noradrenaline (norepinephrine) into presynaptic neurons. Cocaine also inhibits noradrenaline (norepinephrine) reuptake in peripheral sympathetic nerve terminals.

The effect of cocaine is to produce increased motor activity and euphoria. Its effects last for about 30 min when given intravenously. When snorted it can be detected in the circulation after 1 min and peaks after 10 min; there is a further peak after 45 min; this might be due to drug that has been swallowed. With excessive doses cocaine can produce seizures but hallucinations do not occur. The increase in sympathetic activity causes increased vasomotor activity, tachycardia and increases blood pressure. Hyperthermia can occur due to reduced heat loss and increased activity.

The aetiology of myocardial infarction and ischaemia related to cocaine abuse is complex; it is partly due to a surge in sympathetic activity (catecholamine concentrations can be raised up to five times normal). This increased sympathetic activation causes increased oxygen demand and coronary vasospasm. Cocaine use is also associated with dilated cardiomyopathy.

The other well-known side-effect of intranasal cocaine abuse is nasal and palatal destruction. The aetiology of this midline destruction is multifactorial but includes chemical irritation from adulterants, local ischaemia secondary to vasoconstriction, infection, impaired mucociliary transport, and decreased immunity. Cocaine-related nasal destruction has been mistaken for infections, tumours (e.g. angiosarcoma) and granulomatous disease such as Wegener's granulomatosis. Cocaine abuse should be suspected in patients with a palatal or septal perforation of unknown aetiology.

Other stimulant drugs are amfetamines and ecstasy, which cause the release of catecholamines, and serotonin from nerve terminals of the peripheral and central autonomic nervous system. Amfetamines and ecstasy likewise produce adverse cardiovascular effects.

Cocaine has the potential to produce a profound psychological dependence syndrome. Although not as addictive as cigarettes, cocaine is still addictive. This addiction has been linked to the fact that cocaine use results in the release of dopamine in the mesolimbic system (the reason behind the cocaine euphoria). Dopamine receptors are implicated in reward mechanisms and it is via the dopaminergic reward pathway that cocaine is thought to cause addiction.

There is no definitive medical way of aiding cocaine withdrawal other than to abstain from the drug. During withdrawal there is usually intense craving, accompanied by symptoms such as depression, fatigue, irritability, anorexia and sleep disturbances.

References

Benzaquen B S, Cohen V, Eisenberg M J 2001 Effects of cocaine on the coronary arteries. American Heart Journal 142:402–410

Dackis C A, O'Brien C P 2001 Cocaine dependence: a disease of the brain's reward centers. Journal of Substance Abuse and Treatment 21:111–117

Fattinger K, Benowitz N L, Jones R T, Verotta D 2000 Nasal mucosal versus gastrointestinal absorption of nasally administered cocaine. European Journal of Clinical Pharmacology 56:305–310

Smith J C, Kacker A, Anand V K 2002 Midline nasal and hard palate destruction in cocaine abusers and cocaine's role in rhinologic practice. Ear Nose and Throat Journal 81:172–177

32.   Endothelial function

A. F   B. T   C. F   D. F   E. T

The endothelium is a cellular monolayer that lines the blood vessels. Interest in the endothelium has burgeoned in recent years with the realisation that, rather than merely being a barrier to diffusion, the endothelium is an endocrine organ in its own right.

The endothelium is involved in the regulation of vascular tone by the release of vasodilator substances such as nitric oxide, prostacyclin and endothelium-derived hyperpolarising factor (for which no molecular identity exists as yet), and vasoconstrictor substances, for example endothelin. This also has a role in immunological function and the regulation of vascular growth. It is cytotoxic and cytostatic, directly inhibiting mitochondrial respiration, aconitase activity and DNA synthesis.

Nitric oxide is involved in the regulation of vascular growth by inhibiting smooth muscle cell proliferation and migration. It has been shown to inhibit the mitogenesis of fibroblasts and cultured smooth muscle cells. The endothelium also acts to limit thrombus formation. Thrombin, ATP and ADP, as well as activated platelets, also cause the release of prostacyclin from the endothelium, thus inhibiting platelet adherence. Serotonin and ADP released from activated platelets stimulate the endothelium to release nitric oxide, which has potent antiaggregatory and antiadhesive properties. Nitric oxide inhibits expression of P selectin on platelets and suppresses the calcium dependant conformation change in the glycoprotein IIB/IIIA receptor required for fibrinogen binding.

Perhaps of greater relevance to clinical medicine is the fact the endothelial dysfunction as assessed in the coronary and peripheral arteries has been shown to be a prognostic marker for cardiac events and death in patients with known angina, patients with hypertension and in those undergoing vascular surgery. As peripheral artery endothelial function is positively correlated with that in the coronary arteries, the assessment of endothelial function is relatively easy to perform in a laboratory situation, without recourse to coronary angiography.

Treatments that have been shown to improve endothelial function are ACE inhibitors, exercise, spironolactone (in heart failure), vitamin C and statins. It is not known how much of the beneficial clinical effects seen with these treatments are due to an improvement in endothelial function.

At present, methods to assess endothelial function are time consuming and often invasive, and are thus not amenable for use in risk stratification of a population. It is not as yet known if the assessment of endothelial function offers additional prognostic information to traditional risk factor scores. However, surrogate markers (e.g. von Willebrand factor) are released when the endothelium is damaged and could prove to be useful and easily clinically accessible markers of endothelial dysfunction.

References

Anderson T J 1999 Assessment and treatment of endothelial dysfunction in humans. Journal of the American College of Cardiologists 34:631–638

Gokce N, Keaney J F, Hunter L M et al 2002 Risk stratification for postoperative cardiovascular events via noninvasive assessment of endothelial function: a prospective study. Circulation 105:1567–1572

Heitzer T, Schlinzig T, Krohn K et al 2001 Endothelial dysfunction, oxidative stress, and risk of cardiovascular events in patients with coronary artery disease. Circulation 104:2673–2678

Schachinger V, Britten M B, Zeiher A M 2000 Prognostic impact of coronary vasodilator dysfunction on adverse long-term outcome of coronary heart disease. Circulation 101:1899–1906

33.   Endothelin

A. **T**   B. **F**   C. **T**   D. **T**   E. **T**

The major opposition to the vasodilator substances, and the most potent vasoconstrictor substance yet known to man is endothelin 1, a member of a family of structurally similar 21-amino-acid peptides. There are currently three known endothelins: 1, 2 and 3, which are all similar in structure to the snake venom sarafotoxin S6c.

Endothelin 1 is produced and released by the endothelium and its effects are long lasting both in vitro and in vivo. It is released in response to adrenaline (epinephrine), angiotensin I, thrombin and endothelial stress (shear stress, expansion of plasma volume, growth factors and hypoxia). Nitric oxide inhibits the production of endothelin. Endothelin 1 has been shown to transiently increase nitric oxide release, as demonstrated by an increase in forearm blood flow at the start of an endothelin infusion; this increase in forearm blood flow is followed by a long period of intense vasoconstriction. Endothelin has a short half-life. It is synthesised from the preprotein big endothelin and acts in a paracrine nature on membrane bound G-protein-coupled receptors. Very little endothelin 1 is thought to reach the circulation.

There are two endothelin (ET) receptor subtypes known, which are found on the endothelium and on some smooth muscle cells (in the gut and heart). The ETA receptor mediates smooth muscle vasoconstriction and proliferation; it is preferentially activated by endothelin 1. The ETB subtype can be activated by all three isoforms of endothelin and has some protective actions; in the endothelium it has a dual role of clearance and vasodilation whereas in the smooth muscle it also causes vasoconstriction. ETA and ETB receptor antagonists are currently being studied in patients with heart failure, renal disease and pulmonary hypertension. There are likely to be further studies looking at cerebrovascular disease.

Endothelin 1 plasma levels are elevated in chronic heart failure and correlate with haemodynamic severity, symptoms and mortality. Non-selective endothelin receptor antagonists, for example bosentan, show impressive haemodynamic improvements in patients with heart failure. Hypertensive patients with coronary artery disease have increased arterial expression of endothelin 1 and in some hypertensive patients, exaggerated vascular responses to endothelin are found. Studies looking at endothelin receptor antagonists in hypertension are ongoing.

Endothelin also plays a pathological role in pulmonary hypertension, both primary and associated with collagen vascular disease. Bosentan significantly improves exercise capacity, symptoms and functional status in patients with pulmonary hypertension, and has so far proven to be safe in trials.

References

Hurlimann D, Enseleit F, Noll G, Luscher T F, Ruschitzka F 2002 Endothelin antagonists and heart failure. Current Hypertension Reports 4:85–92

Krum H 1998 Effect of endothelin 1 on endothelium derived vascular responsiveness in man. Clinical Science 95:151–156

Rubin L J, Badesch D B, Barst R J et al 2002 Bosentan therapy for pulmonary arterial hypertension. New England Journal of Medicine 346:896–903

Schiffrin E L 2001 Role of endothelin-1 in hypertension and vascular disease. American Journal of Hypertension 14:83S–89S

34.   Complementary medicine

A. F   B. T   C. F   D. F   E. T

The use of alternative therapies is on the increase, especially as more patients are becoming suspicious of taking prescription medications. Herbal medicines, although often benign, have their own range of side-effects and interactions, not to mention problems due to a lack of regulation and evidence to support their use.

Even without considering the pharmacological properties of the actual herb to be taken, it has to be realised that mislabelling has been known to occur and many herbal remedies contain orthodox medicinal products such as non-steroidal anti-inflammatory drugs, sulphonylureas, antidepressants and steroids, as well as occasionally being contaminated with heavy metals.

Guar gum is an agent that has been promoted for many years for weight loss and cholesterol-lowering effects; it is now being looked at for use in drug delivery systems. It is a dietary fibre that is reported to provide a feeling of satiety; it might achieve this by slowing gut transit. It can also chelate bile acids and therefore have some effect in lowering cholesterol. Due to these effects it has been recommended by herbalists as a useful adjunct in diabetes, however, it impairs the absorption of metformin and some other drugs, for example digoxin, paracetamol and bumetanide.

Yohimbine (Yohimbe) is often used as a vitalising agent and has also been recommended as a therapy for erectile dysfunction; it does show promise, although large trials are lacking. Although yohimbine is an α_2-receptor blocker it can cause hypertension if used on its own, and this is seen at lower doses when it is combined with tricyclic antidepressants. Yohimbine is a stimulant drug and can induce panic attacks and mania in patients with bipolar disorders.

Garlic is another commonly used alternative agent. Aged garlic extract is recommended as an agent to prevent cardiovascular disease; it decreases cholesterol and blood pressure and also interferes with platelet function. It has thus has been associated with an increased bleeding risk, e.g. in the postoperative setting.

References

Fugh-Berman A 2000 Herb–drug interactions. Lancet 355:134–138

Steiner M, Li W 2001 Aged garlic extract, a modulator of cardiovascular risk factors: a dose-finding study on the effects of age on platelet functions. Journal of Nutrition 131:980S–984S

Tam S W, Worcel M, Wyllie M 2001 Yohimbine: a clinical review. Pharmacology and Therapeutics 91:215–243

van Nieuwenhoven M A, Kovacs E M, Brummer R J et al 2001 The effect of different dosages of guar gum on gastric emptying and small intestinal transit of a consumed semisolid meal. Journal of the American College of Nutrition 20:87–91

---

35.   Drugs and surgery

A. **T**   B. **F**   C. **T**   D. **T**   E. **F**

Extracts of ginkgo biloba leaves, which contain flavinoids, terpenoids and organic acids (which can act as free-radical scavengers) have been advocated as a therapy for memory disorders including dementia and vascular disease. There are mixed reports in the literature as to the efficacy of ginkgo biloba. However, there are many reports of bleeding associated with this extract, thus it is advised that it should be stopped at least 36 h before surgery.

Cannabis is another alternative therapy that is gaining credence in the treatment of pain (especially spasticity-related pain) and nausea. A recent meta-analysis showed that cannabinoids were better than conventional antiemetics for moderately emetogenic chemotherapy; they were also preferred by the patients, although they had more side-effects. There are no trials as yet looking at perioperative nausea and vomiting.

The risk of postoperative complications is related to the amount of medication that a patient is taking preoperatively. This is more likely to be because the therapies are a marker of risk than because the therapies themselves are detrimental. It is likely that patients who would be considered to be at very high operative risk after being treated with the appropriate medications find themselves in a lower-risk group as a result of the medications, and thus are suitable for surgery. However, when the medications are stopped prior to surgery the patients' physical health deteriorates, thus they tend towards being in a higher risk group. There are obvious reasons for medications being stopped perioperatively, the most common one being ileus after abdominal surgery. However, alternative routes for medications should be considered (e.g. intravenous formulations of ACE inhibitors are available in some countries). The longer a patient is without medication postoperatively, the greater the risk of non-surgical complications. In this particular population, absence of cardiovascular medications for more than 1 day was associated with a 14% event rate.

Beta-blockers are useful in patients with cardiac risk factors undergoing cardiac and vascular surgery, and perhaps in all surgical procedures, probably because of their cardioprotective effects. A reduction in cardiac and all-cause mortality, as well as in cardiac ischaemia, has been shown, and the effect is greatest in those patients with the highest risk.

References

Auerbach A D, Goldman L 2002 Beta-blockers and reduction of cardiac events in noncardiac surgery: scientific review. Journal of the American Medical Association 287:1435–1444

Kennedy J M, van Rij A M, Spears G F et al 2000 Polypharmacy in a general surgical unit and consequences of drug withdrawal. British Journal of Clinical Pharmacology 49:353–362

Le Bars P L, Kastelan J 2000 Efficacy and safety of a Ginkgo biloba extract. Public Health and Nutrition 3:495–499

Tramer M R, Carroll D, Campbell F A et al 2001 Cannabinoids for control of chemotherapy induced nausea and vomiting: quantitative systematic review. British Medical Journal 323:16–21

36.   Drugs of abuse

A. **T**   B. **F**   C. **T**   D. **F**   E. **T**

Gamma hydroxybutyrate is a relatively new drug that has been around for recreational use since the 1980s. It is a naturally occurring metabolite of gamma aminobutyric acid (GABA). Gamma hydroxybutyrate and its analogues (which are widely available) are potent CNS depressants (gamma hydroxybutyrate used to be used to induce anaesthesia); as gamma hydroxybutyrate is now illegal in many countries, use of gamma hydroxybutyrate metabolites is becoming more commonplace. Gamma hydroxybutyrate metabolites produce the same symptoms as the parent compound.

Although few cases of dependency and withdrawal have been reported, chronic usage of gamma hydroxybutyrate can lead to dependency and a withdrawal syndrome characterised by agitation, psychosis and autonomic instability. Gamma hydroxybutyrate is used/misused for its sedative, euphoric and anabolic effects; common adverse effects include a rapid onset of drowsiness, nausea, vomiting, myoclonic seizures, coma of short duration and respiratory depression that might require ventilatory support. Gamma hydroxybutyrate has also has been used as a sleep aid and has been implicated in cases of date rape, usually in combination with alcohol.

Rohypnol (flunitrazepam) is a benzodiazepine that is commonly implicated in cases of date rape; it has a rapid onset and is metabolised rapidly. It is thus is often undetectable by the time the victim seeks medical or police help. It causes disinhibition, relaxation of voluntary muscles and anterograde amnesia for events that happen while under the influence of the drug.

Amfetamines such as 3,4-methylenedioxymethamfetamine (MDMA, Ecstasy), an amfetamine analogue with sympathomimetic properties, are used as stimulants. Although rare, complications such as disseminated intravascular coagulation, rhabdomyolysis, and acute renal failure are recognised. Symptoms of an amfetamine toxic reaction include tachycardia, sweating and hyperthermia. Treatment includes lowering the body temperature and maintaining adequate hydration.

Reference

Teter C J, Guthrie S K 2001 A comprehensive review of MDMA and GHB: two common club drugs. Pharmacotherapy 21:1486–1513

Best-of-5 answers

37. Bupropion (amfebutamone)

Answer: **D**

Bupropion (amfebutamome) is a novel antismoking therapy. It was first marketed as an antidepressant but is similar in structure to the amfetamine-like stimulant diethylpropion. The mechanism of action by which it helps people to stop smoking is not known, although one theory is that it increases dopamine concentrations in the nucleus accumbens, a process that is also involved in nicotine addiction. It is a weak inhibitor of dopamine and noradrenaline (norepinephrine) reuptake, and an even weaker inhibitor of serotonin reuptake.

Bupropion (amfebutamome) has a long half-life of approximately 20 h, it reaches peak plasma concentrations in only 3 h but takes 8 days to reach steady state, thus it is advisable that it is taken for 1–2 weeks before the patient tries to stop smoking. Only 1% of bupropion (amfebutamome) is excreted unchanged in the urine; most of the absorbed dose is metabolised in the liver to further active metabolites. The dose recommended for quitting is 300 mg/day (as 150 mg bd) for 7–9 weeks.

There have been two large trials looking at bupropion (amfebutamome) for smoking cessation. They were both conducted in people who were motivated to quit and both combined treatment with counselling. Both found bupropion (amfebutamome) (300 mg/day) to be significantly better than placebo. One study compared bupropion with a nicotine patch; bupropion (amfebutamome) was significantly better than the patch for continuous abstinence at 12 months and the combination of bupropion (amfebutamome) plus a nicotine patch was no better than bupropion (amfebutamome) alone.

Bupropion (amfebutamome) treatment is not associated with the normal increase in weight seen on stopping smoking; whether this effect is continued into the long term or not is not known. It is also associated with fewer symptoms of withdrawal and craving than placebo. The most serious side-effect reported is epileptiform seizures; although this is uncommon (1/1000), bupropion (amfebutamome) should not be prescribed to patients with epilepsy or patients with an altered seizure threshold. The main side-effects are dry mouth and insomnia. It appears to be free of cardiovascular side-effects, although in combination with nicotine a non-significant increase in blood pressure has been noted. Bupropion (amfebutamome) is contraindicated in pregnancy and in those with eating disorders. It is metabolised using the cytochrome P450 enzyme system and inhibits the action of some of these enzymes (e.g. CYP 2D6). Caution is thus needed if patients are taking medications that are metabolised by this enzyme system such as type Ic antiarrhythmic drugs.

References

Amfebutamone/bupropion for smoking cessation: new preparation. Nicotine replacement therapy is safer. Prescrire International 2001 10:163–167

Bupropion to aid smoking cessation. Drug and Therapeutics Bulletin 2000 38: 73–75

Holm K J, Spencer C M 2000 Bupropion: a review of its use in the management of smoking cessation. Drugs 59:1007–1024

38. Oxidative stress and antioxidants

Answer: **C**

Many studies are being carried out into the potential benefits of antioxidant treatment, especially in cardiovascular disease. An increase in the amount of oxidative stress is seen in states associated with higher levels of cardiovascular disease, for example diabetes, hypertension, smoking and patients with end-stage renal failure. It might be that the increase in cardiovascular disease is the result of a worsening of endothelial function secondary to an increase in oxidative stress (i.e. an increase in the amount of free radicals). Nitric oxide, a molecule that is essential for the maintenance of good endothelial function, is rapidly inactivated by free radicals.

The oxidation of LDL is also thought to be a prominent process in the development of the atherosclerotic plaque; small, dense low-density lipoprotein particles are more prone to oxidation and are prevalent in atherosclerotic plaques. Linking these two findings, smaller sizes of LDL particles are associated with endothelial dysfunction amongst diabetic subjects and oxidised LDL levels correlate with coronary artery endothelial function in patients with coronary spastic angina. It seems that the level of oxidised LDL might also be important clinically; levels have been shown to correlate with the degree of carotid artery stenosis.

Long- and short-term studies have shown that treatment with antioxidants such as vitamins (C and E particularly), beta carotene and allopurinol (which inhibits xanthine oxidase, an important producer of free radicals) improve endothelial function.

A number of epidemiological studies have found an inverse association between levels of antioxidant consumption and cardiovascular disease, although the evidence from randomised controlled trials is mixed. The HOPE and GISSI trials failed to show any long-term benefit of chronic vitamin E ingestion, although chronic administration of vitamin E was seen to decrease the rate of non-fatal MI at 1 year in patients with angiographically proven coronary vascular disease.

In a secondary prevention trial, administration of high-dose vitamin E decreased the incidence of cardiovascular disease in patients receiving haemodialysis. However, vitamin E was found to be of less value than fish oil (n-3 polyunsaturated fatty acids) in a secondary prevention trial, the combination of n-3 polyunsaturated fatty acids and vitamin E was no different from treatment with polyunsaturated fatty acids alone.

The Heart Protection Study compared 40 mg simvastatin to an antioxidant cocktail (600 mg vitamin E, 250 mg vitamin C and 20 mg beta carotene) versus placebo. The patient group selected was at high risk for cardiovascular disease, either having had a cardiovascular event or being at risk because of diabetes or hypertension. The LDL concentration had to be greater than 135 mg/dL. The antioxidant cocktail, although not harmful, showed no benefit but the simvastatin treatment arm showed a significant reduction in morbidity and mortality.

References

Boaz M, Smetana S, Weinstein T et al 2000 Secondary prevention with antioxidants of cardiovascular disease in endstage renal disease (SPACE): randomised placebo-controlled trial. Lancet 356:1213–1218

Brown B G, Zhao X Q, Chait A et al 2001 Simvastatin and niacin, antioxidant vitamins, or the combination for the prevention of coronary disease. New England Journal of Medicine 345:1583–1592

Frei B 1999 On the role of vitamin C and other antioxidants in atherogenesis and vascular dysfunction. Proceedings of the Society of Experimental Biology and Medicine 222:196–204

Gruppo Italiano per lo Studio della Sopravvivenza nell'Infarto miocardico 1999 Dietary supplementation with n-3 polyunsaturated fatty acids and vitamin E after myocardial infarction: results of the GISSI-Prevenzione trial. Lancet 354:447–455

39. COX II inhibitors

Answer: **D**

COX (cyclo-oxygenase) II inhibitors (e.g. celecoxib and rofecoxib) are marketed for chronic pain, although there are preparations in the pipeline for acute pain, and are often prescribed in patients with arthritis, especially if the patient is likely to have a high chance of gastrointestinal bleeding. Normal non-steroidal anti-inflammatory drugs (NSAIDs) inhibit both COX I and COX II, thus the gastric protective effect of COX I is lost when using older NSAIDs. Although drugs such as celecoxib have a lower incidence of gastrointestinal bleeding than normal NSAIDS, the risk is not zero.

Trials comparing COX II inhibitors with conventional NSAIDs have found a higher incidence of cardiovascular events in the COX II arms. It is not known whether this is because of a deleterious effect of the COX II inhibitors, or because of a greater protective effect of NSAIDs (platelet aggregation is COX I mediated). Caution is probably warranted in the presence of active coronary artery disease, however, and the coprescription of aspirin and COX II antagonists carries a significantly higher risk of gastrointestinal bleeding than with COX II inhibitors alone.

Clopidogrel blocks ADP-dependent activation of platelets (ADP activates the GPIIb/IIIa receptor on the surface of platelets, which is the major receptor for fibrinogen). The CURE trial studied patients with a diagnosis of unstable angina, based on ST segment, T wave changes or a positive troponin. They were randomised to receive either clopidogrel plus aspirin or aspirin plus placebo. Clopidogrel plus aspirin significantly reduced the risk of further cardiovascular events (myocardial infarction, angina, heart failure or CVA) or death. There is no evidence that a patient admitted with a clinical diagnosis, whether or not already taking aspirin, will benefit from the addition of clopidogrel if there are no ECG changes or rise in cardiac enzyme levels.

Unfortunately, treatment with clopidogrel and aspirin was associated with a higher bleeding risk than aspirin alone, although there were no more life-threatening bleeding episodes in the clopidogrel group. When clopidogrel alone is compared with aspirin alone, the risk of gastrointestinal bleeding is slightly, but significantly, lower in the clopidogrel group.

Statins are increasingly recognised as having benefits additional to their ability to lower cholesterol levels. They are anti-inflammatory and also improve endothelial function. The MIRACL trial randomised patients with unstable angina or non-Q wave myocardial infarction to atorvastatin or placebo; cholesterol did not have to be elevated for entry into the trial. The atorvastatin group had less recurrent, symptomatic ischaemic events requiring admission in the 4 months follow-up than the placebo group, suggesting that statins have benefits in the short term after a cardiovascular event that are unrelated to their cholesterol lowering effects.

References

Influence of pravastatin and plasma lipids on clinical events in the West of Scotland Coronary Prevention Study (WOSCOPS). Circulation 1998 97:1440–1445

Schwartz G G, Olsson A G, Ezekowitz M D et al 2001 Effects of atorvastatin on early recurrent ischemic events in acute coronary syndromes: the MIRACL study: a randomised controlled trial. Journal of the American Medical Association 285:1711–1718

Yusuf S, Zhao F, Mehta S R et al 2001 Effects of clopidogrel in addition to aspirin in patients with acute coronary syndromes without ST-segment elevation. New England Journal of Medicine 345:494–502

40.   Hypertension

Answer: **E**

Traditionally, beta-blockers have been contraindicated in patients with peripheral vascular disease because the unopposed alpha-adrenergic activity leads to peripheral vasoconstriction. Carvedilol, labetalol and bisoprolol have vasodilator properties and thus are generally well tolerated in peripheral vascular disease.

Both hypertensive encephalopathy and aortic dissection require emergency treatment (as do other signs of end organ damage such as papilloedema, retinal haemorrhages, myocardial ischaemia and heart failure). If a hypertensive emergency exists, treatment with intravenous therapy is preferred. It is also preferable to relatively rapidly lower blood pressure by 20–25% over a couple of hours; more rapid reduction can worsen end-organ damage. Currently, labetalol is recommended for the treatment of a dissecting aortic aneurysm, and it is recommended that the systolic blood pressure is lowered to 110 mmHg or less .

Hypertensive encephalopathy occurs as a result of failure of cerebrovascular autoregulation due to hypertension. The blood pressure at which hypertensive encephalopathy occurs depends on the blood pressure that the patient is used to, patients who are normally normotensive develop encephalopathy at much lower blood pressures than those who are hypertensive. However, in most normotensive people cerebral blood flow is unaltered between mean arterial pressures of 60 and 120 mmHg and the autoregulatory mechanism is usually overcome at mean arterial pressures greater than 180 mmHg, when cerebral oedema ensues. The characteristic MRI feature of hypertensive encephalopathy is occipital hyperintensity on T2-weighted scans consistent with posterior leucoencephalopathy.

Although the HOPE trial showed that the ACE inhibitor ramipril was beneficial in patients with cardiovascular disease, or diabetes and a risk factor for cardiovascular disease, ACE inhibitors have not been shown to be superior to other classes of drug for the treatment of hypertension. The only trial to show a large statistical significance between two classes of antihypertensives was the LIFE study, which compared losartan and atenolol. The STOP2 study compared ACE inhibitors with calcium channel blockers in older patients and found that there was a slightly increased risk of myocardial infarction and heart failure when treated with a calcium channel blocker, however meta-analyses of different antihypertensive drugs have failed to show any difference between the classes.

References

Heintzen M P, Strauer B E 1994 Peripheral vascular effects of beta-blockers. European Heart Journal 15(suppl C):2–7

Vaughan C J, Delanty N 2000 Hypertensive emergencies. Lancet 356:411–417

41. Acute mountain sickness

A. **F**   B. **F**   C. **F**   D. **T**   E. **F**

Acute mountain sickness is diagnosed according to the Lake Louise criteria, which are a gain in altitude accompanied by headache and at least one of the following:

• gastrointestinal symptoms (nausea, vomiting or anorexia)
• fatigue or weakness
• dizziness or lightheadedness
• difficulty sleeping.

Acute mountain sickness rarely progresses to high-altitude pulmonary oedema or high-altitude cerebral oedema. High-altitude cerebral oedema is defined as acute mountain sickness accompanied by mental state change and or ataxia, or mental state change and ataxia after gain in altitude without other features of acute mountain sickness. High-altitude pulmonary oedema is defined as gain in altitude accompanied by at least two of the following: dyspnoea at rest or cough, weakness or decreased exercise tolerance, chest tightness or congestion, together with at least two of the following: crackles/wheeze, central cyanosis, tachypnoea or tachycardia.

Although, strictly, to make a diagnosis of acute mountain sickness the above criteria have to be fulfilled, many people who gain altitude have one or two of the above symptoms without fulfilling the diagnostic criteria. Although altitude is important, it is rare to get acute mountain sickness below 2400 m and the rate of ascent is the most important determinant of whether or not acute mountain sickness ensues at high altitude. In trials comparing intervention with placebo, in the placebo groups, no relationship has been found between altitude and event rate, although a direct relationship between rate of ascent and symptoms of acute mountain sickness is found. The incidence of acute mountain sickness is very low at ascent rates of less than 500 m/day.

Many treatments have been tried for prophylaxis of acute mountain sickness, including nifedepine, furosemide (frusemide), ginkgo biloba and spironolactone; although these treatments might be effective at reducing some component symptoms of acute mountain sickness, they have not proved to be efficacious in preventing the condition. Dexamethasone 8–16 mg/day and acetazolamide 750 mg/day have been shown to be efficacious at preventing acute mountain sickness in people whose ascent rate is greater than 500 m/day. There is much debate as to whether acetazolamide at lower doses is effective in the prevention of acute mountain sickness; many of the studies using lower doses have been carried out at low ascent rates, therefore the event rate has been too low for any firm conclusions to be drawn. Side-effects of dexamethasone include depression on treatment withdrawal; side-effects of acetazolamide include polyuria and peripheral paraesthesia. The best method to prevent acute mountain sickness is slow ascent speeds; if symptoms ensue, they usually abate if altitude is maintained for a day or two before continuing.

High-altitude cerebral and pulmonary oedema are more severe forms of acute mountain sickness and the mainstay of treatment should be to evacuate the patient to lower altitudes. Artificial descent in a hyperbaric chamber has been proven to be effective, although this is not always available. Dexamethasone is usually a good temporising measure for both conditions. If pulmonary oedema is diagnosed, oxygen should be administered where possible and nifedipine has proven to be an effective treatment, probably as a result of reducing pulmonary arterial pressure.

References

Dumont L, Mardirosoff C, Tramer M R 2000 Efficacy and harm of pharmacological prevention of acute mountain sickness: quantitative systematic review. British Medical Journal 321:267–272

Hohenhaus E, Niroomand F, Goerre S et al 1994 Nifedipine does not prevent acute mountain sickness. American Journal of Respiratory and Critical Care Medicine 150:857–860

Medline Plus health information (National Library of Medicine) medical encyclopedia. Online. Available: www.nlm.nih.gov/medlineplus

PSYCHIATRY

True/False answers

42.   Alcohol dependency

A. **F**   B. **F**   C. **T**   D. **T**   E. **T**

Dependency on alcohol is characterised by a cluster of behavioural, physiological and cognitive phenomena. According to the ICD-10 definition, three or more of the following are required for a diagnosis of alcohol dependency:

- compulsion to drink
- difficulties controlling alcohol consumption

- physiological withdrawal
- tolerance to alcohol
- neglect of alternative activities to drinking
- persistent use of alcohol despite evidence of harm.

Withdrawal symptoms include the mental symptoms of depression, anxiety, panic, visual hallucinations and guilt, and the physical symptoms of nausea, tremor, insomnia, sweating and weakness. Alcohol misuse is the term used when harm occurs – physically, economically or socially – secondary to alcohol use but when the criteria for dependency are not fulfilled. Short-term alcohol use increases GABA-ergic function but long-term use leads to reduced GABA-benzodiazepine receptor levels and function. The effect of alcohol on the GABA-benzodiazepine receptor is likely to cause its anxiolytic effect but is also critical in the development of tolerance, dependence and withdrawal. Chronic alcohol consumption also increases the activity of the glutamate system, which remains hyperexcitable for up to a year following abstinence from alcohol.

Up to 80% of heavy drinkers have psychiatric symptoms, often indistinguishable from a diagnosable disorder such as anxiety or depression, but these commonly disappear within weeks or months of abstinence without the need for other medication. Diagnosis of mental illness is thus best undertaken at least 3–4 weeks after abstinence is achieved. However, it is also clear that there are high levels of comorbidity with mental illness and alcohol is used as a form of self-medication, especially in patients with depressive and anxiety disorders.

Withdrawal symptoms start to occur 6–12 h after cessation or reduced consumption. Severity of this withdrawal seems to be related to the rate of fall of blood alcohol level. The peak seizure incidence is at 36 h and peak delirium incidence occurs at 72 h.

Drug treatments for alcohol dependency include benzodiazepines during the acute detoxification phase, disulfiram (Antabuse) and acamprosate. Acamprosate seems to work by restoring normal neuronal NMDA receptor activity. Several trials have shown the efficacy of acamprosate up to 12 months after starting treatment. Double-blind, placebo-controlled trials show that although acamprosate does not affect craving, it is significantly associated with higher abstinence rates and a reduction in relapse rates up to 2 years post-treatment. One study showed that significantly more acamprosate patients than placebo patients remained abstinent at 48 weeks post-treatment (39.9% versus 17.3%, $P = 0.003$). Its other advantages are that it is well tolerated, has no abuse potential and can be used safely in patients with liver dysfunction. It also does not cause adverse reactions when administered with disulfiram, naltrexone or any other medications commonly prescribed to patients with alcohol dependency, such as hypnotics and antidepressants. Acamprosate can be trialled once abstinence is achieved and continued for 1 year. Acamprosate is safe to continue if relapse occurs, although continued alcohol abuse negates its effect.

Psychological treatment includes 'motivational interviewing' which aims to move a patient a step at a time along the 'stages of change' model. This model states that a person goes though a number of stages when giving up an addiction:

1. pre-contemplation (total denial of problem)
2. contemplation (acknowledging problem but does not want to change quite yet)
3. determination ('I'll definitely change tomorrow')
4. action (stopping drinking)
5. relapse prevention.

It must not be forgotten that without a comprehensive package of psychosocial care it is highly likely that a patient will relapse back into drinking after pharmacological detoxification. Packages should address drinking cues and the gap that not drinking leaves, both socially and psychologically.

References

Lingford-Hughes A, Potokar J, Nutt D 2002 Treating anxiety complicated by substance misuse. Advances in Psychiatric Treatment 8:107–716

Mason B 2001 Treatment of alcohol-dependent out-patients with acamprosate: A clinical review. Journal of Clinical Psychiatry 62(suppl 20):42–47

Raistrick D 2000 Management of alcohol detoxification. Advances in Psychiatric Treatment 6:348–354

43.   St John's wort

A. **F**   B. **F**   C. **F**   D. **T**   E. **T**

St John's wort is currently unlicensed in the UK but is bought by many patients over the counter as a homeopathic remedy for depression. Comparison trials show that it is equally effective in the treatment of mild to moderate depression as the tricyclic antidepressant imipramine but has side-effects equivalent to placebo. A recent large-scale study ($n = 340$) comparing St John's wort with placebo and sertraline in patients with moderately severe depression failed to show a treatment effect. However, it also failed to show significant improvement in depression scores in those patients taking sertraline compared with placebo. This low sensitivity to change suggests that the result should be viewed sceptically.

The mode of action of St John's wort is thought to be similar to that of serotonin reuptake inhibitors (SSRIs), thus, like other SSRIs, it can cause the serotonin syndrome. It is therefore important to ask patients whether they take any homeopathic remedies when taking their histories.

Case reports suggest that St John's wort is a potent inducer of hepatic enzymes, perhaps via cytochrome P450 2C9, the activity of which it approximately doubles. As a result, it causes decreased levels of theophylline, digoxin, warfarin, ciclosporin, ethinylestradiol and indinavir. In the last case, HIV patients can develop drug resistance as a result. Reduced ciclosporin levels, secondary to St

John's wort, were reported to have led to rejection of heart transplants in two cases.

References

Ernst E 1999 Second thoughts about safety of St John's wort. Lancet 354:2014–2015

Hypericum depression study group 2002 The effect of *Hypericum perforatum* (St John's wort) in major depressive disorder. Journal of the American Medical Association 287:1807–1814

Jobst K, Wheatley D 2000 Safety of St John's wort (*Hypericum perforatum*). Lancet 355:575–576

44.   Chronic fatigue syndrome

A. **F**   B. **F**   C. **T**   D. **F**   E. **F**

The prevalence of chronic fatigue syndrome is between 0.2 and 2.6%. Female sex is the only demographic risk factor. The diagnosis is made on the presence of at least 6 months of disabling fatigue affecting mental and physical functioning more than 50% of the time. It is associated with other symptoms, for example sleep disturbance, headaches and myalgia, and can only be diagnosed in the absence of other diseases that could cause fatigue or mental illness. Children have a better outcome than adults, with 54–94% showing improvement at 6 years follow-up. Only 20–50% of adults show some improvement and only 6% return to premorbid functioning.

A report on chronic fatigue syndrome (also known as myalgic encephalomyelitis or encephalopathy), commissioned by the Chief Medical Officer of England and Wales, was published in 2002. The report was compiled by a 16-member working party consisting of patients, psychiatrists, physicians and patient representatives. Although six members were unable to endorse the final draft, it did come to some consensus and advocated cognitive behavioural therapy, graded exercise and pacing (despite the latter having only anecdotal evidence) as effective treatments. It also stated categorically that it is no longer acceptable for doctors not to believe in chronic fatigue syndrome and that 'inaction due to ignorance or denial of the condition is not excusable'.

Graded exercise with education about how deconditioning of the body can result in symptoms similar to chronic fatigue syndrome and how deconditioning can worsen symptoms that are already present has shown a benefit up to 1 year later. Cognitive behavioural therapy delivered in specialist centres has a number needed to treat of two. Pacing involves measuring out activities so that the patient doesn't do too much in one go – a balance of activity and rest. In summary, the best evidence advocates symptomatic and rehabilitative treatments. Treatment with antidepressants shows no consistent significant benefit, nor do corticosteroids, bed rest, immunotherapy or dietary supplements.

References

Reid S, Chalder T, Cleare A et al 2000 Extracts from clinical evidence: chronic fatigue. British Medical Journal 320:292–296

Clark C, Buchwald D, MacIntyre A et al 2002 Chronic fatigue syndrome: a step towards agreement. Lancet 359:97–98

Powell P, Bentall R, Nye F, Edwards R 2001 Randomized controlled trial of patient education to encourage graded exercise in chronic fatigue syndrome. British Medical Journal 322:387–389

45. Delirium

A. **T**   B. **T**   C. **F**   D. **T**   E. **F**

Between 9 and 30% of general hospital patients have delirium and this rate increases to 50% in patients on intensive care. Over one-third of cases of delirium go undiagnosed in clinical practice and up to 42% of patients referred to psychiatry for consultation for suspected depression are delirious. Two presentations are typically seen. First, the overactive patient who is up all night and is combative. This can confused with a diagnosis of psychosis or mania. The second presentation, which has a worse outcome (possibly because of under-recognition and under-treatment) is that of a withdrawn and hypoactive patient that can be mistaken for depression or an adjustment disorder. Failure to recognise and treat delirium results in an increase in mortality.

Delirium is characterised by the acute and reversible onset of disturbance in memory (short-term more than long-term because of the core feature of poor attention and concentration), disturbed orientation, changes in mood (which is usually labile but can appear depressed), motor behaviour (either overactive or underactive) , perception (typically visual hallucinations), thinking (often paranoid or depressive) and sleep–wake cycle (awake at night and asleep in the day). The course of delirium characteristically fluctuates but symptoms tend to worsen at night. Deficits in the non-dominant cerebral hemisphere may explain many of the features of delirium and some research suggests that this might distinguish it from dementia and functional psychotic disorders.

There are many causes of delirium and it will often have a multifactorial origin. In general, an elderly patient who is seriously medically ill and who exhibits a change in mental state has a diagnosis of delirium unless proven otherwise. When a diagnosis of delirium has been made it is not possible to diagnose dementia or any other mental illness until the delirium has resolved. Risk factors for delirium include old age; pre-existing cognitive impairment; emergency; certain types of operations, for example hip replacement and long operations; metabolic disturbances; infection; hypoxaemia; visual or auditory impairment; immobility and social isolation. Delirium is worsened and triggered by drugs with anticholinergic properties and by benzodiazepines, except in patients in alcohol or drug withdrawal where benzodiazepines are the treatment of choice.

The treatment of delirium is to identify and try to treat or remove the causes. Conventional or atypical antipsychotics will relieve the symptoms but typically haloperidol is used and titrated to response because it is relatively safe in renal, liver and lung impairment, does not interact with many other drugs and is less sedative than most. Extrapyramidal side-effects occur less than would be expected. Between 0.5 mg oral and 100 mg intravenous haloperidol over a 24-h period can be used, depending on circumstances and the patient.

Because of the fluctuation in mental state of patients with delirium it is possible for consent to be obtained from a patient during a lucid interval. Otherwise, emergency treatment is given under common law. Interestingly, the benzodiazepine antagonist flumazenil has been given to patients in hepatic failure who are delirious. This has restored mental capacity for a short period of time to enable patients to make decisions about treatment.

References

Meager D 2001 Delirium: optimizing management. British Medical Journal 322:144–149

Meager D 2001 Delirium: the role of psychiatry. Advances in Psychiatric Treatment 7:433–443

46.   Nicotine addiction

A. **T**   B. **F**   C. **F**   D. **T**   E. **T**

Smoking causes significant mortality and morbidity; 120 000 deaths a year are caused by cigarette smoking and half of all smokers will die as a result of their addiction. As a result, the Royal College of Physicians has produced guidelines regarding smoking cessation and specialist services are being set up around the country to provide expert treatment of nicotine addiction.

Nicotine acts as an agonist at the nicotinic acetylcholine receptors of the autonomic ganglia, adrenal medulla and neuromuscular junction and nicotinic receptors in the brain. It is eliminated by direct renal excretion.

Although not carcinogenic itself, nicotine is highly addictive, as characterised by craving, compulsion to use, development of tolerance, persistent use despite harm, high relapse rates and a withdrawal syndrome. Withdrawal symptoms include irritability, poor concentration, anxiety, hunger, depressed mood and craving. Nicotine has a half-life of 2 h. Symptoms of withdrawal develop within 12 h, and therefore will be present in a smoker by morning, and last 3 weeks. Tolerance to adverse affects of smoking, such as nausea, increased blood pressure and heart rate occurs within days. Relapse rates match those for alcoholics and heroin addicts. Nicotine administration in dependent animals leads to the stimulation of the reward pathway with release of dopamine in the nucleus accumbens.

Treatment for nicotine addiction includes brief interventions, group meetings, bupropion (amfebutamone) and nicotine replacement therapy. Buproprion (amfebutamone) is an atypical antidepressant that inhibits neuronal uptake of dopamine and noradrenaline (norepinephrine). It should be started 2 weeks prior to the patient quitting and, in placebo-controlled trials, is equally effective as the various nicotine replacement therapies, such as patches. It has a small risk of inducing seizures (1 in 1000). Its effect appears to be independent of its antidepressant qualities. Nicotine replacement therapy can be delivered by several methods: chewing gum, transdermally as patches, as an inhalator, as a nasal spray, sublingually or as lozenges. Unfortunately, none of these methods deliver the nicotine and thus reward as quickly as cigarettes. The use of nicotine replacement therapy approximately doubles the cessation rates. Side-effects of patches include, nausea, headaches, flu-like symptoms, palpitations, insomnia with vivid dreams and gastrointestinal disturbance.

A 5-min intervention of advice to smokers is shown to increase abstinence rates by 3% above control levels at 6 months and specialist smoking cessation clinics increase quit rate at 1 year by 17% above control. Some studies have shown that patients with a history of major depression find it harder to abstain from smoking than those who do not. There is evidence that in these patients the cessation of smoking can lead to a relapse of depressive illness.

References

Britton J, Jarvis J 2000 Bupropion: a new treatment for smokers. British Medical Journal 321:65–66

Lancaster T 2000 Effectiveness of interventions to help people stop smoking: findings from the Cochrane Library. British Medical Journal 321:355–357

Luty J 2002 Nicotine addiction and smoking cessation treatments. Advances in Psychiatric Treatment 8:42–48

Niaura R, Abrams D 2001 Stopping smoking: a hazard for people with a history of major depression? Lancet 357:1900–1901

Best-of-5 answers

47. Psychosis

Answer: **C**

This patient exhibits symptoms and signs of neuroleptic malignant syndrome. This is a rare syndrome but has a mortality of up to 10%. It occurs in patients taking neuroleptic medications, particularly high potency ones such as haloperidol, although it can happen with all neuroleptics, including atypical agents such as quetiapine, risperidone and clozapine. The risks might be higher in those patients also taking lithium. Abrupt discontinuation of antiparkinsonian agents or the use of dopamine-depleting agents has also been reported as responsible. Onset is usually in the first 10 days of treatment and young males are more likely to be affected, although it has been seen in all ages and in women.

There are two theories as to the development of neuroleptic malignant syndrome; the first is a neuroleptic-induced alteration of central neuroregulatory mechanisms and the second is an abnormal reaction of predisposed skeletal muscle to neuroleptics (by influencing calcium ion transport) or a direct toxic effect. Neuroleptic malignant syndrome has many features in common with malignant hyperthermia, including hyperthermia, rigidity and raised creatinine phosphokinase levels.

Neuroleptics are dopamine antagonists. The hyperthermia that occurs in neuroleptic malignant syndrome might be caused by blockade of hypothalamic dopamine receptors. Bromocriptine, a dopamine agonist, has been shown to be effective in the treatment of the hyperthermia associated with neuroleptic malignant syndrome. Blockade of dopamine receptors in the corpus striatum probably causes muscle rigidity.

Clinically, the patient presents with acute onset of muscle rigidity with generalised lead pipe tone, altered level of consciousness, hyperpyrexia > 38.5°C and autonomic instability. The patient can then develop renal failure secondary to rhabdomyolysis or cardiovascular collapse. The diagnosis of neuroleptic malignant syndrome can be hard to make and many features of it remain controversial. There is still no single set of criteria in general use and some clinicians believe that there is a spectrum of clinical severity and or signs. Clinical research studies of neuroleptic malignant syndrome commonly use the presence of three major, or two major and four minor symptoms as necessary for a diagnosis. Fever, rigidity and raised CPK level are major signs and tachycardia, abnormal arterial pressure, tachypnoea, altered consciousness, diaphoresis and leucocytosis are the minor signs.

The differential diagnosis includes other causes of rhabdomyolysis, neuroleptic-induced heatstroke, serotonin syndrome, acute lethal catatonia and anaesthetic-induced malignant hyperthermia. In neuroleptic-induced heatstroke there is an absence of extrapyramidal signs and sweating and a history of physical exertion or exposure to high temperature without adequate fluid intake. Acute lethal catatonia is rare. Symptoms and laboratory findings are similar to neuroleptic malignant syndrome but there will be a history for the preceeding 2–3 weeks of depressive symptoms. Serotonin syndrome can be differentiated from neuroleptic malignant syndrome by its more rapid onset and progression, association with combinations of serotonergic drugs and presence of hyperkinesia, hyperreflexia and myoclonus rather than lead pipe rigidity and bradykinesia.

Patients with neuroleptic malignant syndrome will have a raised white cell count (up to 30×10^9/L) and a very high CPK level (> 1000 IU/L) representing myonecrosis from intense muscle contracture.

Lumbar puncture is normal as is cerebral CT. Symptoms last for 1–2 weeks after the drug is stopped, and longer if a depot neuroleptic was responsible. Treatment is to stop all neuroleptics and then manage symptomatically to reduce the temperature and prevent secondary complications. Dantrolene, bromocriptine and diazepam have all been used to help with symptoms. Electroconvulsive therapy can improve some of the symptoms such as sweating and level of consciousness. Rechallenge with the agent thought to be responsible for neuroleptic malignant syndrome does not necessarily result in a recurrence of it.

References

Adnet P, Lestavel P, Krivosic-Horber R 2000 Neuroleptic malignant syndrome. British Journal of Anaesthesia 85:129–135

Gillman P 1999 The serotonin syndrome and its treatment. Journal of Psychopharmacology 13:100–109

Hasan S, Buckley P 1998 Novel antipsychotics and the neuroleptic malignant syndrome; a review and critique. American Journal of Psychiatry 155:1113–1136

48.   Lithium toxicity

Answer: **A**

Lithium acts as a mood stabiliser and is the treatment of choice for patients with mania. It is also used as prophylaxis and maintenance treatment of bipolar affective disorder, recurrent major depression and as an adjunct to antidepressants in refractory depression. There is evidence that lithium treatment reduces the risk of suicide in patients with recurrent depression.

Lithium has a very narrow therapeutic range (0.5–1.2 mmol/L); levels above 1.5 mmol/L lead to toxicity. In acute mania, levels of 1.2 mmol/L are recommended and for maintenance, 0.8 mmol/L. The lithium level is approximately proportional to the lithium dose, thus doubling the dose will double the level. Regular monitoring of serum lithium level is important, initially weekly until levels are stable and then every 6 months.

Lithium commonly causes side-effects, most of which are benign. Side-effects encountered early in therapy include a fine tremor, which is related to the peak serum level and gastrointestinal effects such as nausea, vomiting and diarrhoea. Later on in treatment, patients can develop benign ECG changes, including T-wave flattening or inversion. It is thus prudent to perform a baseline ECG prior to beginning therapy, especially in the elderly.

Lithium will induce hypothyroidism in 5% of patients, although 30% will have elevated TSH levels. This usually becomes evident after 6–18 months of treatment and is why regular thyroid function tests are important. Lithium less commonly affects the parathyroid gland and can increase calcium levels.

Lithium is excreted unchanged by the kidneys. It is transported in competition with sodium by sodium–potassium active transport in the proximal tubule. Lithium's effect on the kidney is to cause an initial diuresis and polyuria with related polydipsia. This is usually mild but occasionally nephrogenic diabetes insipidus develops. Lithium has been reported to cause interstitial nephritis in studies on renal biopsies but this is not usually clinically significant. However, it is recommended that renal function is monitored regularly. Dermatological effects include the development of acne and exacerbation of psoriasis. Other side-effects of lithium include oedema, weight gain and leucocytosis. At toxic levels, patients develop impaired consciousness with increased tendon reflexes, a coarsening of their tremor, slurred speech, choreiform movements and fits. Severe toxicity can lead to coma and death. Treatment of acute intoxication, as in the case of overdose, is with fluid and electrolyte replacement and in severe cases, haemodialysis.

References

Cookson J 2001 Use of antipsychotic drugs and lithium in mania. British Journal of Psychiatry 178(suppl 41):148–156

Dunner D 2000 Optimizing lithium treatment. Journal of Clinical Psychiatry 61(suppl 9):76–80

49. Psychiatric drugs and weight gain

Answer: **B**

Schizoaffective disorder is a severe mental illness in which the patient has symptoms of schizophrenia and a mood disorder within the same illness event. It is often a life-long, chronic illness and patients will need several types of psychiatric medication to keep symptoms under control. Patients with schizophrenia or schizoaffective illnesses commonly have problems with obesity because most antipsychotics cause weight gain. In turn, obesity increases the risk of the development of several illnesses, including type 2 diabetes and heart disease.

The novel antipsychotics include olanzapine, risperidone, clozapine, quetiapine and sulpiride. They differ from the typical antipsychotics such as haloperidol and chlorpromazine by their action in that typicals are primarily dopamine D2 receptor antagonists whereas the atypical antipsychotics act at numerous receptors, including dopamine D1 and D4, alpha adrenergic, muscarinic, histaminergic and serotonin receptors. The advantage this gives the atypical compounds is that they cause far fewer extrapyramidal side-effects or tardive dyskinesias and thus drug therapy is more likely to be complied with. However, it has recently been realised that the novel atypicals cause substantially more weight gain than the older, typical antipsychotics. Trials have shown that a person taking olanzapine will gain, on average, 4.2 kg within 10 weeks and 11.8 kg in 1 year. Only clozapine causes more weight gain, with an average of 4.5 kg in 10 weeks. By contrast, haloperidol causes only 1.1 kg weight gain in the same time period and risperidone 2.1 kg. The mechanism for this weight gain is not clearly understood. However, schizophrenia is associated with abnormal phospholipid metabolism and clozapine commonly causes increased triglyceride levels.

Fluoxetine, an antidepressant with selective serotonin reuptake inhibitor properties usually causes weight loss rather than gain. Zopiclone is a hypnotic and is licensed for short-term use in patients with insomnia. It does not cause weight gain. Carbamazepine, which is licensed as a mood stabiliser as well as an anticonvulsant, can cause weight loss secondary to a reduction in appetite.

References

Allison D, Mentore J, Heo M et al 2000 Review: most antipsychotic drugs are associated with weight gain. Evidence Based Medicine 3:58

Green I, Patel JK, Goisman RM 2000 Weight gain from novel antipsychotic drugs: need for action. General Hospital Psychiatry 22:224–235

Peet M 2002 Essential fatty acids: theoretical aspects and treatment implications for schizophrenia and depression. Advances in Psychiatric Treatment 8:223–229

50. Depression in older people

Answer: **B**

Depression in older people is an important predictor of suicide and suicide rates in the elderly are higher than in any other age group. Older men are more at risk than women of committing suicide, the ratio being three to one. The government has made reduction of suicide rates a priority for the health service. In its Green Paper 'Our Healthier Nation', it proposed a reduction of 17%, from 1996 figures, of suicide by 2010.

Depression presents slightly differently in older people than in the young. According to the ICD-10 definition, a diagnosis of depression is made on the basis of at least 2 weeks of two out of the following three symptoms: low mood, loss of interest and pleasure in things (anhedonia) and low energy levels. The severity of the depression depends on how many other symptoms are present, including low self-esteem, feelings of guilt, suicidal ideation, poor concentration, change in appetite (can be increased or decreased) and sleep disturbance (classically early morning wakening). Patients with psychotic depression can present with delusions of guilt, poverty and nihilism, for example that they are to blame for children starving in Africa, that they have no money or that they have no internal organs. Patients with psychotic depression can also experience auditory hallucinations that are usually derogatory in nature.

Older patients are less likely to verbalise suicidal ideas, which is why they should be specifically asked about such ideas. Older patients, especially males, also tend to present with complaints of physical illness in the form of somatisation or hypochondriasis rather than depression. This is perhaps because they are less able to verbalise depressed mood or admit to suicidal thoughts. Older patients who present following a suicide attempt should always be taken seriously as this is a much stronger predictor of future completed suicide than in younger age groups. The ratio of attempts to completed suicide in the elderly is 4:1 compared with 200:1 in younger groups. Studies suggest that up to 90% of older patients who attempt suicide have a diagnosis of depression. There is little evidence that suicide in older patients is ever a rational act taken in response to an irreversible and understandable situation.

References

Cattell H 2000 Suicide in the elderly. Advances in Psychiatric Treatment 6:102–108

World Health Organization 1998 Pocket guide to the ICD-10 classification of mental and behavioural disorders. Churchill Livingstone, London, p 131–137

51. Dementia

Answer: **B**

Lewy-body dementia accounts for up to 20% of all cases of dementia. The age of onset ranges from 50 to 83 years, with slightly more males than females being affected. Mean survival is similar to Alzheimer's disease although some patients show a rapid progression of disease, with death within 2 years. Post-mortem examination shows senile plaques (as in Alzheimer's disease) and neuronal inclusions, or Lewy bodies, in the substantia nigra, paralimbic and neocortical areas.

The core features of Lewy-body dementia are fluctuating cognitive function with confusion and variation in attention and alertness, visual hallucinations that are typically well formed and motor features of parkinsonism. Two-thirds report visual hallucinations but hallucinations can occur in other sensory modalities too. Patients might develop a psychosis and 40% develop major depression. Recurrent falls and syncope occur in up to one-third and are supportive of a diagnosis of Lewy-body dementia; 70% develop parkinsonism. Neuroleptics should be avoided as these patients are extremely sensitive to them and can develop irreversible parkinsonism.

Frontotemporal dementia was previously known as Pick's disease. The terminology has changed because not all patients with this syndrome have 'Pick-like' histological changes. Patients with frontotemporal dementia present with profound personality and behavioural changes, such as stereotypical movements (which develop over time) and a blunting of emotions or disinhibition. Poor insight into loss of emotional and cognitive abilities is exemplified by a lack of concern when difficulties are encountered. This might be preceded by anxiety, depression and hypochondriasis. Stereotypical movements include hand rubbing and stereotypical speech with perseveration and echolalia. Frontotemporal dementia is the second most common cause of presenile dementia after Alzheimer's disease. Age of onset is between 45 and 65 years, with a mean duration of illness of 8 years.

Patients with vascular dementia commonly have other indications of or risk factors for vascular disease, such as high blood pressure, heart disease, diabetes and hypercholesterolaemia. Classically, the dementia progresses in a stepwise fashion, is fluctuating in course and there might be focal neurological signs. However, there is increasing debate as to whether this is a separate disease entity because it often coexists with Alzheimer's disease and, in fact, they both share the above risk factors as well as having similar clinical pictures.

Alzheimer's disease presents with minor forgetfulness, which is usually most marked for recent events. Eventually only the earliest learned memories, such as date of birth, are retained. Personality traits tend to become more pronounced. Later there might be features of temporal and parietal lobe damage, such as dysphasia and dyspraxia. Although visual hallucinations are more common with patients who have Lewy-body dementia, hallucinations can occur in Alzheimer's disease. Delusions, which are usually paranoid and unsystematised, might also be present. Visuospatial problems, which often only come to light in new surroundings, are also common.

The patient who presents with a dementia associated with alcohol use will usually have a history of heavy alcohol abuse with other physical evidence of harm. Patients often present with a frontal lobe picture. CT scans show brain atrophy with enlargement of the lateral ventricles and subarachnoid spaces. MRI scans show loss of grey matter in both cortical and subcortical areas. Patients who are thiamine deficient, as can occur in long-term abusers of alcohol, can develop Korsakov's syndrome, in which short-term memory is poor and the individual is unable to lay down new memories, although remote memory is preserved. The patient might fill-in gaps in their memory by confabulating; such stories can be convincing until the information given by the patient is checked out. This syndrome is caused by haemorrhagic lesions in the mamillary bodies and, at post-mortem, haemorrhages can also be found in the region of the third ventricle, periaqueductal grey matter and thalamic nuclei.

References

Gelder M, Mayou R, Cowen P et al 2000 Cognitive impairment syndromes with specific psychological dysfunctions. Oxford Textbook of Psychiatry, 3rd edn. Oxford University Press, Oxford, p 314–316, 449–450

McKeith I 2002 Dementia with Lewy bodies. British Journal of Psychiatry 180:144–147

Snowden J, Neary D, Mann D 2002 Frontotemporal dementia. British Journal of Psychiatry 180:140–143

Stewart R 2002 Vascular dementia: a diagnosis running out of time. British Journal of Psychiatry 180:152–155

MISCELLANEOUS
True/False answers

52. **Visual impairment in older people**

   A. F   B. F   C. T   D. T   E. T

Visual impairment becomes increasingly common with advancing age and is associated with a reduced quality of life, as well as being a risk factor for accidents, including falls. Despite the fact that visual loss is insidious in older people, there is no evidence that screening an older, asymptomatic population allows effective intervention to reduce the burden of visual impairment. Screening can, however, allow those with impaired vision to receive support to allow them to circumvent some of the problems that impaired vision brings.

   Cataract surgery is a highly effective procedure in all age groups but outcomes are not quite as good in older people. A recent survey of cataract surgery in the UK revealed that one-third of patients undergoing cataract surgery had comorbid ocular disease, including glaucoma, macular degeneration and diabetic retinopathy. Comorbid disease was more common in older than in younger people and the presence of comorbid disease predicted a threefold increase in the chance of not achieving a visual acuity of at least 6/12 after cataract surgery. Older people have a higher incidence of technical complications, including eye infection and rupture of the posterior capsule.

   A number of drugs have become available for controlling the intraocular pressure in glaucoma. Dorzolamide is a carbonic anhydrase inhibitor that reduces the production of aqueous humour. Brimonidine is an alpha$_2$ agonist with similar effects. Latanoprost is a prostaglandin F$_2$ agonist that increases aqueous humour outflow. It can be used in conjunction with beta-blockers or the above drugs, or can be used alone when beta-blockers are contraindicated.

   Macular degeneration is the most common cause of visual loss in older people and it is not currently reversible. A recent cross-sectional study has suggested that it is much less common in patients taking statins; whether statin therapy given early in the course of the disease can actually halt or reverse the condition remains to be seen. Vitamin E, when given alone over a 4-year period, did not have any effect on the progression of early macular degeneration in a recent randomised, placebo-controlled trial. However, a combination of vitamins C, E, beta-carotene and zinc did reduce progression from moderate to advanced disease in a 6-year trial involving over 3000 patients.

References

Age-related Eye Disease Study Group 2001 A randomised, placebo-controlled clinical trial of high-dose supplementation with vitamins C and E, beta carotene, and zinc for age-related macular degeneration and vision loss. Archives of Ophthalmology 119:1417–1436

Fielder A R, Bentley C, Moseley M J 1999 Recent advances: ophthalmology. British Medical Journal 318:717–720

Hall N F, Gale C L, Syddall H et al 2001 Risk of macular degeneration in users of statins: cross sectional study. British Medical Journal 323:375–376

Taylor H R, Tikellis G, Robman L D et al 2002 Vitamin E supplementation and macular degeneration: randomised controlled trial. British Medical Journal 325:11–14

Wong T Y 2001 Effect of increasing age on cataract surgery outcomes in very elderly patients. British Medical Journal 322:1104–1106

53.   Thyroid eye disease

A. **F**   B. **T**   C. **T**   D. **F**   E. **F**

Thyroid eye disease is a common eye disorder that usually accompanies clinical and biochemical signs of thyroid dysfunction. It classically accompanies Graves' disease but can also occur in patients who are euthyroid, as well as in patients with autoimmune thyroiditis. Symptoms include grittiness and eye pain, blurred vision, diplopia, reduced colour saturation and watering eyes. Signs include lid lag and retraction, proptosis, chemosis, reduced ocular movements, failure of conjugate gaze, and optic nerve problems including disc pallor, enlarged blind spot and reduced visual acuity or fields.

Most cases of thyroid eye disease are self limiting, the mean duration being about 1 year. The pathogenesis of the condition is unclear but inflammation of periorbital fat and soft tissue appears to be the central pathological process. Deposition of glycosaminoglycans and inflammation of the extraocular muscles then leads to proptosis, stretching or compression of the optic nerve, and reduced ocular muscle movement. Failure of the lid to cover the eye puts the eye at high risk of corneal abrasion. Chronic inflammation can lead to fibrotic changes, with permanent proptosis, shortening of extraocular muscles and permanent disability. Surgical intervention is necessary if there are signs of optic nerve compromise or if the cornea is threatened, and surgery is also indicated for chronic 'burnt-out' disease with residual fibrosis of the extraocular muscles. Orbital decompression surgery is carried out urgently for optic nerve involvement; decompression or lateral tarsorrhaphy are carried out to protect the cornea.

Radioiodine therapy appears to be associated with a higher incidence of thyroid eye disease than surgery; most eye disease associated with radioiodine is mild and self-limiting and covering the radioiodine treatment with steroids can prevent the observed excess of thyroid eye disease. Steroids also form the mainstay of treatment for established active thyroid eye disease; normalisation of thyroid function, for example with carbimazole, is not sufficient to treat established eye disease. A number of other immunosuppressant medications, including methotrexate and ciclosporin, have been used as steroid-sparing agents with some success. Patients who are at high risk for severe eye disease are: older patients, males, smokers, diabetics, those with prolonged disease, those with rapid progression of signs at onset and those with reduced visual acuity. These patients should be monitored more closely than others.

References

Bartalena L, Marcocci C, Bogazzi F et al 1998 Relation between therapy for hyperthyroidism and the course of Graves' ophthalmopathy. New England Journal of Medicine 338:73–78

Denniston A, Dodson P, Reuser T 2002 Diagnosis and management of thyroid eye disease. Hospital Medicine 63:152–157

Best-of-5 answers

54. Sexually transmitted diseases

Answer: **D**

The clinical scenario described is of secondary syphilis. The causal organism is the spirochaete *Treponema pallidum*. *Treponema pertenue* causes yaws, one of the tropical non-venereal treponematoses, which also includes pinta (*Treponema carateum*) and endemic syphilis (see references for more details). Syphilis is characterised by intermittent periods of disease and latency. Early syphilis can be classified into primary (initial chancre on genitalia, anus or lips/mouth) and secondary infection with systemic manifestations, as in the case described. Early manifestations can be followed by a period of latency for many years. Late complications include tertiary gummatous syphilis (gummas of almost any tissue, but in particular the skin, mucosal surfaces and bone), cardiovascular syphilis (aortitis and aneurysm formation) and neurosyphilis.

Haemophilus ducreyi and *Calymmatobacterium granulomatis* cause the tropical sexually transmitted infections chancroid and granuloma inguinale (donovanosis), respectively. Although herpes simplex virus can cause erythema multiforme and systemic illness, genital lesions are characterised by intense pain, in particular during primary infection.

During the 1980s and early 1990s, rates of all sexually transmitted infections fell in the UK, almost certainly because of the publicity surrounding HIV infection, together with the safer sex message. Over the last few years, however, rates of gonorrhoea diagnosed at genitourinary medicine clinics have climbed sharply and several localised outbreaks of syphilis have been noted in larger cities, e.g. Bristol and Manchester. Rates of chlamydial infection are also rising rapidly. These figures suggest that the safer sex message has not penetrated the current generation of sexually active adults; the highest numbers of infected individuals are in the 16–24-year-old age bracket.

Worldwide, sexually transmitted disease imposes a huge burden on populations in the developing world; the effect of HIV infection on the demographics of many sub-Saharan countries are well known, with falling life expectancy and infection rates of over 25% of the population. Worldwide, it is estimated that over 300 million cases of treatable sexually transmitted infection occur each year; not only do these infections impose their own burden of morbidity, infertility and early death, but they facilitate transmission of HIV.

References

Arya O P 1996 Tropical STDs. Medicine 24:18–21

Hughes G, Fenton K A 2001 Epidemiology of STIs: UK. Medicine 29:1–2

Mabey D 2001 Epidemiology of STIs: worldwide. Medicine 29:3–5

55.   Driving and the DVLA

Answer: **D**

According to the DVLA, 'the DVLA is legally responsible for deciding if a person is medically unfit to drive. They need to know when driving license holders have a condition which may now or in the future, affect their safety as a driver'. It is a doctor's duty to advise that a patient should contact the DVLA but if the patient refuses or the doctor knows that he or she continues to drive, and thus pose a risk, then the doctor should inform the patient's relatives and, if this has no effect, the DVLA with notification to the patient that this has been done.

DVLA notification is required in a number of illnesses but this does not necessarily mean that restrictions on driving will be made. Examples include epilepsy, chronic neurological disorders, tumour or injury affecting the brain, diabetes (unless managed by diet alone), field of vision deficits, alcohol/drug misuse, dementia and chronic renal failure. In general, the DVLA wants to know about chronic or progressive illnesses that can potentially affect the patient's ability to drive. Notification is not necessary following angina, angioplasty or coronary artery bypass grafting, although there is guidance on how long a patient should not drive for (when asymptomatic, 2 weeks and

4 weeks respectively). Notification is required if the patient has a pacemaker implanted. It is also not necessary after a stroke or TIA unless there is residual neurological deficit although, again, driving should be ceased for 1 month after the event. These guidelines are for ordinary drivers and do not include those in charge of lorries or buses, for whom restrictions are much tighter.

References

DVLA 2001 At-a-glance guide to current medical standards of fitness to drive. Drivers Medical Unit, DVLA, Swansea, p 2–31

INFECTIOUS DISEASES

True/False answers

56. Antibiotic resistance

A. **T**   B. **T**   C. **T**   D. **F**   E. **T**

Somewhat surprisingly, *Streptococcus pyogenes* is always sensitive to penicillin. However, *S. pyogenes* strains resistant to other commonly used antibiotics, such as the macrolides (e.g. erythromycin), have been isolated. Globally, resistance to first-line antibiotics has been documented for almost all common community-acquired pathogens (e.g. respiratory tract infections, infectious diarrhoea, HIV, tuberculosis, malaria and gonorrhoea). For example, *Streptococcus pneumoniae*, the most common cause of community-acquired pneumonia worldwide, is increasingly resistant to penicillin in many countries of the world (e.g. Spain and the USA). *Salmonella typhi*, the cause of typhoid fever, has been adept at escaping first-line antibiotic regimens over the past 30 years. Most strains are now resistant to chloramphenicol, the traditional therapy, and increasingly to other antibiotics, including the quinolones (e.g. ciprofloxacin). Multidrug-resistant strains have emerged. Fortunately, resistance to helminthic infections, which are a leading cause of chronic ill health in resource-poor countries, is yet to cause public health concern.

Microbes become resistant to antimicrobial agents as a result of Darwinian selection pressure applied by humans in the shape of antimicrobial therapy. In the community, resistance is fuelled by overuse of antimicrobial agents in human medical and veterinary practice. A good example of this is the prescribing of antibiotics for viral upper respiratory tract infections in children. In the 1980s, such practice resulted in a dramatic increase in the carriage of penicillin-resistant pneumococci in Icelandic children, following the introduction of a clonal strain. A subsequent decrease in the prescribing of antibiotics by Icelandic doctors resulted in reduced resistance. The

UK Department of Health has recently made various recommendations about antimicrobial resistance (see references). In particular, it advises no prescribing of antibiotics for simple coughs, colds or viral sore throats, limiting the prescribing of antibiotics for uncomplicated urinary tract infections in women to 3 days and limiting over-the-phone prescribing.

In hospitals, although the selection of resistance by antibiotic pressure is initially important (e.g. third-generation cephalosporins have been associated with the colonisation of patients by vancomycin-resistant enterococci), it is the spread of resistant organisms that appears to be at the crux of the problem. Standard infection control practice (i.e. hand washing and use of gloves for contact with bodily fluids) is likely to be the key effective infection control intervention. The presence of a hospital infection control team will not necessarily control hospital microbial resistance. It is how this team is resourced and how it deploys resources that is important. Likewise, a microbiological surveillance programme will be successful only if the information is used to guide appropriate infection control interventions. For example, there is increasing evidence that combining surveillance (i.e. the microbiological detection of MRSA colonisation) with isolation (including the use of gowns, gloves and masks) of colonised and infected patients can control the spread of resistant microbes. The problem with this approach in the UK is that few, if any, hospitals are resourced to employ such a strategy. The control of antibiotic prescribing (i.e. minimising inappropriate and broad-spectrum use by employing, for example, protocols, early intravenous to oral switch, infection pharmacists, alert antibiotic status and computer-based information systems), including the use of novel approaches such as rotating antibiotic protocols, used alone, is unlikely to control microbial resistance. A multi-strategy approach combining all of above interventions, however, might have a positive benefit.

A positive blood culture for *Staphylococcus aureus*, whether methicillin resistant or not, should trigger a careful reassessment of the patient's history and examination. In particular, it is important to consider skin sources (e.g. bed-sores and wound infection), intravenous line sites (especially if central), endocarditis and bone/joint sepsis. Other potential sources include the respiratory and urinary tracts, but infection at the other sites should be excluded first. In the UK, severe MRSA infections have 'traditionally' been treated with intravenous vancomycin or teicoplanin with, depending on the clinical circumstances, switch to oral combination therapy (e.g. rifampicin plus trimethroprim). Linezolid, the first oxazolidinone antibiotic, has recently been licensed in the UK for use against Gram-positive bacteria, including MRSA. It acts by interfering with bacterial protein synthesis at the RNA/ribosome level. Importantly, both intravenous and oral formulations are available, with the latter providing almost 100% bioavailability. Resistance has already been documented, however, and to avoid inappropriate use it is important to discuss the use of this valuable agent with an experienced microbiologist or infectious disease physician.

References

Barlow G D, Nathwani D, Davey P 2001 Appropriate antimicrobial prescribing. Report on a joint symposium between the Royal College of Physicians, Edinburgh and the Royal Pharmaceutical Society of Great Britain. Proceedings of the Royal College of Physicians, Edinburgh 31:310–316

Farr B M, Salgado C D, Karchmer T B, Sherertz R J 2001 Can antibiotic-resistant nosocomial infections be controlled? Lancet, Infectious Diseases 1:38–45

Standing Medical Advisory Committee Sub-Group on Antimicrobial Resistance 1998 The path of least resistance. Department of Health, London

WHO 2000 Overcoming antimicrobial resistance. World health report on infectious diseases 2000. Online. Available: www.who.int/infectious-disease-report/2000/index-rpt2000_text.html

57. Influenza

A. F   B. F   C. T   D. F   E. T

Influenza viruses have two surface glycoproteins, haemagglutinin and neuraminidase. Inhaled (zanamivir) and oral (oseltamivir) neuraminidase inhibitors have recently become available for the treatment of influenza infection. These agents have been shown to reduce the duration of illness by 1–3 days, the incidence of complications and the need to prescribe antibiotics. They are also effective prophylactic agents, for example to prevent household transmission or in nursing home outbreaks. Although neuraminidase inhibitors are undoubtedly an improvement over amantadine and rimantadine, which have activity against influenza A alone, the potential for the development of resistance means that these agents should be used cautiously. In the UK, the National Institute for Clinical Excellence (NICE) recommends that they should be prescribed only for at-risk adults when influenza is circulating in the community and if they are able to commence treatment within 48 h of the onset of symptoms. The role of neuraminidase inhibitors in patients admitted to hospital with severe illness is yet to be established. Patients with influenza pneumonia requiring admission to intensive care units are often found to have secondary bacteraemia with a respiratory pathogen, in particular with *Staphylococcus aureus*.

Influenza vaccine contains inactivated virus and is therefore not contraindicated in immunocompromised or pregnant patients. It should not be given, however, to those with egg hypersensitivity. Patients with significant chronic respiratory or heart disease, chronic renal failure, diabetes mellitus or immunosuppression due to disease or treatment, as well as those over 65 years of age and residents of residential or nursing homes and other long-term facilities should receive annual vaccination. Patients with chronic lung disease (as well as those with homozygous sickle-cell disease, asplenia or severe splenic dysfunction, immunosuppression (including HIV), significant chronic heart, renal or liver disease, coeliac disease and diabetes mellitus) should also receive pneumococcal vaccination.

Influenza is spread by aerosol, has a short incubation period of 1–4 days and is highly infectious. Although it is not always possible in the busy hospital setting, ideally, patients with suspected or confirmed influenza should be either isolated or cohort nursed with other infected patients.

Enzyme immunoassay of a nasopharyngeal aspirate sample is the rapid diagnostic method of choice in the acute hospital setting. Tracheal aspirates, blind protective specimen brush sampling or bronchoalveolar lavage samples may be used in ventilated patients.

References

Gubareva L V, Kaiser L, Hayden F G 2000 Influenza virus neuraminidase inhibitors. Lancet 355:827–835

Oliveira E C, Marik P E, Colice G 2001 Influenza pneumonia: a descriptive study. Chest 119:1717–1723

Salgado C D, Farr B M, Hall K K, Hayden F G 2002 Influenza in the acute hospital setting. Lancet Infectious Diseases 2:145–155

58.   Lyme disease

A. **F**   B. **F**   C. **T**   D. **T**   E. **T**

Lyme borreliosis (Lyme disease) is caused by the spirochaete *Borrelia burgdorferi*. *Borrelia recurrentis* and *Borrelia duttoni* cause louse-borne and tick-borne relapsing fevers, respectively. Lyme disease is transmitted by the bite of ticks of the *Ixodes* genus. In the USA the white-footed mouse is an important reservoir; a variety of small mammals and birds are important in Europe. Erythema migrans, which can be accompanied by systemic viral-like symptoms, is the characteristic cutaneous feature of early Lyme borreliosis and is seen in 90% of cases. Central clearing is often said to be a typical feature, but is not always present. Other cutaneous manifestations include borrelial lymphocytoma and acrodermatitis chronica atrophicans (long-standing discoloration of extensor surfaces). Non-cutaneous manifestations include carditis, neurological complications (lymphocytic meningitis, cranial nerve palsies, radiculoneuropathy and rarely encephalomyelitis) and rheumatological disease (arthralgia and chronic arthritis). The latter appears to be more common in the USA. Differences in the clinical presentations seen in Europe and the USA might be due to infection with genospecies of different virulence. In endemic areas, when the presentation includes erythema migrans, the diagnosis is clinical. Extracutaneous disease is usually diagnosed serologically in the presence of a suitable clinical history. To limit the number of false positives, a positive initial 'screening' ELISA or immunofixation test is followed by an immunoblot. Early erythema-migrans-associated Lyme disease in the absence of serious neurological or cardiac manifestations can be treated with oral antibiotics (amoxicillin or doxycycline) for 14–21 days. There is no evidence that antibiotic therapy hastens resolution of seventh cranial nerve palsy but an oral regimen should be prescribed to prevent further neurological complication. Lyme arthritis can be treated initially with oral antibiotics (as above for 28 days) or, if persistent, with intravenous ceftriaxone therapy for 14–28 days. Meningitis, radiculopathy or third degree heart block require parenteral therapy for 14–28 days. A Jarisch–Herxheimer-type reaction can occur in some patients after commencing antibiotics and is treated symptomatically.

References

Nadelman R B, Wormser G P 1998 Lyme borreliosis. Lancet 352:557–565

Wormser G P, Nadelman R B, Dattwyler R J et al 2000 Practice guidelines for the treatment of Lyme disease. Clinics in Infectious Diseases 31(suppl 1):S1–S14

59.   The systemic inflammatory response syndrome

A. **F**   B. **F**   C. **F**   D. **T**   E. **T**

The systemic inflammatory response syndrome is the early stage of an acute infectious process and is clinically defined as the presence of two or more of the following criteria:

- heart rate > 90/min
- respiratory rate > 20/min
- temperature < 36°C or > 38°C
- white cell count < 4×10^9/L or > 12×10^9/L.

Sepsis is present if a patient with the systemic inflammatory response syndrome has suspected or microbiologically proven infection. In some patients, with or without appropriate therapy, sepsis can progress to severe sepsis, which is defined as sepsis plus evidence of organ hypoperfusion (e.g. metabolic acidosis, oliguria or acute confusion) and/or hypotension (systolic BP < 90 mmHg). Subsequently, septic shock can develop and is defined as sepsis-associated hypotension despite adequate fluid resuscitation. In patients with suspected infection, the likelihood of a positive blood culture and death is low in patients without the systemic inflammatory response syndrome. Each extra criterion that is present increases the risk of death or a positive blood culture; the risk is higher still in those with severe sepsis and septic shock. These definitions can be used therefore to assess the severity of sepsis on admission and determine appropriate initial management. For example, a patient with symptoms and/or signs of infection but with no positive criteria is at low risk of death and, depending on the clinical circumstances, could be managed with oral antibiotics and discharged early from hospital, whereas a patient with all four criteria is at higher risk of death and will require more aggressive therapy.

   The systemic inflammatory response syndrome criteria should not be confused with the recently updated British Thoracic Society criteria for the severity assessment of patients with community-acquired pneumonia. These state that patients with two or more of the following parameters should be defined and managed as having severe community-acquired pneumonia:

- respiratory rate ≥ 30/min
- systolic BP < 90 mmHg or diastolic BP ≤ 60 mmHg
- the presence of new confusion (MSQ ≤ 8/10)
- urea > 7.0 mmol/L.

References

Jeljaszewicz J 1996 The epidemiology of the systemic inflammatory response syndrome. Current Opinion in Infectious Diseases 9:261–264

Members of the American College of Chest Physicians/Society of Critical Care Medicine Consensus Conference Committee 1992 Members of the American College of Chest Physicians/Society of Critical Care Medicine consensus conference: definitions of sepsis and organ failure and guidelines for the use of innovative therapies in sepsis. Critical Care Medicine 20:864–874

60. Microbes, cancer and chronic diseases

A. **F**   B. **F**   C. **F**   D. **T**   E. **F**

Table 60.1 provides examples of cancers or chronic diseases that have been associated with or shown to have a microbial aetiology. Human herpesvirus 8 has been associated with Kaposi's sarcoma, whereas human herpesvirus 6 has recently been shown to be the third most common cause of heterophile-negative infectious mononucleosis (it also causes roseola infantum in children) after cytomegalovirus and Epstein–Barr virus, which is the most common cause. The last has also been associated with nasopharyngeal carcinoma, which is common in the Canton Chinese population, and Burkitt's lymphoma, which most commonly occurs in young boys of the African tropical belt region. Chronic infection with hepatitis B and/or C virus is associated with the development of hepatocellular carcinoma, a major public health concern in many endemic and resource-poor countries. Hepatitis E virus infection causes acute hepatitis and is epidemiologically and clinically similar to hepatitis A. One difference is that infection in pregnancy is associated with a high mortality due to acute liver failure. Finally, an organism not mentioned in the table, but under much scrutiny at present, is *Chlamydia pneumoniae*. This has been associated with atherosclerosis using a variety of laboratory techniques (e.g. serology, culture and polymerase chain reaction). However, the exact role of this bacterium in the pathogenesis of vascular disease, and the implications for treatment (if any) are yet to be determined.

A number of treatment options are available for Kaposi's sarcoma. Classic Kaposi's sarcoma in immunocompetent patients usually responds well to local therapies (e.g. cryotherapy, radiation, lasers or intralesional/topical chemotherapy), although recurrence can occur. Endemic African Kaposi's sarcoma generally responds to systemic therapy (alpha interferon or cytotoxic chemotherapy), if such

Table 60.1   Chronic diseases and cancers associated with specific microbes

Disease	Microbe
Peptic ulcer disease, gastritis and gastric carcinoma	*Helicobacter pylori*
Cervical, vulval and anal carcinoma	Human papillomavirus 16 and 18
Hepatocellular carcinoma	Hepatitis B and C viruses
Kaposi's sarcoma	Human herpesvirus 8 (HHV8)
Burkitt's lymphoma, nasopharyngeal carcinoma	Epstein–Barr virus (EBV)
Whipple's disease	*Tropheryma whippelii*
Adult T cell leukaemia, tropical spastic paraparesis	Human T cell lymphotropic virus type 1 (HTLV-1)
Creutzfeldt–Jakob disease	Prion protein*

* Considered to be a 'transmissible agent'

treatments are available. Iatrogenic Kaposi's sarcoma due to immunosuppressive therapy usually regresses following a reduction or cessation of treatment. Treatment of AIDS-associated Kaposi's sarcoma is palliative and does not appear to affect survival. Patients can respond to commencement or intensification of highly active antiretroviral therapy. If the patient does not respond to antiretroviral therapy and has early Kaposi's sarcoma with a CD4 count greater than 200/mm^3, alpha interferon therapy is recommended. If the CD4 count is < 200/mm^3 or there is advanced Kaposi's sarcoma, pegylated liposomal doxorubicin is the treatment of choice. Other treatment options, of varying efficacy, include antiherpesvirus therapy with foscarnet or cidofovir, other cytotoxic agents, thalidomide and angiogenesis inhibitors.

References

British Medical Association, Royal Pharmaceutical Society of Great Britain 2001 *Helicobacter pylori* infection. British National Formulary, September 42:37

Cassell G H 1998 Infectious causes of chronic inflammatory diseases and cancer. Emerging Infectious Diseases 4:475–487

Lorber B 1996 Are all diseases infectious? Annals of Internal Medicine 125:844–851

61. Severe sepsis and protein C

A. **T**   B. **F**   C. **F**   D. **T**   E. **T**

The systemic inflammatory response syndrome is the human body's response to infection. It can occur in response to a variety of microbes but is most commonly as a result of either Gram-positive (e.g. *Streptococcus pneumoniae, Staphylococcus aureus* and *Streptococcus pyogenes*) or Gram-negative (e.g. *Eschericia coli, Pseudomonas aeruginosa* and *Neisseria meningitidis*) bacteria. Sepsis is usually triggered by components of the bacterial cell wall. In Gram-positive bacteria this is usually peptidoglycan and lipoteichoic acid, whereas in Gram-negative bacteria, lipopolysaccharide (an endotoxin) is the culprit. Additionally, some Gram-positive bacteria produce exotoxins capable of producing severe sepsis-like conditions (e.g. staphylococcal and streptococcal toxic shock syndromes). These molecules trigger release of cytokines and cause activation of neutrophils (which adhere to vascular endothelium, thereby resulting in inflammation and vascular damage), the complement system and both the intrinsic and extrinsic coagulation pathways. Ultimately this can result in the characteristic features of severe sepsis with vasodilatation, diffuse endovascular injury, microvascular thrombosis, subsequent tissue ischaemia and, if progressive, multiorgan failure and death. This response also explains the Jarisch–Herxheimer reaction, which classically occurs in some spirochaete infections (e.g. *Borrelia recurrentis, Treponema pallidum* and *Borrelia burgdorferi*), as a result of the release of cell wall components following commencement of antibacterial therapy.

Biochemically, sepsis is characterised by the release of proinflammatory cytokines, for example, TNF-α, interleukin-1, interleukin-6 and chemokines from monocytes and macrophages. The therapeutic reduction of such cytokines by the use of, for example, monoclonal antibodies has been attempted but is yet to be proven useful in acute infections. Down-regulatory molecules (anti-inflammatory cytokines) such as interleukin-10 and transforming growth factor-β are also secreted. The subsequent release of tissue factor from monocytes and vascular endothelium triggers the production of thrombin and the formation of fibrin clots. Both the proinflammatory cytokines and thrombin impair endogenous fibrinolytic activity by inhibiting tissue plasminogen activator through the release of plasminogen activator inhibitor-1 from platelets and vascular endothelium and activation of thrombin-activatable fibrinolysis inhibitor. Additionally, thrombin has considerable proinflammatory activity.

Protein C exerts antithrombotic effects by inactivating factors Va and VIIIa and thereby limiting the production of thrombin. It facilitates fibrinolysis by inactivating plasminogen activator inhibitor-1 and preventing the activation of thrombin-activatable fibrinolysis inhibitor. It also produces anti-inflammatory actions by inhibiting the production of proinflammatory cytokines and thrombin and limiting the rolling action of monocytes and neutrophils on vascular endothelium. In severe sepsis, however, protein C activation is inhibited by the inflammatory response in the majority (80%) of patients. In a recent multicentred, cluster randomised controlled trial, administration of a 96-h infusion of a recombinant form of activated protein C was shown to reduce D-dimer and interleukin-6 levels and improve survival in patients with severe sepsis. Unsurprisingly, the main adverse event was serious bleeding, although this was not significantly different ($P = 0.06$) from that in the placebo group.

References

Bernard G R, Vincent J-L, Laterre P-F et al 2001 Efficacy and safety of recombinant human activated protein C for severe sepsis. New England Journal of Medicine 344:699–709

Friedland J 1998 Cytokines in infectious diseases. Journal of the Royal College of Physicians, London 32:195–198

62. Viral infections in pregnancy

A. **F**   B. **T**   C. **F**   D. **T**   E. **T**

Viral infections in pregnancy that can have important fetal consequences include rubella, cytomegalovirus (CMV), parvovirus B19, varicella zoster virus (VZV) and measles. Acute infections with rubella, parvovirus B19, cytomegalovirus (rarely) and measles can all present with a non-specific rash. Clinically significant chickenpox usually presents with the typical vesicular rash and is therefore readily identifiable. Acute HIV infection can also present with a non-specific rash and has obvious implications for both mother and fetus. Pregnant women with non-vesicular rashes should be investigated at least for rubella (IgM and IgG) and parvovirus B19 (IgM) and other causes of rash, depending on the clinical history and initial investigations.

There is a high risk of adverse fetal outcome (90%) if rubella infection occurs in the first 11 weeks of pregnancy. This decreases to 20% (mainly deafness) at weeks 11–16 and to a minimal risk of deafness after week 16. There is no risk of adverse fetal outcome after week 20. There is no specific intervention but further obstetric investigation and termination of pregnancy should be discussed if infection occurs early in pregnancy. It should be remembered, however, that the vaccination programme means that only a small percentage of adult females in the UK are susceptible.

Infection with parvovirus B19 in the first 20 weeks of pregnancy can lead to intrauterine death (excess risk 9%) or hydrops fetalis (3%). Intrauterine blood transfusions can reduce the risk of death in the latter. Approximately half the adult female population is susceptible.

The risk of congenital varicella syndrome is 1% if infection occurs in the first 12 weeks of pregnancy and 2% between weeks 13 and 20. If congenital infection does occur, abnormalities can include reddened zoster-like scars, growth retardation, limb deformity with hypoplasia, microcephaly and cataracts. There is a 20% risk of potentially life-threatening neonatal chickenpox if infection occurs in the 4 days before or the 2 days after delivery. Pregnant women who develop chickenpox and present within 24 h of the onset of rash should be prescribed oral aciclovir (there is no evidence of adverse events in pregnancy). Patients with pneumonitis or complicated infection require admission to hospital for intravenous aciclovir and close observation. One in ten adult females is susceptible to VZV infection.

CMV infection is usually asymptomatic and therefore rarely presents in pregnancy. There is no specific intervention. Measles can cause intrauterine death and preterm delivery (as can all acute systemic infections) but there is no associated congenital syndrome. Infection in pregnancy rarely occurs in developed countries.

Hand, foot and mouth disease is usually caused by Coxsackie A viruses and is not associated with fetal complications. Infectious mononucleosis is usually caused by Epstein–Barr virus, which has no adverse fetal effects. It should be remembered, however, that CMV, toxoplasmosis and HIV occasionally cause glandular fever-like illness.

Pregnant women exposed (15 min in the same room or face-to-face contact) to a non-specific non-vesicular rash illness should be assessed for rubella immunity status (patient is immune if she has received two previous doses of vaccine or two documented positive antibody screening tests or one previous dose of vaccine followed by a positive antibody screening test). If susceptibility is possible, rubella-specific IgM (primary or reinfection) and IgG (recent or past infection or immunisation) tests should be performed. If IgG is unequivocally positive and IgM negative, the patient is immune. If neither is positive, the patient is susceptible and repeat testing at a later stage should be performed to assess the possibility of seroconversion. If both are positive the case should be discussed with a virologist, who might order further specialised tests. Patients should also be investigated for their parvovirus B19 immunity status (IgM and IgG). Pregnant women exposed to chickenpox or shingles should undergo urgent VZV IgG testing if there is no clear history of previous chickenpox. VZV IgG negative patients should then be offered VZV-specific immunoglobulin within 10 days of the exposure. This attenuates the infection and is likely to reduce the increased risk of severe chickenpox in pregnant women.

References

Morgan-Capner P, Crowcroft N S, on behalf of the PHLS Joint Working Party of the Advisory Committees of Virology and Vaccines and Immunisation 2002 Guidelines on the management of, and exposure to, rash illness in pregnancy (including consideration of relevant antibody screening programmes in pregnancy). Communicable Disease and Public Health 5:59–71

Nathwani D, Maclean A, Conway S, Carrington D 1998 Varicella infection in pregnancy and the newborn. Journal of Infection 36:59–71

Yeung S, Davies E Gm 2001 Infection in the fetus and neonate. Medicine 29:78–83

Best-of-5 answers

63. Infection in the homeless and intravenous drug users

Answer: **D**

Table 63.1 highlights some of the specific infections that have been associated with homelessness and intravenous drug use. *Coxiella burnetii* (Q-fever) and *Borrelia burgdorferi* (Lyme disease) are both infections of rural or semirural areas and are associated with exposure to sheep or cattle (Q-fever) and tick-bites (Lyme disease). Neither is likely, therefore, to be associated with homelessness, which is mainly a problem of urban areas. The high prevalence of heavy tobacco use, alcohol abuse and intravenous drug use, all of which predispose to weakened immunity and specific infections, is higher in homeless persons. Additionally, other important factors predisposing to infection include poor nutrition, lack of access to personal hygiene, clean clothes and dentistry, physical trauma and burns, exposure to cold temperatures and close proximity of living on the streets and in shelters. Measures that could be employed to reduce infections in the homeless and drug users include vaccination (e.g. hepatitis A and B, diphtheria (homeless only), tetanus, influenza, pneumococcal and BCG), assessment and investigation for pulmonary tuberculosis, needle exchange programmes for drug users, availability of foot care in shelters/homes, weekly boil washing of clothes to kill and prevent body lice, ivermectin (200 mg/kg) for scabies and access to free condoms and sexual health advice.

Clostridium novyi is a Gram-positive anaerobic toxin-producing bacillus that has recently been linked with an outbreak of severe and often fatal infection in Glasgow drug users. Most patients presented with pain, severe inflammation and oedema (sometimes necrosis) at the injection site associated with high white cell counts and severe sepsis or septic shock. All patients had been 'popping', which is the injection of heroin into subcutaneous skin or muscle tissue. Drug users presenting in this way should be treated aggressively with high-dependency/intensive-care support and intravenous antibiotics. A combination regimen of high-dose benzylpenicillin and clindamycin should provide the necessary anaerobic activity but will also cover other organisms such as *Staphylococcus aureus* and *Streptococcus pyogenes*. As with necrotising fasciitis, extensive tissue debridement might be necessary and early discussion with a surgeon is therefore vital.

Although anthrax has been documented in drug users, the history of pain would be against this. Additionally, *Bacillus anthracis* is an aerobic organism and is therefore less likely to occur at the site of 'popping', which creates an anaerobic environment. All the other suggested organisms are not particularly associated with intravenous drug use.

Table 63.1 **Infections associated with homelessness and intravenous drug use (IDU)**

	Infection	Risk factor
Homeless	*Respiratory tract:* common organisms that cause respiratory tract infections, tuberculosis and *Pneumocystis carinii* (HIV positive only)	Smoking, alcoholism, IDU and close proximity of living
	Bloodborne: HIV and hepatitis B/C	IDU with sharing of equipment
	Skin: In particular infections of the feet such as *Tinea pedis* and cellulitis, which can eventually lead to ulcers, osteomyelitis and gangrene. Cutaneous (mainly) and classic diphtheria are also recognised in this group	Poor/dirty footwear, inadequate foot-care, exposure to cold and moisture, minor trauma, venous stasis (sitting/standing), peripheral neuropathy (alcohol), peripheral vascular disease (smoking)
	Infestations and related infections: human body lice (*Pediculosis humanus*) and head lice (*Pediculosis capitis*) and scabies (*Sarcoptes scabiei*). The human body louse transmits *Bartonella quintana* (urban trench fever), which can present as a recurrent febrile illness with headache and leg pains and/or endocarditis	Poor hygiene and close proximity of living
IDU	As above, depending on whether homeless or not, but specifically including:	
	Bloodborne: right-sided endocarditis and pulmonary abscesses (usually *Staphylococcus aureus* but occasionally other bacteria or fungi)	IDU, poor injection practices and infection at the site

References

Raoult D, Foucault C, Brouqui P 2001 Infections in the homeless. Lancet, Infectious Diseases 1:77–84

Scottish Centre for Infection and Environmental Health. Information available online: www.show.scot.nhs.uk/scieh

64. Anthrax

Answer: **D**

The Gram-positive aerobic spore-forming bacterium, *Bacillus anthracis*, causes anthrax. It is one of the few clinically important Gram-positive bacilli (others worth remembering are *Listeria monocytogenes*, *Clostridia* species, *Corynebacterium diptheriae*, *Actinomyces israelii* and *Nocardia asteroides*). In its natural state, anthrax is usually a disease of wild or farm animals with humans acquiring infection, most commonly cutaneous, from spore-contaminated animal products (e.g. hides and wool). Inhalational anthrax (wool-sorters' disease) is rare and used to occur due to aerosolised spores in hide or wool processing factories. Epidemics are still occasionally seen in developing countries.

Cutaneous anthrax is characterised by the initial appearance of a painless itchy papule progressing to a vesicle (with or without satellite vesicles) surrounded by non-pitting oedema (which may be massive). The lesion subsequently ulcerates and forms the typical black eschar. Without antibiotic treatment mortality can be as high as 20%. Surgical intervention should be avoided, however, as this can promote bacteraemia.

The differential diagnosis includes acute skin infections (often painful) due to *Staphylococcus aureus* or *Streptococcus pyogenes*, orf (usually sheep farmers/handlers), *Mycobacterium marinum* infection in tropical fish keepers, insect bites and ecthyma gangrenosum due to *Pseudomonas aeruginosa* bacteraemia in neutropenic patients.

Inhalational anthrax is characterised by an initial influenza-like illness for 2–3 days followed by sudden deterioration with dyspnoea (some patients have stridor due to lymphadenopathy and oedema of the chest wall and neck) and signs of severe sepsis progressing to septic shock. Symptoms or signs of meningitis appear to be relatively common. A widened mediastinum on the chest radiograph of a patient with this scenario should arouse suspicion of the diagnosis.

Diagnosis should be based on the Gram-stain and culture of skin (vesicle fluid or eschar), blood or cerebrospinal fluid. Serological tests are available but are only of use retrospectively.

The initial antimicrobial treatment of a suspected case of anthrax is detailed in Table 64.1. As with all antibiotic regimens, therapy should be tailored according to the results of subsequent microbiological investigation. Because of the significant risk of late germination of anthrax spores, if a patient has had aerosol exposure, both treatment and prophylactic regimens should be continued for 60 days. Although penicillin is the traditional drug of choice, resistant strains of anthrax have been developed for bioterrorism. An effective vaccine is available but is in limited supply and will only be available to aerosol-exposed persons on public health department advice.

References

Swartz M N 2001 Recognition and management of anthrax – an update. New England Journal of Medicine 345: 1621–1626

Public Health Laboratory Service. Information available online: www.phls.co.uk

Table 64.1   Initial antimicrobial therapy for suspected cases of anthrax

Nature of Illness	Treatment
Cutaneous	*Mild*: oral ciprofloxacin 500 mg twice daily *Severe*: as for inhalational anthrax
Inhalational, meningitic or gastrointestinal	Intravenous ciprofloxacin 400 mg twice daily
Post-exposure prophylaxis	Oral ciprofloxacin 500 mg twice daily *or* Oral doxycycline 100 mg twice daily

65.   Arboviruses

Answer: **B**

Yellow fever virus is a zoonotic flavivirus that affects monkeys. It is transmitted to humans by the bite of *Aedes* (Africa) and *Haemagogus* (Central and South America) species of mosquito. Most of these mosquitoes prefer to breed in tree-holes and people can be exposed during occupational or recreational activities in forests (jungle yellow fever) or if their villages lie close to jungle areas. *Aedes aegypti*, an urban mosquito often implicated in the transmission of dengue fever, is also capable of transmitting yellow fever. Person-to-person transmission (urban yellow fever) can occur if an infected person returns to an urban area.

The severity of infection can range from asymptomatic or a mild febrile illness to fatal haemorrhagic fever. Typically it is characterised by an initial severe influenza-like illness 3–6 days after an infected mosquito bite. Following a short period of remission, recrudescence then occurs in about 15–25% of cases with fever, vomiting, epigastric pain, jaundice, renal failure and haemorrhage. Treatment is supportive. Diagnosis is by detection of virus or viral antigen by polymerase chain reaction or ELISA, respectively, or by serology. Yellow fever is endemic in much of sub-Saharan Africa and Central and South America, but not in Asia. A live vaccine is available and is considered mandatory for travel to most endemic countries.

Dengue fever, dengue haemorrhagic fever and dengue shock syndrome are caused by a flavivirus (dengue virus serotypes 1 to 4) that is endemic in much of the tropical and subtropical belt of the Americas, Africa and Asia. It is an infection of urban living with transmission to humans occurring via the bite of *Aedes* mosquitoes. Most cases of dengue, however, are asymptomatic or mild and usually occur in children. Older children and adults can develop classical dengue with influenza-like symptoms, arthralgia, retro-orbital pain and a maculopapular rash. Dengue haemorrhagic fever and shock syndromes are characterised by severe plasma leakage and haematological upset; thrombocytopenia and, in particular, a haematocrit increase of 20% are the key haematological features. These syndromes occur in 2–4% of children or adults suffering a second dengue infection. The pathophysiological response is not fully understood but is thought to be due to a complex interaction of viral and host factors. Treatment is supportive, with patients often responding to aggressive intravenous fluid management. A tetravalent vaccine is currently being investigated but is not available to travellers or, more importantly, as a control measure in endemic countries.

West Nile virus is a flavivirus of the same serocomplex as Japanese encephalitis virus. It is a zoonosis of birds and is transmitted to humans (dead-end hosts) via the bite of *Culex* mosquitoes. It hit the headlines in 1999 because of an outbreak of West Nile encephalitis in New York. This was the first time the virus had been identified in the Western hemisphere; it is usually enzootic in Southern and Eastern Europe, Africa and Asia. It is likely that it was transported to the USA by migrant birds. Clinically, infection is often mild, but life-threatening encephalitis (not hepatitis) can develop. In the New York outbreak, 7% of hospitalised patients died. Death appeared to be significantly associated with diabetes mellitus and advanced age (over 75 years). Advanced age was also significantly associated with developing severe neurological disease. Treatment is supportive and a vaccine is not currently available.

Other than malaria chemoprophylaxis, travellers can reduce the risk of mosquito-borne infections by wearing appropriate clothing (tightly woven light-coloured long-sleeved shirts, trousers and socks), regular use of mosquito repellents (e.g. diethyltoluamide and/or essential oils such as eucalyptus) and sleeping under insecticide-impregnated bednets.

References

Guzmán M G, Goustavo K 2001 Dengue: an update. Lancet Infectious Diseases 2:33–42

Lanciotti R S, Roehrig J T, Deubal V et al 1999 West Nile virus confirmed as cause of an encephalitis outbreak in the New York region. Science 286:2333–2337

Monath T P 2001 Yellow fever: an update. Lancet Infectious Diseases 1:11–20

66.   Meningococcal disease

Answer: **C**

The history and signs in the clinical scenario are highly suggestive of meningococcal disease. Given that the diagnosis is not in doubt and that the patient has a significantly depressed conscious level, a lumbar puncture should not be performed. Other contraindications to lumbar puncture include other signs of raised intracranial pressure and/or focal neurological signs (if a lumbar puncture is considered clinically essential in such patients, a CT scan of the brain should be performed first), shock and coagulopathy. Although the first four of the investigations listed in the question should all be performed, the one most likely to provide early microbiological confirmation is a blood culture (positive in 50% of invasive meningococcal disease cases). Theoretically, meningococcal PCR of an admission blood sample could provide rapid evidence. In practice in the UK, however, this test is currently performed in few laboratories and the result, therefore, could take several days to get back to the clinician. Additionally, false positives have been reported. Acute and convalescent meningococcal serology is available but is a retrospective diagnostic tool. Because a proportion of the healthy population (approximately 30%) carry meningococci as commensal organisms, a positive throat swab provides only circumstantial evidence but will be positive in about 50% of patients with meningococcal disease. A Gram-stain of skin tissue fluid aspirated from a purpuric lesion has been used successfully as a rapid diagnostic tool in some centres (about two-thirds are positive in meningococcal sepsis). Urinary meningococcal antigen is currently a research tool.

Guidance on the prevention of meningococcal disease in healthcare staff has recently been published. These guidelines state that:

> Chemoprophylaxis is recommended only for those healthcare workers whose mouth or nose is directly exposed to infectious respiratory droplets/secretions within a distance of 3 feet from a probable or confirmed case of meningococcal disease. This type of exposure is most likely to occur in staff who undertake airway management during resuscitation without wearing a mask or other mechanical protection. In most cases this would imply a clear perception of physical contact with droplet/secretions. Droplets and facial secretions are considered to be infectious from the onset of acute illness until completion of 24 hours treatment with systemic antibiotics. Oral antibiotics such as rifampicin 600 mg twice daily for 2 days or ciprofloxacin 500 mg as a single dose are recommended for prophylaxis.

The guidelines also encourage the wearing of masks by healthcare workers performing procedures prone to respiratory droplet/secretion exposure on patients with suspected meningococcal disease.

References

Begg N, Cartwright K A V, Cohen J et al 1999 Consensus statement on diagnosis, investigation, treatment and prevention of acute bacterial meningitis in immunocompetent adults. Journal of Infection 39:1–15

Stuart J M, Gilmore A B, Ross A et al 2001 Preventing secondary meningococcal disease in health care workers: recommendations of a working group of the PHLS Meningococcus Forum. Communicable Disease and Public Health 4:102–105

GASTROENTEROLOGY
True/False answers

67. *Helicobacter pylori*

A. **T**   B. **F**   C. **T**   D. **F**   E. **F**

Helicobacter pylori is a spiral bacterium found in the stomach. It was first recognised in 1975 but not cultured until 1982. It infects only gastric-type mucosa and thus can also cause infection in the oesophagus and duodenum in the presence of gastric metaplasia. Infection is associated with a number of conditions including gastritis, peptic ulcer disease, gastric cancer and low-grade B cell lymphoma of the mucosa-associated lymphoid tissue (MALToma). The mode of acquisition of *H. pylori* is not currently known but might result from water-borne infection or from oral-oral transmission. Acquisition in adulthood is low (< 1% per annum).

A number of tests are available for the diagnosis of *H. pylori* infection, including breath tests, serum antibody measurement and tests involving gastric biopsies (urease tests, culture and histology). Serological tests can remain positive for some time after eradication, limiting their usefulness. The urease test and the urea breath test rely on urease production by the bacterium. In the case of the urease test, conversion of urea to ammonia and carbon dioxide by *H. pylori* in a biopsy specimen leads to a pH and colour change. In the urea breath test, radiolabelled urea is broken down, leading to the liberation of radiolabelled carbon dioxide, which can be detected in breath samples.

Current treatment regimens involve acid suppression (usually with a proton pump inhibitor) and combinations of antibiotics (usually amoxicillin, metronidazole or clarithromycin). Resistance develops rapidly with single antibiotic regimens so two antibiotics are usually used. Successful eradication can be confirmed by the non-invasive urea breath test and reduces recurrence of ulceration. The majority of MALTomas occur in combination with *H. pylori* infection. Regression of early disease has been described following eradication. The role of *H. pylori* eradication in non-ulcer dyspepsia currently remains unproven.

The outcome of *H. pylori* infection depends on a number of factors. Duodenal ulceration is more common in men and smokers. Patients with duodenal ulcer usually develop antral gastritis. Antral gastritis tends to cause hypergastrinaemia (stimulating acid secretion) and reduces somatostatin production (impairing inhibition of acid secretion) leading to enhanced gastric acid production, duodenal gastric metaplasia and, ultimately, ulceration. Patients with gastric ulcer or cancer tend to have severe pangastritis with atrophy. Atrophy of the corpus mucosa leads to a reduction in the parietal cell mass and hypochlorhydria. Genetic polymorphisms in the interleukin-1β gene might play a role in determining the outcome of infection. Interleukin-1β is a potent inhibitor of gastric acid secretion and polymorphisms leading to enhanced interleukin-1β production are associated with an increased risk of gastric atrophy and cancer. The mechanism of this effect is not certain but acid suppression by interleukin-1β could allow more extensive gastric colonisation with associated atrophy.

References

El-Omar E M 2001 The importance of interleukin 1 beta in *Helicobacter pylori* associated disease. Gut 48:743–747

Goodwin C S, Mendall M M, Northfield T C 2002 *Helicobacter pylori* infection. Lancet 349:265–269

68. Pancreatic cancer

A. **F**   B. **F**   C. **T**   D. **F**   E. **T**

Pancreatic cancer is the fifth most common cause of cancer death in the Western world. It has a very poor prognosis, largely as a result of the high rate of advanced disease at presentation (incurable in > 80% at diagnosis). As chemotherapy and radiotherapy are ineffective, surgery is the only treatment with significant survival benefit.

Risk factors for pancreatic cancer include smoking, diabetes mellitus and family history. Whereas 25% of cases are estimated to be due to smoking, 5–10% are thought to be related to a genetic predisposition. Pancreatic cancer is associated with germline mutations in *BRCA2* (also increased risk of male and female breast cancer), familial atypical multiple mole melanoma syndrome (multiple atypical naevi, familial clustering of cutaneous malignant melanoma and increased risk of extracutaneous cancers such as pancreatic and breast cancers), hereditary pancreatitis, hereditary non-polyposis colorectal cancer and Peutz–Jeghers syndrome. Hereditary pancreatitis is an autosomal dominant condition in which a mutation in the cationic trypsinogen gene leads to autoactivation of trypsinogen within the pancreas leading to recurrent abdominal pain and pancreatitis from childhood. Also patients have a dramatically increased risk of pancreatic cancer, particularly in smokers (150-fold increase in smokers, 40-fold in non-smokers). As a result, 40% of patients will have developed pancreatic cancer by age 70. In Peutz–Jeghers syndrome, patients have multiple hamartomatous polyps of the gastrointestinal tract, pigmented lesions in the lips, oral mucosa and digits. The risk of any cancer is approximately 50%, particularly gastrointestinal, gynaecological, breast and pancreatic.

The identification of high-risk groups raises the possibility of screening for pancreatic cancer. Unfortunately, none of the currently available screening modalities has a high-enough sensitivity and specificity and some (particularly ERCP) are invasive with high risks. Examples include detection of K-ras mutations, CA 19-9, endoscopic ultrasound, spiral CT, magnetic resonance cholangiopancreatography and positron emission tomography.

Reference

Efthimiou E, Crnogorac-Jurcevic T, Lemoine N R, Brentnall T A 2001 Inherited predisposition to pancreatic cancer. Gut 48:143–147

69.   Microsatellite instability in colorectal cancer

A. T   B. F   C. F   D. T   E. T

Hereditary non-polyposis colorectal cancer is an autosomal dominant condition with a penetrance of between 80 and 85%. It makes up 5–10% of colorectal cancers in the Western world. In addition to colorectal cancers (70% of which are proximal to the splenic flexure) patients also have an increased risk of certain extracolonic carcinomas (endometrial, ovarian, gastric, pancreatic, small bowel, hepatobiliary, ureteric and renal pelvis). Compared with women, men with hereditary non-polyposis colorectal cancer more commonly develop cancer (91% versus 69%) and colorectal cancer (74% versus 30%). In women with hereditary non-polyposis colorectal cancer, endometrial cancer is more common than colorectal cancer (42% versus 30%). In the Muir–Torre syndrome, features of hereditary non-polyposis colorectal cancer are accompanied by sebaceous adenomas and carcinomas and keratoacanthomas.

Patients frequently have germline mutations in mismatch repair genes: six have been identified thus far (*hMSH2, hMSH6, hMLH1, hPMS1, hPMS2* and *hMLH3*); 70% of cases have mutations in either *hMSH2* or *hMLH1*. A second somatic mutation in a mismatch repair gene results in what is known as microsatellite instability. Microsatellites are repetitive sequences of one to five base pairs, which are prone to errors in replication. These are normally repaired by mismatch repair genes but, in the absence of an effective repair system, errors occur resulting in multiple copies of differing length – microsatellite instability. Instability is found in 90% of hereditary non-polyposis colorectal cancer but only 10–15% of sporadic colorectal cancers. Whereas in hereditary non-polyposis colorectal cancer, microsatellite instability is caused by a combination of a germline mutation in one copy of a mismatch repair gene and a somatic mutation in the other, in sporadic colorectal cancers mutations in mismatch repair genes are rarely found. Microsatellite instability probably results from hypermethylation of the promoter region of *hMLH1*, with resultant lack of hMLH1 protein.

References

Cole T R P, Sleightholme H V 2000 ABC of colorectal cancer. The role of clinical genetics in management. British Medical Journal 321:943–946

Goel A, Arnold C N, Boland C R 2001 Multistep progression of colorectal cancer in the setting of microsatellite instability: new details and novel insights. Gastroenterology 1497–1502

Wheeler J M D, Mortensen N J McC 2000 DNA mismatch repair genes and colorectal cancer. Gut 47:148–153

70. Non-alcoholic steatohepatitis

A. **F**   B. **F**   C. **F**   D. **T**   E. **T**

Non-alcoholic steatohepatitis is the term used to describe patients with liver biopsy histological changes indistinguishable from alcoholic hepatitis but in the absence of a history of alcohol abuse. It is part of the spectrum of non-alcoholic fatty liver disease that extends from simple steatosis through steatohepatitis to cirrhosis. Non-alcoholic steatohepatitis is not as uncommon as was previously thought and might not have a completely benign prognosis.

Although the prevalence of non-alcoholic steatohepatitis in the general population is not known, in high-risk groups (such as severely obese patients) the prevalence could be as high as 25%. The natural history of non-alcoholic steatohepatitis is also unclear at present, although in one study cirrhosis was found on index biopsy or progression to cirrhosis had occurred over a median of 8 years of follow-up in 3.4% of patients with simple steatosis and 25% of patients with non-alcoholic steatohepatitis.

Epidemiological factors associated with non-alcoholic steatohepatitis include obesity (particularly increased waist:hip ratio), hyperlipidaemia (particularly hypertriglyceridaemia) and type II diabetes mellitus. The pathogenic mechanism of development of non-alcoholic steatohepatitis is not clear although it is thought to involve two 'hits'. The first is thought to be steatosis, which sensitises the liver to a second 'hit' that causes inflammation, necrosis and fibrosis. Insulin resistance seems to be involved in the development of steatosis and is found even in the absence of diabetes mellitus or impaired glucose tolerance. Studies in the *ob/ob* leptin-deficient mouse show an improvement in steatosis with metformin, a drug known to improve insulin sensitivity. The second 'hit' is likely to involve oxidative stress and could involve bacterial overgrowth, found in 50% of non-alcoholic steatohepatitis patients compared with 22% of controls.

The majority of patients with non-alcoholic steatohepatitis are asymptomatic and hepatomegaly is the only common clinical finding. Serum transaminases are elevated to two to fours times normal and aspartate transaminase is usually lower than alanine transaminase. Slight elevations in alkaline phosphatase are found frequently, serum ferritin is elevated in more than half of patients and transferrin saturation is elevated in approximately one in six patients. Ultrasonography often reveals a hyperechoic liver. Ultimately, the diagnosis is a histological one and biopsies will show macrovesicular steatosis and necrotic and inflammatory changes.

The rate of progression of non-alcoholic steatohepatitis to cirrhosis is not clear but patients with cryptogenic cirrhosis have a similar rate of obesity and diabetes mellitus as patients with non-alcoholic steatohepatitis, whereas rates are lower in patients with primary biliary cirrhosis and hepatitis C. However, these patients do not have histological evidence of non-alcoholic steatohepatitis. It remains to be seen what proportion, if any, of cases of cryptogenic cirrhosis are related to non-alcoholic steatohepatitis. Several factors help to predict the presence of non-alcoholic steatohepatitis and cirrhosis, including age > 50 years, obesity, ALT more than twice normal, serum triglycerides > 1.7 mmol/L, hypertension, AST > ALT and increased waist:hip ratio. Several treatments have been shown to lead to improvements in liver biochemistry, such as weight loss, ursodeoxycholic acid and vitamin E. Unfortunately, large controlled studies with serial biopsies are lacking. At present it seems reasonable to treat non-alcoholic steatohepatitis with moderate, sustained weight loss and treatment of diabetes mellitus and hyperlipidaemia.

References

Day C P 2002 Non-alcoholic steatohepatitis (NASH): where are we now and where are we going? Gut 50:585–588

Reid A E 2001 Nonalcoholic steatohepatitis. Gastroenterology 121:710–723

71. Genetics in inflammatory bowel disease

A. **T**   B. **F**   C. **F**   D. **T**   E. **T**

In recent years, the understanding of genetic involvement in inflammatory bowel disease (IBD) has been advanced dramatically. Concordance rates in twin studies for Crohn's disease are 35% for monozygotic and 7% for dizygotic twins, compared with 11% and 3%, respectively, for ulcerative colitis. Indeed, siblings of patients with Crohn's disease have a 20- to 35-fold increased risk for developing Crohn's disease.

Susceptibility loci for IBD have been identified on chromosomes 1, 5, 6 (*IBD 3*), 12 (*IBD 2*: more strongly associated with ulcerative colitis), 14, 16 (*IBD 1*) and 19. A susceptibility gene, *NOD2*, within the IBD1 locus on chromosome 16 has recently been discovered to be specific for Crohn's disease. *NOD2* is found on chromosome 16q12 and encodes for a protein containing two copies of the caspase recruitment domain (a domain involved in apoptosis), a nucleotide binding region and a region of ten leucine-rich repeats (a feature of proteins involved in the molecular recognition of bacterial products). Intracellular binding of NOD2 to bacterial endotoxins results in activation of nuclear factor-κB (NF-κB) and ultimately the production of inflammatory cytokines.

A number of polymorphisms within the *NOD2* gene, particularly in the leucine-rich repeat region, are now recognised. Homozygotes and compound heterozygotes for a number of these polymorphisms have a markedly increased risk of developing Crohn's disease (relative risk of between 10 and 30). *NOD2* polymorphisms also seem to be strongly associated with ileal disease (all homozygotes and compound heterozygotes within one study had ileal disease) and protective against fistulising disease. The mechanism by which *NOD2* mutations are involved in Crohn's disease is currently unknown. Mutant NOD2 protein binds less strongly to bacterial endotoxin leading to impaired activation of NF-κB, although it is unclear why this would increase the risk of a disease in which NF-κB and inflammatory cytokines are produced in excess.

References

Ahmad T, Armuzzi A, Bunce M et al 2002 The molecular classification of the clinical manifestations of Crohn's disease. Gastroenterology 122:854–866

Elson C O 2002 Genes, microbes, and T cells – new therapeutic targets in Crohn's disease. New England Journal of Medicine 346:614–616

Parkes M, Jewell D 2001 Ulcerative colitis and Crohn's disease: molecular genetics and clinical implications. Expert Reviews in Molecular Medicine 19: 1–18. Online. Available: www.ermm.cbcu.cam.ac.uk/010039lxh.htm

Best-of-5 answers

72. Screening for colorectal cancer

Answer: **C**

There are 30 000 new cases of colorectal cancer in the UK each year; average 5-year survival is just 40%. Spread through the bowel wall or further has occurred in 90% at diagnosis, resulting in poorer survival. As the majority arise from premalignant adenomatous polyps, an opportunity exists to prevent the development of colorectal cancer by polyp removal. A number of screening techniques are available to allow identification of early cancers and polyps. These include faecal occult blood testing, sigmoidoscopy (either rigid or flexible), colonoscopy, barium enema and CT colonography.

Biennial faecal occult blood testing of normal risk individuals is the only method of screening to reduce colorectal cancer mortality (by 15–18%) in randomised controlled trials but has low sensitivity and specificity. Sensitivity is increased by rehydrating samples but results in a lower specificity. Patients with positive tests require further investigation with either flexible sigmoidoscopy or colonoscopy; 2% of screened individuals require further investigation but only 11% of these have colorectal cancer and 37% have colorectal polyps. Randomised controlled trials of flexible sigmoidoscopy are currently under way, including once only flexible sigmoidoscopy at age 55–64. Colonoscopic screening has not been subjected to randomised controlled trials. Barium enema has a low sensitivity (48% of polyps > 1 cm are detected) and CT colonography currently has a low specificity (83%), although this will undoubtedly improve. Both of these radiological methods require bowel preparation and, when lesions are found, endoscopic removal of polyps is still required.

Screening has major resource implications and is not entirely risk-free or universally acceptable. Faecal occult blood screening would generate approximately 60 000 colonoscopies per year in the UK and once-only flexible sigmoidoscopy would generate 270 000 additional flexible sigmoidoscopies per year in the UK. Both tests are associated with a complication rate (perforation in 1–2 per 1000 colonoscopies and 1 per 10 000 flexible sigmoidoscopies) and colonoscopy has a mortality of 1–3 per 10 000 procedures. Compliance with colorectal cancer screening is low (45% for flexible sigmoidoscopy, 38% for faecal occult blood screening).

References

Ransohoff D F, Sandler R S 2002 Screening for colorectal cancer. New England Journal of Medicine 346:40–44

Rhodes J M 2000 Colorectal cancer screening in the UK: joint position statement by the British Society of Gastroenterology, the Royal College of Physicians, and the Association of Coloproctology of Great Britain and Ireland. Gut 46:746–748

UK Flexible Sigmoidoscopy Screening Trial Investigators 2002 Single flexible sigmoidoscopy screening to prevent colorectal cancer: baseline findings of a UK multicentre randomised trial. Lancet 359:1291–1300

73. Oesophageal cancer

Answer: **C**

Although squamous cell carcinomas made up the majority of oesophageal cancers in the 1970s, a subsequent dramatic increase in the number of oesophageal adenocarcinomas means that these are now the most common oesophageal neoplasms. Risk factors associated with squamous cell carcinomas include smoking and alcohol consumption; smoking, obesity, gastroesophageal reflux symptoms (with increased length and severity of symptoms) and Barrett's oesophagus are important in oesophageal adenocarcinoma.

Oesophageal cancer is associated with poor outcome. Even in those in whom curative surgery is attempted, 2-year survival is only 20–30% as a result of surgical mortality, locally advanced disease or undetected metastatic disease. The majority of tumours are squamous cell or adenocarcinoma. It is vital that patients are staged accurately to ensure that those with advanced disease do not undergo aggressive attempted curative therapy with little hope of benefit. Recent advances in the staging of oesophageal cancer include the development of endoscopic ultrasound (which is highly accurate for T and N staging) and PET scanning (which appears to have greater diagnostic accuracy for distant nodal involvement and metastases). Nevertheless, CT remains the most important and accessible investigation for determining regional spread and the presence of distant metastases.

A recent study suggests that surgical outcome can be improved with preoperative chemotherapy (cisplatin and 5-fluorouracil) with 2-year survival of 43% with preoperative chemotherapy and 34% with surgery alone. No increase in complications occurred as a result and resection was more commonly microscopically complete.

Palliative therapy for oesophageal cancer includes endoscopic stent insertion, chemotherapy, radiotherapy and laser therapy. Successful palliation of dysphagia with endoscopic stents can now be performed with relatively low complication rates.

Reference

Medical Research Council Oesophageal Cancer Working Party 2002 Surgical resection with or without preoperative chemotherapy in oesophageal cancer: a randomised controlled trial. Lancet 359:1727–1733

74. Crohn's disease

Answer: **C**

Crohn's disease is an idiopathic chronic inflammatory condition affecting any part of the gastrointestinal tract (from mouth to anus). It runs a remitting and relapsing course causing symptoms such as diarrhoea and abdominal pain. Traditionally, treatment has been medical and surgical. Medical treatments have included aminosalicylates, corticosteroids, antibiotics (metronidazole and ciprofloxacin) and dietary therapy (elemental diet). Steroid-dependent and steroid-resistant cases are treated with immunosuppressive therapy, including azathioprine, 6-mercaptopurine and methotrexate. Leucopenia with azathioprine and 6-mercaptopurine can now be predicted by genotyping and phenotyping an enzyme involved in their metabolism, thiopurinemethyl transferase; low activity is associated with leucopenia, although the tests are not yet widely available. Surgical therapy is indicated for strictures causing obstructive symptoms, failure to respond to medical therapy and the development of complications. Attempts should be made to preserve bowel length to prevent the development of short bowel syndrome.

More recently, interest has developed in biological therapies. Crohn's disease is characterised by a type 1 T helper cell immune response. This results in elevations in certain proinflammatory cytokines, such as tumour necrosis factor alpha (TNF-α). Monoclonal antibodies against this cytokine have been developed and are now frequently used in the treatment of Crohn's disease and rheumatoid arthritis. Infliximab is an IgG1 murine–human chimeric monoclonal antibody against this cytokine. It is effective in the treatment of chronic active and fistulising Crohn's disease. Evidence suggests that repeated treatment with infliximab is effective in chronic active Crohn's disease but studies of repeated treatment in fistulising disease are awaited. Infliximab is expensive, can only be given intravenously and is associated with a number of adverse effects (development of anti-dsDNA antibodies and human antichimeric antibodies, which reduce its efficacy, delayed-type hypersensitivity and reactivation of tuberculosis). Recent guidance on its use by NICE has recently recommended that it be made available only for patients with severe active Crohn's disease in whom the disease is refractory to corticosteroids and immunomodulating drugs (or if intolerance or toxicity is experienced) and in whom surgery is inappropriate.

References

Hanauer S B, Feagan B G, Lichtenstein G R et al 2002 Maintenance infliximab for Crohn's disease: the ACCENT 1 randomised trial. Lancet 359:1541–1549

Present D H, Rutgeerts P, Targan S et al 1999 Infliximab for the treatment of fistulas in patients with Crohn's disease. New England Journal of Medicine 340:1398–1405

75. Familial adenomatous polyposis (FAP)

Answer: **D**

Familial adenomatous polyposis is an autosomal dominant condition occurring in 1 in 8000 of the population with a penetrance approaching 100%. It is caused by mutations in the *APC* gene on chromosome 5q21; 30% of cases are due to new mutations in this gene. The APC protein binds and inactivates beta-catenin, a key molecule in the development of colorectal cancer. APC protein resulting from mutations causing familial adenomatous polyposis has fewer beta-catenin binding sites than wild-type protein. Mutations in this gene are thought to be an early event in the development of sporadic colorectal cancers. Turcot's syndrome (characterised by polyps and carcinomas of the colon and glioblastomas) is also caused by a mutation in APC.

Familial adenomatous polyposis is characterised by the presence of multiple (hundreds to thousands) colorectal polyps. It can also be associated with a number of extracolonic mutations: congenital hypertrophy of the retinal pigment epithelium, epidermoid cysts and benign craniofacial and long bone tumours (Gardner's syndrome), desmoid tumours (usually retroperitoneal or involving the abdominal wall), upper gastrointestinal polyposis and rarely non-medullary thyroid cancers and hepatoblastomas. After prophylactic colectomy, most disease-related mortality is due to desmoid tumours and duodenal carcinomas. An attenuated form of familial adenomatous polyposis also exists (attenuated APC). Trials of chemoprophylaxis are underway using agents such as aspirin.

Phenotypic differences can occur between and within kindreds. Differences between kindreds probably result from different sites of APC mutation. For example, severe colorectal disease is associated with germline mutations between codons 1250 and 1464 (including the most common mutation at codon 1309), mild disease with truncating germline mutations at the 5' and 3' regions of the APC gene, desmoid tumours with germline mutations between 1403 and 1578 and congenital hypertrophy of the retinal pigment epithelium with mutations between 463 and 1387. Differences within kindreds probably result from environmental factors (desmoids are associated with pregnancy and intra-abdominal surgery).

References

Cole T R, Sleightholme H V 2000 ABC of colorectal cancer. The role of clinical genetics in management. British Medical Journal 321:943–946

Houlston R, Crabtree M, Phillips R et al 2001 Explaining differences in the severity of familial adenomatous polyposis and the search for modifier genes. Gut 48:1–5

76. Hepatitis C virus

Answer: **B**

Hepatitis C virus is a RNA virus estimated to have infected 200 000 to 400 000 people in the UK. It can be transmitted parenterally, sexually and vertically. The most common route is parenteral via transfusion (blood or blood products) or intravenous drug use. Risk of sexual transmission is low, except in the presence of co-infection with HIV (11.7% of HIV-infected homosexuals with no history of blood transfusion or intravenous drug use are seropositive). Risk of vertical transmission is < 6% and breast feeding appears to be safe.

Only 10% of patients infected with hepatitis C virus develop an acute icteric illness. The majority develop chronic disease, chronic active or persistent hepatitis, cirrhosis and hepatocellular carcinoma. High-level viraemia, genotype 1, immune deficiency, excess alcohol consumption and co-infection with hepatitis B or HIV can all increase the rate of disease progression. Median time from infection to cirrhosis seems to be 30 years. Progression of fibrosis is more rapid in those infected when older than 40, men and in those with excess alcohol consumption. Although blood transfusion is thought to lead to more active disease, patients infected with anti-D immunoglobulin have recently been shown to have a relatively benign course with no evidence of cirrhosis or hepatocellular carcinoma. Viral clearance is more common in patients with the HLA DRB1*01 allele and in those describing an icteric illness.

Chronic infection is usually asymptomatic, although non-specific symptoms can occur. Extrahepatic manifestations include mixed essential cryoglobulinaemia, thyroiditis and the sicca syndrome. Hepatocellular carcinoma develops in between 1 and 7% of patients with hepatitis C and cirrhosis annually.

The diagnosis of hepatitis C infection is made using a combination of tests including antibody tests (ELISA and radioimmunoassay), polymerase chain reaction (measuring viral RNA) and liver biopsy (allowing measurement of inflammation and fibrosis). Liver biochemistry correlates poorly with liver biopsy findings. The hepatitis C virus can also be genotyped. At least six genotypes have now been identified.

Response rates to antiviral treatment are currently unsatisfactory. At present, regimes utilise interferon alpha and ribavirin. Contraindications to interferon use include depressive illness and psychosis, neutropaenia, thrombocytopaenia and decompensated cirrhosis. For ribavirin, contraindications include end-stage renal disease, anaemia and pregnancy. Increasing length of interferon monotherapy improves sustained response (14% with 6 months treatment and 35% with 12–18 months treatment). Combination therapy also improves response rates (48-week monotherapy 19%, 24-week combination therapy 35%, 48-week combination therapy 43%). Length of treatment will depend on genotype and viral load. Patients with mild histological disease should undergo repeat biopsy (possibly at 2–3 years) and be offered treatment if disease is progressing. Patients with moderate disease should be offered treatment. Serious side-effects of interferon therapy are rare but include neuropsychiatric disturbances, autoimmune hepatitis, renal and cardiovascular disease. Haemolysis is the major adverse effect of ribavirin therapy.

References

Barrett S, Goh J, Coughlan B et al 2001 The natural course of hepatitis C virus infection after 22 years in a unique homogenous cohort: spontaneous viral clearance and chronic HCV infection. Gut 49:423–430

Booth J C, O'Grady J, Neuberger J et al 2001 Clinical guidelines on the management of hepatitis C. Gut 49(suppl 1):i1–i21

NEPHROLOGY

True/False answers

77. Diabetic nephropathy

A. **T**   B. **T**   C. **F**   D. **T**   E. **T**

Diabetic nephropathy is the single most common cause of end-stage renal disease in the Western world. Although type 1 (insulin-dependent) and type 2 (non-insulin-dependent) diabetes mellitus are distinct conditions in terms of their aetiology and epidemiology, no major differences have been identified between the nephropathies seen in these conditions, thus they can be considered together. There are a number of distinct phases in the evolution of the disease:

- *Hyperfiltration* – characterised by renal enlargement, intrarenal hypertension and a high glomerular filtration rate. These phenomena have been linked with the development of microalbuminuria but are partly reversible by tight glycaemic and blood pressure control. Early microalbuminuria is usually associated with a raised glomerular filtration rate and a normal filtration rate in this context might indicate that renal function has already been lost.
- *Silent phase* – very few patients develop microalbuminuria during the first 10 years of disease, although during this time histological

abnormalities might be seen, including glomerular hypertrophy and thickening of the basement membrane.

- *Microalbuminuria* – the normal urinary protein excretion rate is up to 300 mg/24 h, about 10% of which is albumin. Albumin excretion rates of 20–200 μg/min are defined as microalbuminuria. The presence of microalbuminuria predicts the development of overt renal disease and is also associated with an increased risk of cardiovascular and microvascular complications, as well as all-cause mortality.
- *Overt nephropathy* – albumin excretion rates of > 200 μg/min or 300 mg/24 h are dipstick positive and defined as overt nephropathy. Once this has developed, there is usually an inexorable decline in renal function (decrease in glomerular filtration rate by 1–24 mL/min/year). The rate of progression of nephropathy is heavily influenced by blood pressure control.

Risk factors for the development of diabetic nephropathy are hypertension, poor glycaemic control, male sex, genetic factors (such as ACE gene polymorphisms), hyperlipidaemia, dietary protein intake and smoking. Hypertension is of particular importance; the rate of decline in patients with overt nephropathy strongly correlates with hypertension. Furthermore, in normoalbuminuric type 1 diabetics, small increases in blood pressure have been correlated with the development of microalbumniuria. In terms of glycaemic control, it has been noted that HbA1c levels correlate with the development of nephropathy. Polymorphisms in the ACE gene, which cause an elevated circulating ACE level, are known to be associated with an increased risk of ischaemic heart disease. One study has noted an association of the DD genotype with increased risk of diabetic nephropathy in type 2 diabetes. Raised plasma triglycerides and low levels of high density lipoprotein have also been correlated with the development of diabetic nephropathy.

References

Cooper M E 1998 Pathogenesis, prevention and treatment of diabetic nephropathy. Lancet 352:213–219

Foggensteiner L, Mulroy S, Firth J 2001 Management of diabetic nephropathy. Journal of the Royal Society of Medicine 94:210–217

78.   Renal stones

A. **F**   B. **F**   C. **F**   D. **F**   E. **T**

Renal stones are extremely common, affecting approximately 10% of the population at some time in their lives. Stone formation is thought to occur in urine when concentrations of, for example, calcium and oxalate reach saturation. Initially, small amounts of crystalloid associate to form nuclei, which then grow and aggregate on surfaces such as collecting ducts and epithelial cells. A number of factors can promote stone formation, including elevated levels of urinary calcium, sodium, oxalate, urate, cystine, a low urinary pH, low urine flow and bacterial products. Nephrocalcin is an acidic protein of renal tubular origin that is known to inhibit stone formation. In some people who form stones, this protein lacks the amino acid γ-carboxyglutamic acid, thus reducing its ability to prevent nucleation. Prothrombin fragment-1 (crystal matrix protein) is found in many renal stones. It is derived from the cleavage of prothrombin and has been shown to inhibit calcium oxalate crystal formation in animal models.

Calcium stones are radio-opaque and their formation is promoted by hypercalciuria (> 4 mg of urinary calcium per kg of body weight per day). Between 30 and 50% of patients with hypercalciuria will have idiopathic hypercalciuria, a familial disorder affecting both sexes equally, in which urinary calcium concentration is elevated despite normal concentrations of blood calcium. A number of pathogenic mechanisms have been postulated, which might occur individually or in combination, including high intestinal calcium absorption, increased renal filtered load, increased bone resorption, defective tubular calcium reabsorption with an inappropriately high phosphate excretion (thus inducing activation of 1,25 dihydroxy vitamin D), and elevated phospholipid–arachidonic acid concentrations in serum with associated raised urinary prostaglandin E2 concentrations. There are rarer genetic causes of hypercalciuria, including a recently described mutation in the gene encoding the CLCN5 chloride channel in some Japanese families and mutations of the calcium receptor gene (which regulates parathyroid hormone secretion), as seen in autosomal dominant hypercalciuria hypocalcaemia.

Investigations should aim at determining size, location and type of stone. Intravenous pyelography remains the gold standard for imaging, although ultrasonography, which has the advantage of being non-invasive, can indicate the location of the stone and the degree of obstruction. Other investigations that should be performed include blood levels of calcium, phosphate, uric acid, alkaline phosphatase and bicarbonate and urinary levels of calcium, urate, creatinine, citrate and oxalate, as well as urinary pH, microscopy and culture.

Once a kidney stone forms there is a 50% chance that a second stone will form within 5–7 years in the absence of treatment. Standard preventive therapy has involved the reduction of urinary supersaturation by maintenance of adequate fluid intake. In the case of calcium-containing stones, a reduction in dietary calcium was considered to be a logical way of reducing urinary calcium and thus relative supersaturation. However, a recent study does not support this but rather suggests that the use of a normocalcaemic (1200 mg/day) diet with reduced animal protein and salt is more efficacious in terms of prevention of stone recurrence. Preventive strategies should also involve the avoidance of drugs that promote stone formation. For calcium stones this includes loop diuretics, glucocorticoids, acetazolamide, theophylline and calcium-containing antacids. Drugs that promote uric acid stone formation include thiazide diuretics, salicylates, probenecid and allopurinol. Specific therapies for calcium stones include thiazide diuretics, which increase distal tubular calcium resorption.

Most symptomatic upper urinary tract stones are small and pass spontaneously if less than 5 mm in diameter. For stones between 5 mm and 2 cm, extracorporeal shock-wave lithotripsy is the preferred therapeutic option. For larger or complex stones a percutaneous nephrolithotomy or ureteroscopy might be required.

References

Bhil G, Meyers A 2001 Recurrent renal stone disease – advances in pathogenesis and management. Lancet 358:651–656

Borghi L, Schianchi T, Meschi T et al 2002 Comparison of two diets for the prevention of recurrent stones in idiopathic hypercalciuria. New England Journal of Medicine 346:77–84

Morton A R, Iliescu E A, Wilson J W 2002 Investigation and treatment of recurrent kidney stones. Canadian Medical Association Journal 166:213–218

79.   Anaemia in chronic renal failure

A. **F**   B. **T**   C. **F**   D. **F**   E. **T**

Anaemia can occur in association with both acute and chronic renal failure. Both are associated with erythropoietin deficiency and a shortening of red cell survival. Erythroid suppression is greater in acute renal failure, probably as a result of the more marked reduction in erythropoietin secretion because of acute renal injury and associated cytokine activation (secondary to inflammation and infection) that is often seen in the acute setting. Anaemia is usually present when glomerular filtration rate decreases to < 35 mL/min, and worsens as the filtration rate reduces further. The anaemia of chronic renal failure is usually normochromic and normocytic. Although in most cases erythropoietin deficiency is the cause, potential exacerbating factors such as iron deficiency, hypothyroidism, haemolysis and vitamin B_{12}/folate deficiency should be excluded, particularly if there is microcytosis (iron deficiency, aluminium toxicity), macrocytosis (vitamin B_{12}/folate deficiency, haemolysis) or an elevated reticulocyte count (haemolysis).

Erythropoietin is a glycopeptide synthesised by fibroblast-like interstitial cells in the kidney (and to a much lesser extent in the liver). The isolation of the human erythropoietin gene in 1983, followed by its cloning and the production of recombinant human erythropoietin, has revolutionised the treatment of anaemia in chronic renal failure. Erythropoietin is usually given subcutaneously two or three times a week (dose range 25–1500 units/kg/week). The current recommended target for patients with end-stage renal failure, suggested by the National Kidney Foundation-Dialysis Outcomes Quality Initiative, are a haematocrit of 33–36% and a haemoglobin of 11–12 g/L. Correction of anaemia with erythropoietin has led to improvements in quality of life of patients with end-stage renal failure, particularly in terms of exercise capacity, cognitive function, sexual function, sleep disturbance and bleeding tendencies related to uraemia.

Perhaps one of the most important aspects of normalising haemoglobin levels is the reduction of cardiac output (resulting from the decrease in anaemia-induced peripheral vasodilation). This can lead to a reduction in left ventricular hypertrophy, which can have significant long-term benefits because left ventricular hypertrophy is associated with a 2.9-fold increase in mortality in patients with end-stage renal failure.

Failure to respond to erythropoietin therapy can be due to inadequate dosage or, more commonly, persistent iron deficiency. However, even with adequate iron stores, other factors can lead to erythropoietin hyporesponsiveness, including concurrent infection/inflammation, aluminium excess, hyperparathyroid osteitis fibrosa, folate deficiency, ACE-inhibitor therapy and haemoglobinopathies. Adverse effects are minimal but an increase in blood pressure has been described in up to 23% of patients with chronic renal failure. The mechanism of action is unclear because hypertension does not occur in anaemic patients without renal failure treated with erythropoietin. It is thought that the extracellular volume status of patients with renal failure could contribute to any hypertension that is seen. However, the erythropoietin receptors on endothelial cells might have a different reactivity in renal patients. Neutralising antibodies were very rarely seen with erythropoietin treatment (three reported cases in 10 years) but in 2000–2001 a series of 21 cases have been described (possibly due to a slight modification in production processes). In these patients there was not only resistance to erythropoietin but also a pure red cell aplasia. Discontinuation of erythropoietin and, in some cases, the use of immunosuppressive therapy, led to the disappearance of antierythropoietin antibodies and improvement of red cell aplasia.

References

Casadevall N, Nataf J, Viron B et al 2002 Pure red cell aplasia and anti-erythropoietin antibodies in patients treated with recombinant EPO. New England Journal of Medicine 346:469–475

Macdougall I C, Cooper A 2002 The inflammatory response and EPO sensitivity. Nephrology, Dialysis, Transplantation 17(S1):48–52

Valderrabano F 2002 Anaemia management in chronic kidney disease patients: an overview of current practice. Nephrology, Dialysis, Transplantation 17(S1):13–18

80. Autosomal dominant polycystic kidney disease

A. **T**   B. **T**   C. **T**   D. **T**   E. **T**

Autosomal dominant polycystic kidney disease is a systemic disorder that primarily affects the kidneys. The formation of fluid-filled cysts in both kidneys, together with interstitial fibrosis, results in end-stage renal failure in late middle age. Diagnostic ultrasonographic criteria in at risk individuals (i.e. positive family history) include two cysts, either unilateral or bilateral, in those < 30 years of age, two cysts in both kidneys in patients aged 30–59 years, and at least four cysts in each kidney in those > 60 years of age. The disease is also associated with a number of extra-renal manifestations, including cardiovascular manifestations (mitral valve prolapse, mitral/tricuspid incompetence, dilation of the aortic root, thoracic aortic arterial dissections and coronary artery aneurysms), intracranial aneurysms in approximately 8%, and cyst formation in other organs such as the liver, spleen, ovaries, thyroid and pineal gland.

Polycystic kidney disease is also common, with 1 in 1000 caucasians affected. Linkage studies have shown that the disease is genetically heterogeneous; two disease loci have been mapped and identified, on chromosome 16 (*PKD1*, found in 85% of affected families) and chromosome 4 (*PKD2,* found in 15% of affected families). Several unlinked families have also been identified, suggesting the existence of a further locus, as yet uncharacterised. PKD1 and PKD2 are clinically similar, with polycystic liver disease and intracranial aneurysms being described in both. However, there does seem to be a difference in terms of severity of renal disease; the average age of onset of end-stage renal failure is 53 years for PKD1 and 69 years for PKD2.

The *PKD1* gene encodes a large integral membrane protein, polycystin-1. It has a large extracellular region, 11 membrane-spanning domains, and a short cytoplasmic tail, which has been shown to interact with polycystin-2. The precise location of polycystin-1 remains controversial but recent studies have indicated that it might be located at desmosomal junctions. *PKD2* encodes a smaller protein polycystin-2, which shows homology to the pore forming units of several cation channels. Recent work has shown that polycystin-2 is localised to the endoplasmic reticulum, but tethered close to the surface membrane of the cell by its association with polycystin-1. Cell culture systems have shown that polycystin-2 can act as a high-conductance cation channel, permeable to calcium, with opening probability enhanced by calcium elevation on the cytosolic side of the membrane. Thus, it has been proposed that it is a novel calcium channel, with properties that allow it to mediate calcium-induced calcium release. The precise functional relationship between polycystin-1 and polycystin-2 is as yet unknown, as is the mechanism by which dysfunction of calcium release leads to the disease phenotype.

References

Cahalan M D 2002 The ins and outs of polycystin-2 as a calcium release channel. Nature Cell Biology 4:E56–E57

Harris P C 2002 Molecular basis of polycystic kidney disease. Current Opinion in Nephrology and Hypertension 11:309–314

Peters D J, Breuning M H 2001 Autosomal dominant polycystic kidney disease: modification of disease progression. Lancet 354:1439–1444

81. Renal vasculitis

A. **F**   B. **T**   C. **T**   D. **F**   E. **T**

Wegener's granulomatosis and microscopic polyangiitis are primary systemic vasculitides predominantly affecting small vessels. Immune deposits are usually scanty or absent and antineutrophil cytoplasmic antibodies (ANCA) present at diagnosis. ANCA causing a diffuse granular cytoplasmic pattern of immunofluorescent staining (cANCA) were first described in the early 1980s in association with Wegener's granuolomatosis. Proteinase 3, a serine protease found in the azurophilic granules of neutrophils, was subsequently identified as the target antigen for these antibodies. The antibody is thought to bind near the catalytic domain of the molecule and interfere with its inactivation by α_1-antitrypsin.

Myeloperoxidase-specific ANCA, giving a perinuclear pattern of immunofluorescent staining (pANCA), has been found in association with microscopic polyangiitis, pauci-immune glomerulonephritis without systemic manifestations and in a minority of patients with Wegener's granulomatosis. These antibodies have a high specificity for the autoimmune vasculitides and levels can correlate with disease activity. However, the relationship is not a reliable one; cANCA can remain high in patients with quiescent disease. Infection in these individuals can subsequently induce a severe disease flare. It is thought that proteinase-3 is not expressed on the cell surface of resting neutrophils and is therefore inaccessible to cANCA. However, following infection and neutrophil activation, proteinase-3 is transported to the cell surface where cANCA can bind and stimulate degranulation of neutrophils, thus inducing inflammation. Control of infection can therefore reduce disease relapses.

Renal involvement is common in the ANCA-associated vasculitides occurring in approximately 80% of patients with Wegener's granulomatosis and 90% of patients with microscopic polyangiitis. These patients often present clinically with a rapidly progressive glomerulonephritis. In the early stages, histopathological and immunohistochemical examination of the kidney reveals pauci-immune, segmental fibrinoid necrosis. This can rapidly progress to a widespread necrotising glomerulonephritis with crescent formation.

The treatment of systemic vasculitides with renal involvement has not been standardised but some trial evidence is available. Following presentation, induction of remission is usually attempted using a combination of cyclophosphamide and corticosteroids. Overall, data indicates that daily oral cyclophosphamide is more efficacious than monthly pulsed intravenous cyclophosphamide in induction of sustained remission, but is associated with increased adverse effects. The CYCLOPS study is currently comparing the efficacy of daily oral versus pulsed cyclophosphamide in patients with renal vasculitis. In patients with severe renal disease, delayed time to diagnosis increases the risk of development of renal failure. The addition of pulsed methyl prednisolone and/or plasma exchange to cyclophosphamide and oral prednisolone has been advocated to increase the chances of renal recovery. The pooled analysis of a number of small trials has shown that plasma exchange seems to be of benefit in these patients. The MEPEX trial is currently comparing rates of renal recovery for patients with an initial creatinine over 500 μmol/L between the addition of 3 g of methylprednisolone and seven plasma exchanges, as well as daily oral cyclophosphamide and prednisolone. The results of both these trials are awaited.

References

Levy J 2001 New aspects in the management of ANCA-positive vasculitis. Nephrology, Dialysis, Transplantation 16:1314–1317

Proceedings of the 10th International Vasculitis and ANCA workshop 2002 Cleveland Clinic Journal of Medicine 69(suppl 2)

Savage C O S 2001 ANCA-associated renal vasculitis. Kidney International 60:1614–1627

Update on all European vasculitis trials run by EUVAS, including CYCLOPS and MEPEX. Online. Available: www.vasculitis.org

Best-of-5 answers

82.   Treatment of early diabetic nephropathy

Answer: **B**

Microalbuminuria rarely occurs within the first 5–10 years in type 1 diabetes, or before puberty, therefore screening should start with onset of puberty or after 5 years disease duration. In type 2 diabetes, the precise onset of disease is often unclear and annual screening should therefore begin at diagnosis. Once microalbuminuria has been detected, the patient should have urinary albumin/creatinine ratio, or an albumin excretion rate estimated every 3–6 months. In addition, serum creatinine, urea and electrolytes should be measured at least every 6 months.

The target blood pressure that should be aimed for in diabetics has not been clearly defined. The British Hypertension Society recommends a target BP of < 140/80 mmHg, or 125/75 mmHg in type 1 diabetic patients with > 1 g/day proteinuria. Both the UKPDS and HOT trials have shown that this often requires multiple antihypertensive medications. ACE inhibitors remain the first choice, although blood pressure reduction with any of the standard antihypertensive agents (beta-blockers, diuretics, dihydropyridine calcium antagonists, alpha-blockers) is beneficial. In microalbuminuric type 1 diabetics with controlled hypertension, two studies have shown a 63% reduction in progression to overt proteinuria with captopril treatment, showing an additional renoprotective effect above and beyond antihypertensive properties. This association is much less clear in type 2 diabetes. However, more recent studies support a blood pressure-independent renoprotective effect of angiotensin II receptor antagonists in type 2 diabetics with microalbuminuria.

A number of meta-analyses have shown a beneficial effect of dietary protein-restriction on the progression of diabetic nephropathy in type I diabetics, but precise levels of restriction are unclear. There are no prevention studies to show whether lipid-lowering interventions in diabetics affect decline in renal function. However, dyslipidaemia is a risk factor for the development and progression of renal dysfunction in primary renal disease. Several studies have indicated that both total cholesterol and triglyceride concentrations are significant predictors of coronary artery disease in diabetics. In addition, microalbuminuria is associated with an increase in cardiovascular mortality in diabetic patients; these facts provide the rationale for aggressive treatment of dyslipidaemia in diabetics with nephropathy. Current recommendations in the UK are to maintain total cholesterol < 5.0 mmol/L and LDL cholesterol < 3.0 mmol/L.

The high cardiovascular risk in diabetic patients with microalbuminuria or overt nephropathy also argues strongly for the use of aspirin as a primary prevention strategy.

References

Foggensteiner L, Mulroy S, Firth J 2001 Management of diabetic nephropathy. Journal of the Royal Society of Medicine 94:210–217

Parving H H, Lehnert H, Brochner-Mortensen J et al 2001 The effect of irbesartan on the development of diabetic nephropathy in patients with type 2 diabetes. New England Journal of Medicine 345:870–878

Waugh N R, Robertson A M 2000 Protein restriction for diabetic renal disease. Cochrane Database System Review 2:CD002181

83.   Transplant failure

Answer: **E**

Since the first renal transplant in 1954, graft survival has greatly improved and now runs at 88% at 1 year and 60% at 10 years post-transplantation for cadaveric grafts, and 95% and 70%, respectively, for grafts obtained from living donors. Most of this has been due to improvements in immunosuppression therapy and in better matching of donor organ and recipient.

Chronic rejection and death with functioning graft remain the leading causes of late loss of renal allografts. Mechanisms of chronic rejection in the kidney are not fully understood and there appear to be a number of contributing factors, both immunological and non-immunological. This has led to the use of a more inclusive term chronic allograft nephropathy. This is characterised histologically by obliterative intimal fibrosis (transplant arteriopathy) duplication of the glomerular basement membrane (chronic transplant glomerulopathy), tubular atrophy and interstitial fibrosis. Contributory factors include number of HLA mismatches, production of alloantibodies against HLA class I or II of the donor, recurrent episodes of acute rejection, delayed graft function, hypertension and hyperlipidaemia. The role of calcineurin inhibitor (ciclosporin and tacrolimus) toxicity in chronic allograft nephropathy remains controversial but there is evidence to suggest that the use of mycophenolate instead of the calcineurin inhibitors might reduce the incidence of the condition.

One of the major barriers to transplantation in recent years, and an increasing problem, is that of inadequate supply of donor organs. There are currently some 6000 patients waiting for renal transplants (figures for December 2001). The number of cadaveric brainstem-dead donors has not increased at the same rate as numbers of those on the waiting list, possibly due to improved road safety and a reduced trust/willingness of the public to donate organs following various high profile cases on the handling of tissue and organs in some pathology departments. The NHS organ register, launched in 1994, was aimed at promoting organ donation in the UK, allowing individuals to register their willingness to donate organs when they renew their passport or driving licence. The efficacy of this measure is questionable. The adoption of an opting-out system of organ donation (that is, potential organ donors are presumed to consent unless they have specifically registered a wish not to donate) has been proposed and its implementation in a number of European countries (Belgium, France and Germany) has led to an increase in number of organ donors. The paucity of supply of cadaveric grafts has led to the increasing use of living grafts (both from related and unrelated donors) and these now makes up 20% of UK transplants. The better survival of grafts from living donors is due to a higher quality of graft and optimal retrieval conditions. A good immunological match does not appear to be as important in grafts from living donors. The use of non-heart-beating donors is also being developed. This requires very rapid organ retrieval to minimise damage due to warm ischaemia but might provide a means of increasing organ availability. Work also continues on the development of xenotransplantation, as this would provide an almost limitless supply of organs.

Recurrence of the original disease in the graft is difficult to quantify because in many cases the original disease leading to end-stage renal failure is unknown. The main recurrences are focal segmental glomerulosclerosis (30–40%), membranoproliferative glomerulonephritis (approximately 30%) and haemolytic uraemic syndrome (approximately 50%).

References

Andrews P A 2002 Renal transplantation. British Medical Journal 324:530–534

Halloran P F, Melk A, Barth C 1999 Rethinking chronic allograft nephropathy. Journal of the American Society of Nephrology 10:167–181

84. Transplant immunosuppression

Answer: **D**

Ciclosporin or tacrolimus (FK506) are used as the mainstay treatments for prevention of acute rejection, usually in combination with azathioprine and corticosteroids. Their mechanism of action (following intracellular activation by binding to cyclophyllin or FK binding protein) is to inhibit calcineurin, a phosphatase that activates nuclear factor of activated T cells (NF-AT). Activated NF-AT normally binds to AP1 to form a complex that can induce the transcription of genes required for T cell activation, including the interleukin-2 gene. Interleukin-2 is a cytokine produced mainly by T cells. It causes T cell and NK cell proliferation and activation, and B cell proliferation and antibody synthesis. In comparison with both the initial formulation of ciclosporin and the new microemulsion formulation of ciclosporin, tacrolimus is associated with a lower incidence of acute rejection, although 1-year survival of patient and allograft are similar. Tacrolimus also appears to have a more favourable cardiovascular profile (in terms of incidence of hypertension and hyperlipidaemia) but is associated with an increased risk of glucose intolerance and even frank diabetes mellitus.

Mycophenolate mofetil is a prodrug that is rapidly converted into mycophenolic acid by plasma esterases following oral administration. It blocks purine synthesis by inhibition of the enzyme IMPDH, thus inhibiting the proliferation of B and T cells. Studies comparing the use of mycophenolate versus azathioprine in combination with ciclosporin and prednisolone showed a lower incidence of acute rejection at 6 months with mycophenolate and its use longer term might lead to a reduction in chronic rejection.

Rapamycin (Sirolimus) is a macrolide antibiotic originally derived from the actinomycete *Streptomyces hygroscopicus*. Rapamycin blocks the proliferation of lymphocytes by inhibiting the signal transduction pathway triggered by ligation of the interleukin-2 receptor. The use of rapamycin instead of azathioprine in ciclosporin-based regimens has been shown to produce a significant reduction in the incidence of acute rejection. Preliminary data suggest even more benefit when used in combination with tacrolimus rather than ciclosporin. The main adverse effect associated with the use of rapamycin appears to be that of dyslipidaemias but it is less nephrotoxic than ciclosporin or tacrolimus.

Selective inhibition of the interleukin-2 receptor with monoclonal antibodies has now been introduced into immunosuppressive regimes by some centres. Daclizumab (a humanised monoclonal antibody) and basiliximab (also known as Simulect, a chimeric monoclonal antibody) appear to have good safety profiles and reduce the incidence of acute rejection when added to immunosuppressive regimens containing ciclosporin and corticosteroids. The cost effectiveness of their widespread use remains controversial.

References

Margreiter R 2002 Efficacy and safety of tacrolimus compared with ciclosporin microemulsion in renal transplantation: a randomised multicentre study. Lancet 359:741–746

Pascual M, Theruvath T, Kawai T et al 2002 Strategies to improve long-term outcomes after renal transplantation. New England Journal of Medicine 346:580–590

Saunders R N, Metcalfe M S, Nicholson M L 2001 Rapamycin in renal transplantation: a review of the evidence. Kidney International 59:3–16

85.   Membranous glomerulonephritis

Answer: **B**

Membranous glomerulonephritis is the most common cause of adult onset nephrotic syndrome in the world. In spite of its overall good prognosis, it remains the third most common cause of end-stage renal failure within the primary glomerulonephritis group because of its frequency. In industrialised countries, the most common variant is idiopathic membranous glomerulonephritis. However, it can occur secondary to infections (such as hepatitis B and malaria, less commonly hepatitis C, filariasis and leprosy), in association with malignancies (found in up to 20% of patients > 50 years of age) and in systemic lupus erythematosus (class V lupus nephritis). A number of drugs have also been associated with membranous glomerulonephritis including gold, penacillamine, non-steroidal anti-inflammatory agents and toxins such as hydrocarbons and formaldehyde.

   The rule of thirds applies to idiopathic membranous glomerulonephritis in terms of prognosis; one-third of patients will undergo spontaneous remission, one-third will remain proteinuric and one-third will progress to end-stage renal failure. A number of factors are known to predict worse outcome including advanced age, male sex, severity of initial proteinuria and renal insufficiency and some histopathological changes such as tubular interstitial damage and glomerulosclerosis.

   Evaluation of a nephrotic patient with membranous glomerulonephritis should include regular monitoring of renal function and blood pressure, urine protein excretion measurement, serum albumin and cholesterol levels and exclusion of any secondary causes of membranous nephropathy. Blood pressure should be controlled, preferably with ACE inhibitors or angiotensin II receptor blockers. Several studies have shown that ACE inhibitors seem to have a renoprotective effect in addition to their antihypertensive actions and should therefore be used in patients with persistent proteinuria. Patients with nephrotic range proteinuria of any cause often have elevated lipid levels, which should be treated appropriately. Moderate dietary protein restriction has been associated with a reduction in proteinuria and progression rate as a function of initial urinary protein level. In patients who are severely nephrotic (proteinuria > 10 g/24 h) and hypoalbuminaemic, serious consideration should be given to prophylactic oral anticoagulation with warfarin because the risk of thromboembolic episodes, particularly renal vein thrombosis, is high.

   Disease-specific therapy is reserved for those patients who show progressive proteinuria or decline in renal function, and are therefore likely to fall into the 'poor prognosis' group. There is no definitive protocol for treating membranous glomerulonephritis but, overall, evidence indicates that oral corticosteroids alone are not of benefit. However, some studies have shown that corticosteroids used in combination with cytotoxic drugs might be of use. The most convincing trials of this approach have been those employing a regimen of 3 days of intravenous methyl prednisolone (1 g/day), followed by high-dose oral prednisolone for 1 month alternating with 1 month of oral chlorambucil. At 10 years, 88% of the treatment group had complete or partial remissions of nephrotic syndrome, versus 47% of controls. Other studies combining steroids and chlorambucil have confirmed their efficacy in patients with declining renal function. Ciclosporin has been used as an alternative to steroids and chlorambucil. Overall, the data obtained from a number of trials, both controlled and uncontrolled, indicate that ciclosporin can effectively induce remission in 20–30% of patients with progressive idiopathic membranous glomerulonephritis. A recent small trial of mycophenolate mofetil showed it to be effective in reducing proteinuria in patients with membranous glomerulonephritis but larger long-term trials are awaited. Pentoxifylline (oxpentifylline), which suppresses TNF-α production, has been used in a pilot study of patients with membranous glomerulonephritis. Urinary TNF-α excretion is known to correlate with proteinuria in membranous nephropathy, and pentoxifylline did seem to significantly reduce proteinuria (from 11 g/day to 1.8 g/day) in this study. It might, therefore, provide an adjunct to steroid and immunosuppressants in patients with membranous glomerulonephritis.

References

Cattran D C 2001 Idiopathic membranous glomerulonephritis. Kidney International 59:1983–1994

Ducloux D, Bresson-Vautrin C, Chalopin J 2001 Use of pentoxifylline in membranous nephropathy. Lancet 357:1672–1673

Ponticelli C, Passerini P 2001 Treatment of membranous nephropathy. Nephrology, Dialysis, Transplantation 16(S5):8–10

Torres A, Dominguez-Gil B, Carreno C et al 2002 Conservative versus immunosuppressive treatment of patients with idiopathic membranous nephropathy. Kidney International 61:219–227

86. Renal cell carcinoma

Answer: **A**

Renal cell carcinoma accounts for approximately 85% of all primary renal neoplasms. Clinical presentation is variable and often late; approximately 25% of individuals have distant metastases and a further 30% have locally advanced disease at presentation. Classic symptoms include macroscopic haematuria, flank pain/mass and weight loss. More obscure presentations include recurrent fevers, acute varicocele (usually left sided, secondary to left renal vein thrombosis/obstruction by tumour), hepatic dysfunction in the absence of metastatic disease ('Stauffer's syndrome', thought to be due to cytokine production by the tumour) and ectopic hormone production (ACTH, renin, erythropoietin, parathyroid-like hormone, gonadotropin, glucagons and insulin). Common sites of metastases include lung (75%), lymph nodes, bone and liver.

Most renal cell carcinomas are sporadic, but the study of rarer hereditary renal cancer syndromes has allowed the identification of several tumour suppressor genes and oncogenes involved in the majority of sporadic renal cancers. Factors suggesting a hereditary cause include first-degree relatives with the disease, bilateral tumours, or onset before the age of 40 years. Several kindreds with clear cell carcinoma have been identified with consistent abnormalities on the short arm of chromosome 3. In addition, patients with tuberose sclerosis, autosomal dominant adult polycystic kidney disease and von Hippel–Lindau disease are at increased risk of developing renal cell carcinoma. Renal cell carcinomas develop in about a third of patients with von Hippel–Lindau disease and are a major cause of death. Renal cysts are also common in this condition.

Genetic analysis of kindreds with clear cell type renal cell carcinoma and patients with von Hippel–Lindau has allowed the identification and characterisation of the *VHL* gene, a renal cell carcinoma susceptibility gene located at 3p25-26. The VHL protein (pVHL) has been cloned and is expressed at high levels in both the kidney and the cerebellum. It is thought to act as a tumour suppressor, similar to APC and p53. Patients with von Hippel–Lindau disease inherit one mutated copy of the *VHL* gene and subsequently undergo a second hit in the normal copy of the *VHL* gene in certain tissues. Recent work has shown that pVHL functions as a ubiquitin ligase, targeting proteins for degradation. One of its target proteins is hypoxia-inducible factor-1, which acts to increase the transcription of genes such as vascular endothelial growth factor and transforming growth factor (TGF) beta-1. Both of these factors are potently proangiogenic and provide additional therapeutic targets in patients with renal cell carcinoma, both sporadic and von Hippel–Lindau associated. In a murine model of renal cell carcinoma, TGF-β neutralising antibodies have been shown to cause tumour regression. Humanised neutralising antibodies against vascular endothelial growth factor have been tested in animal models and are currently in phase I and II clinical trials in patients with metastatic renal cancers.

Radical nephrectomy is the preferred treatment in patients with organ-confined disease. However, because curative surgery is almost impossible in disseminated disease, the benefits of surgery to a patient with metastatic disease have been disputed. However, two recent clinical trials have confirmed a survival advantage for patients who have undergone radical nephrectomy prior to the administration of immunotherapy in the form of interferon alpha. Interferon alpha has been widely studied in metastatic renal cell carcinoma and produces a variable response rate. In the US, interleukin-2 is used in the treatment of metastatic renal cell carcinoma, with an overall response rate of 17% and a 5–7% complete response rate. However, interleukin-2 administration is associated with a high incidence of side-effects. Other therapeutic possibilities include immunisation with dendritic cell/tumour cell hybrid vaccines, which have shown promise in pilot studies.

References

Flanigan R C, Salmon S E, Blumenstein B A et al 2001 Nephrectomy followed by interferon alfa2b compared with interferon alone for metastatic renal cell cancer. New England Journal of Medicine 345:1655–1659

Karumanchi S A, Merchan J, Sukhatme V P 2002 Renal cancer: molecular mechanisms and newer therapeutic options. Current Opinion in Nephrology and Hypertension 11(1):37–42

Kugler A, Stuhler G, Walden P et al 2000 Regression of human metastatic renal cell carcinoma after vaccination with tumour cell-endritic cell hybrids. Nature Medicine 6:332–326

GENETICS

True/False answers

87.   Proteomics

A. **F**   B. **F**   C. **T**   D. **F**   E. **T**

The human genome project has revealed that the human genome consists of only 40 000–60 000 genes, potentially making sequencing and investigation of function a realistic target.

Gene expression is primarily controlled at a transcriptional level through coordinate binding of transcription factors, interactions with cofactors such as histone acetylases or deacetylases and through signal transduction pathways. A second level of control occurs at the level of mRNA splicing, which removes the intron-derived sequences and joins the coding exons together. Alternative splicing sequences allow different exons to be included or excluded from the transcript and, hence, ultimately different proteins to be created from a single gene. The final level of regulation occurs following translation of mRNA into a polypeptide in which modifications such as cleaving of leader sequences and attachment of phosphate or acetyl groups promote the final functional form of the protein and direct it to its ultimate destination. Different splicing and post-translational modification means that one gene potentially results in several (in humans, at least three to six) functionally different proteins. Examination of the genome alone cannot predict the functional relevance of proteins in different biological milieu. The human genome project has concentrated on identifying genes; the major challenge now is to complement this with understanding of protein function.

Proteomics involves the identification of proteins within the body and the determination of their role in physiological and pathophysiological conditions. Two-dimensional gel electrophoresis is the mainstay of protein separation techniques and allows separation on the basis of charge and molecular mass. Differences between healthy and diseased samples can thus be revealed. One example in which proteomics has led to advancement in clinical diagnosis is with Creutzfeldt–Jakob disease. Cerebrospinal fluid analysis using 2-dimensional gel electrophoresis has revealed two proteins, p130 and p131, which are members of the 14-3-3 family, which can discriminate between Creutzfeldt–Jakob disease and other forms of dementia.

References

Banks R E, Dunn M J, Hochstrasser D F et al 2000 Proteomics: new perspectives, new biomedical opportunities. Lancet 356:1749–1756

88.   DNA microarrays

A. **F**   B. **T**   C. **F**   D. **T**   E. **T**

DNA microarrays (microarrays, cDNA arrays, gene expression arrays, gene chips) consist of thousands of individual gene sequences bound to a 1–2 cm square glass or silica slide. They allow the simultaneous detection of thousands of specific DNA or RNA sequences, unlike conventional techniques, which use a single DNA probe. mRNA from samples (e.g. body tissues or fluids) can be reverse transcribed into fluorescently labelled cDNA and then incubated with the DNA microarray under conditions that allow each gene on the array to hybridise with its complementary cDNA in the sample. After washing unhybridised cDNA away, the microarray can be analysed. The intensity of fluorescence at each DNA spot corresponds to the level of gene expression in that position on the microarray slide. By adding two different samples (e.g. control and patient), each labelled with a different fluorescent tag, it is possible to see the differences in gene expression in disease compared with normal samples.

Oligonucleotide arrays consist of slides with short oligonucleotide sequences arranged on them. mRNA from samples is converted to cDNA, which is then used as a template to generate fluorescent complementary RNA (cRNA), which in turn can be hybridised with the array producing fluorescence signals with intensity corresponding to the level of expression of mRNA within the sample.

DNA microarrays have limited clinical application at present. However, once genetic variants to common conditions have been identified, the technology is in place to type large numbers of patients and this will have profound implications for both prophylaxis and tailored treatment approaches.

References

Aitman T J 2001 DNA microarrays in medical practice. British Medical Journal 323:611–615

Brugarolas J, Haynes B F, Nevins J R 2001 Towards a genomic-based diagnosis. Lancet 357:249–250

89. The cell cycle

A. **F**   B. **T**   C. **T**   D. **T**   E. **T**

Cell proliferation is a highly organised and regulated process. The eukaryotic cell cycle consists of two main phases:

interphase – during which the cell grows and DNA is synthesised
mitosis – when the single cell divides to produce two daughter cells.

Interphase itself is subdivided into three phases, with two gap phases (G1 and G2) separated by an S-phase during which DNA is synthesised. Within the G1 phase is the restriction point. This is the point at which the cell no longer requires mitogens to undergo cell division. Early G1 phase (before the restriction point) is growth dependent. If growth factor stimulus is sufficient during this phase the cell will progress through the restriction point. Late G1 (after the restriction point) is growth factor independent. If growth factor stimulus is insufficient during early G1, the cell exits the cell cycle and enters G0, a quiescent state. The cell can be stimulated to exit G0 and return to the cell cycle at early G1 by reintroduction of mitogens.

Checkpoints during the cell cycle assess whether the cell is competent to progress through replication. Control is overseen in particular by a series of proteins, the cyclins, cyclin-dependent kinases and cyclin-dependent kinase inhibitors. These in turn are under the influence of cell signalling pathways that transmit and integrate external cellular signals, for example from membrane bound receptors.

Cell cycle control is essential to prevent inappropriate cell proliferation. The critical role of checkpoints within the cell cycle is highlighted when control is lost. Genes involved in cell cycle control tend to be oncogenes whose mutation leads to aberrant cell growth or cell death (apoptosis). One such oncogene, *rb*, produces the retinoblastoma protein (pRb), which regulates the G1/S transition. Differences in phosphorylation of pRb determine whether it binds the E2F family of transcription factors and consequently whether transition from G1 to S-phase is inhibited or promoted.

p53 is stabilised in response to DNA damage, for example due to ultraviolet (UV) irradiation or chemical damage, and accumulates in the nucleus. p53 can induce apoptosis in this situation but it can also work by inducing cell cycle arrest at the G1 phase – a vital barrier to the proliferation of cells with damaged DNA. Loss of normal p53 function, which is present in 50% of cancers, removes this block on uncontrolled cell proliferation.

Reference

Sampath D, Plunkett W 2001 Design of new anticancer therapies targeting cell cycle checkpoint pathways. Current Opinons in Oncology 13(6):484–490

IMMUNOLOGY
True/False answers

90.   Intravenous immunoglobulin

A. **F**   B. **T**   C. **T**   D. **F**   E. **T**

Intravenous immune globulin is used in the treatment of immune deficiencies (primary and secondary) and in autoimmune disorders, including idiopathic thrombocytopenic purpura, Guillain–Barré syndrome, chronic inflammatory demyelinating polyneuropathy, myasthenia gravis, Kawasaki disease, steroid-resistant dermatomyositis and antineutrophil cytoplasmic antibody (ANCA)-positive vasculitis. It is prepared from pooled plasma samples obtained from between 5000 and 10 000 donors and contains intact IgG molecules with a distribution of subclasses corresponding to that seen in normal human serum. It also contains cytokines, CD4, CD8 and HLA molecules. The half-life of infused immunoglobulin is 3 weeks. Its immunomodulatory response in inflammation and autoimmune conditions is thought to be mediated via a number of mechanisms.

Fc receptors are expressed on the surface of most immune system cells and bind to the Fc portion of antibody. Broadly speaking, they can be activatory (FcγRI, IIA, III) or inhibitory (FcγRIIB). The blockade of Fc receptors on macrophages is thought to be one mechanism by which intravenous immunoglobulin prevents platelet consumption in idiopathic thrombocytopenic purpura. More recent work in animal models suggests that it might also exert its effects by upregulating the inhibitory receptor, FcγRIIB, thus reducing macrophage activity and subsequent clearance of opsonised platelets.

IgG can bind a number of complement components (the C_H2 part of the Fc portion binds Clq and the Fab portion between C_H1 and V_L domains to C3b and C4b). This ability is important in its use in the management of dermatomyositis. The administration of intravenous immunoglobulin in dermatomyositis is associated with decreased plasma levels of membrane-attack complex and a reduction in amounts of C3b and membrane attack complex deposited in endomysial capillaries.

In Kawasaki disease, the administration of intravenous immunoglobulin is associated with a reduction in interleukin-1 levels and an increase in plasma interleukin-1 receptor antagonist. Similarly, in Guillain–Barré syndrome, a reduction in interleukin-1β has been noted following treatment.

Immunoglobulin can interact with idiotypes (serologically defined constituents of the variable region) of autoantibodies. Thus anti-idiotype antibodies can neutralise autoantibodies against factor VIII in autoimmune haemophilia and suppress ANCA levels in patients with vasculitis.

References

Jayne D R, Chapel H, Adu D et al 2000 Intravenous immunoglobulin for ANCA-associated systemic vasculitis with persistant disease activity. Quarterly Journal of Medicine 93:433–439

Kazatchkine M D, Kaveri S V 2001 Immunomodulation of autoimmune and inflammatory diseases with intravenous immune globulin. New England Journal of Medicine 345:747–755

Samuelsson A, Towers T L, Ravetch J V 2001 Anti-inflammatory activity of IVIG mediated through the inhibitory Fc receptor. Science 291:484–486

91. Monoclonal antibodies

A. **F**   B. **F**   C. **T**   D. **F**   E. **T**

A monoclonal antibody is derived from a single B cell clone. Initially, these clones were created by fusing murine B cells with lymphoma cells. Therapeutic monoclonal antibodies have been modified to contain only a murine-variable fragment (chimeric antibodies) or a murine complementarity-determining region (humanised antibodies) in order to minimise allergies and adverse reactions. A number of monoclonal antibodies are now licensed for use in the UK:

- *Infliximab* is a chimeric antibody that binds to both free and membrane bound TNF-α. A number of controlled clinical trials have shown significant clinical improvement and induction of remission in patients with fistularising and resistant Crohn's disease. Infliximab is also licensed for use in refractory rheumatoid arthritis. A large, double-blind, placebo-controlled trial using infliximab in combination with methotrexate versus methotrexate alone in 428 patients with rheumatoid arthritis found that patients in the infliximab group had a significant clinical improvement by standard criteria when compared to controls, although a number went onto develop anti-dsDNA antibodies during the course of treatment. Infliximab has also been used in the treatment of Behçet's disease and Wegener's granulomatosus.
- *Etanercept* (a recombinant IgG1 Fc fragment fused to two p75 TNF receptors) is another anti-TNF agent used in the treatment of refractory rheumatoid arthritis. It is given as a twice-weekly subcutaneous injection.

Several monoclonal antibodies have been used in oncology/haematology in the treatment of malignancies:

- *Rituximab* (a chimeric IgG1 that recognises CD20 expressed on B cells) is used in the treatment of refractory low-grade or follicular B cell lymphoma. It binds to CD20+ B cells and induces destruction either by apoptosis or removal by antibody-dependent cellular cytotoxicity. Normal CD20+ B cells are able to regenerate from early pre-B cells (CD20–).
- *Trastuzumab* is a humanised IgG1 antibody that targets the extracellular domain of the HER2 growth receptor (which has

intrinsic tyrosine kinase activity). The overexpression of the *HER2* gene predicts a worse prognosis in breast cancer. Trials in HER2-positive breast cancer patients who progress despite standard chemotherapy, have shown that 4% of patients achieve a complete response and a further 11% a partial response with use of weekly infusions of trastuzumab.

- *Abciximab* is a chimeric monoclonal antibody that blocks the platelet membrane glycoprotein IIb/IIIa receptor, preventing binding of fibrinogen/von Willebrand factor and thus inhibiting platelet crosslinking and aggregation. It has been found to be of particular benefit in patients with unstable angina or myocardial infarction undergoing coronary angioplasty (reduced death, infarction, revascularisation procedures in the EPILOG trial).
- *Basiliximab* is an IgG1k chimeric antibody that targets CD25 and can be used in renal transplantation in the prophylaxis of acute rejection.

References

Bell S, Kamm M A 2000 Antibodies to TNFα as treatment for Crohn's disease. Lancet 355:858–860

Breedveld F C 2000 Therapeutic monoclonal antibodies. Lancet 355:735–740

Cobleigh M A, Vogel C L, Tripathy D et al 1999 Multinational study of efficacy and safety of humanised anti-HER2 monoclonal antibody in women who have HER-2 overexpressing metastatic breast cancer that has progressed after chemotherapy. Journal of Clinical Oncology 17:2639–2648

Drewe E, Powell R J 2002 Clinically useful monoclonal antibodies in treatment. Journal of Clinical Pathology 55:81–85

Pisetsky D S, St Clair E W 2001 Progress in the treatment of rheumatoid arthritis. Journal of the American Medical Association 286:2787–2790

92.   Pathogenesis of autoimmune disease

A. **F**   B. **T**   C. **F**   D. **T**   E. **T**

Autoimmune diseases, although individually rare, affect a significant proportion of the population. The clinical spectrum of autoimmunity is vast and ranges from diseases that are relatively cell or organ specific, such as type I diabetes mellitus, to those that are systemic, such as systemic lypus erythematosus. Precise mechanisms of pathogenesis remain obscure but it is clear that a low level of autoreactivity in B and T cell repertoires is physiological. For disease to occur, pathways of control must become aberrant. This is likely to require a combination of susceptibility factors, probably genetic, and an environmental trigger, possibly an infectious agent. This process might require a specific mixture of inflammatory cytokines and, once tissue injury has occurred, is likely to be self-perpetuating.

A few autoimmune diseases, such as autoimmune lymphoproliferative syndrome and the syndrome of polyglandular endocrinopathy with candidiasis and ectodermal dysplasia, are due to single gene mutations. However, most autoimmune diseases are polygenic, with multiple susceptibility genes working in concert to produce the abnormal phenotype. It is likely that autoimmune genetic polymorphisms occur in the normal population and only when present with other susceptibility genes does autoimmunity arise.

Patients with autoimmune lymphoproliferative syndrome have a defect in the gene encoding the Fas protein or its receptor. Fas (CD95) is a member of the nerve growth factor/tumour necrosis factor receptor superfamily and can initiate a signal transduction cascade leading to apoptosis. It is expressed at high levels in activated lymphocytes and acts as a major pathway for the peripheral deletion of antigen-primed lymphocytes. Mice homozygous for the *lpr* or *gdl* mutation (leading to non-functional Fas or FasL proteins, respectively) have increased numbers of B and T cells, autoantibodies and develop lymphadenopathy and immune-complex-mediated glomerulonephritis. Further evidence that aberrant mechanisms of apoptosis can lead to autoimmunity comes from the overexpression of the proto-oncogene *bcl-2*. *Bcl-2* encodes a 24-kDa membrane-associated protein, which protects cells from apoptosis. Transgenic overexpression of Bcl-2 in B cells prevents apoptosis, blocks peripheral self-tolerance and can predispose to autoantibody production and immune-mediated glomerulonephritis.

A reduction in the activation threshold of T and B cells can lead to the development of autoimmunity. Upon antigen binding to the B cell receptor, the net effects of positive and negative regulatory molecules determine B cell activation thresholds. If the balance between these inputs is disturbed then autoimmunity can result. A decrease or absence of negative regulators, for example, CD32 (FcγRIIB, a single chain transmembrane glycoprotein expressed on B cells, macrophages, neutrophils and other cells of the myeloid lineage), or CD22 (a B cell-specific negative regulator) or of downstream molecules in the inhibitory pathway such as Lyn and SHP-1 leads to B cell hyperactivity, autoantibody production and even SLE in murine models. Conversely, overexpression of B cell activators, for example, CD19 (a cell surface glycoprotein expressed exclusively on B cells, in a complex with CD21 (complement receptor 2), CD81, and Leu 13) can also lead to autoimmunity in mouse models. In addition, upregulation of CD19 has been noted in patients with systemic sclerosis. Thus by lowering the activation threshold on B cells, CD19 overexpression could contribute to the breakdown of tolerance and the development of autoimmune disease.

The complement system is known to be important in facilitating the disposal of immune complexes by the mononuclear phagocytic system. Immune complexes, which fix complement, are transported in the blood (bound to erythrocytes via complement receptor 1) to the spleen and liver where they are disposed of by phagocytic cells. Hereditary complement deficiencies (particularly early complement components, such as C1q, C2 and C4) predispose to the development of SLE, presumably due to the accumulation of immune complexes. This is supported by the observation that C1q-deficient mice have a significantly reduced splenic uptake of immune complexes compared with controls and develop lupus.

Cytokines appear to have variable effects in different autoimmune diseases. TNF-α overexpression appears to contribute to the inflammatory component of disease in patients with rheumatoid arthritis who benefit from treatment with TNF-α blockade. However, in approximately 10% of patients treated with anti-TNF therapies, antinuclear antibodies develop and, in a smaller proportion, SLE. The role of cytokines is therefore far from clear.

References

Bolland S, Ravetch J V 2000 Spontaneous autoimmune disease in FcgRIIB-deficient mice results in strain-specific epistasis. Immunity 13:277–285

Davidson A, Diamond B 2001 Autoimmune disease. New England Journal of Medicine 345(5):340–350

Kamradt T, Mitchison N A 2001 Tolerance and autoimmunity. New England Journal of Medicine 334:655–664

O'Shea J J, Ma A, Lipsky P 2002 Cytokines and autoimmunity. Nature Reviews. Immunology 2:37–45

93.   Immunotherapy for cancer

A. **T**   B. **F**   C. **T**   D. **F**   E. **T**

It has been known for a number of years that, in some circumstances, the immune system is capable of recognising and removing tumour cells. Cytotoxic T cells are one of the critical effector cells in this response. This interaction relies upon the recognition, by T cells, of antigen presented on the surface of a class I major histocompatibility complex (MHC). In addition, a costimulatory signal is required and, in the absence of this, T cells might become tolerant to the antigen. Antigen-presenting cells, such as dendritic cells and macrophages, capture and process tumour antigens released during cell lysis and present them in the context of MHC class II antigens to antigen-specific CD4 T helper cells. These T cells then produce a number of cytokines, such as interleukin-2 and granulocyte–macrophage colony stimulating factor (GM-CSF), that stimulate further CD8 T cells and CD4 T cells to proliferation and activation.

Despite these measures, some tumour cells manage to avoid recognition and removal by the immune system. Possible mechanisms include loss of expression of MHC class I antigens, loss of expression of costimulatory molecules, and poor recognition of tumour antigens by T cells due to the fact that they are self-antigens. Tumour cells can also counterattack the immune system, producing immunosuppressive cytokines, such as transforming growth factor β and interleukin-10, or by expressing apoptosis-inducing molecules on their surface (for example, Fas ligand).

The ideal tumour target antigen should be strongly immunogenic and expressed exclusively on tumour cells. In reality, most tumour antigens are expressed to some degree on normal tissues, making the immune response generated somewhat non-specific. Whole irradiated tumour cells combined with an immunological adjuvant, such as BCG, have been used as anticancer vaccines. Clinical studies in patients with colorectal cancer have shown this to be safe and moderately effective, at least in terms of recurrence-free survival in patients with an initial low tumour load. Whole-cell tumour vaccine trials in patients with melanoma and renal cells carcinoma continue.

The immunogenicity of whole-cell tumour vaccines can also be increased by genetically modifying the cells, for example by adding genes that encode proimmunogenic cytokines. A GM-CSF-secreting renal cell carcinoma vaccine has been developed and has shown some promise in early human studies. Antigenic peptides derived from cancer antigens used alone or in combination with adjuvants or cytokines are also potential vaccines. Candidate tumour antigens include MAGE-3 and NY-ESO-1 (cancer-testis antigens), and Melan-A/MART 1, tyrosinase and gp100 (melanocyte differentiation antigens).

Dendritic cell vaccines are now being developed in cancer immunotherapy. Dendritic cells are potent antigen-presenting cells and can be generated from patient's peripheral blood monocytes or CD34+ haemopoeitic stem cells. They can then be loaded with tumour antigens and injected into patients, where they interact with antigen-specific CD4 T cells to produce an immune response. Dendritic cell vaccines are being developed and trialled in melanoma and metastatic renal cell carcinoma. The introduction of tumour-antigen-encoding genes into dendritic cells could provide a renewable source of antigen for presentation.

A graft versus leukaemia effect has been noted if allogeneic lymphocytes are infused into patients with chronic myeloid leukaemia. It is thought that donor T cells recognise host MHC antigens, as well as tumour antigens. However, these T cells might also recognise healthy host cells (graft versus host disease). To overcome this, donor T cells can be modified so as to sensitise cells to specific drugs. If a graft versus host response does then occur, the lymphocytes can be specifically eliminated. Other approaches involve the selection and expansion of allogeneic T cells, which are more selectively toxic to tumour cells prior to infusion into the host.

References

Armstrong A, Eaton D, Ewing J C 2001 Cellular immunotherapy for cancer. British Medical Journal 323:1289–1293

Jager E, Jager D, Knuth A 2002 Clinical cancer vaccine trials. Current Opinion in Immunology 14:178–182

Pardoll D M 2002 Spinning molecular immunology into successful immunotherapy. Nature Reviews, Immunology 2:227–238

94.   Regulatory T cells

A. **F**   B. **T**   C. **T**   D. **F**   E. **T**

T cells that were able to suppress immune responses were first described in the 1970s. They were initially proposed to mediate their effects via secreted antigen-specific factors. Failure to identify these factors over the ensuing years led to some questions over the very existence of suppressor T cells. However, in the past decade their presence has been confirmed and they have gradually been characterised.

T regulatory or suppressor cells make up a minor population of CD4+ T cells (approximately 10%) and coexpress the interleukin-2 receptor (IL-2R) α chain (CD25). CD4+CD25+ T cells are also the only T cells to express cytotoxic T lymphocyte antigen 4. As well as occurring naturally as part of the T cell population, oral administration of antigen can also induce suppressor T cells. They are powerful inhibitors of T cell activation both in vitro and in vivo.

The mechanism by which suppression is mediated is unclear, but it seems that cell-to-cell contact is required. Early in vitro studies have indicated that when cultured with CD25– T cells, inhibition of these cells could be achieved, but required activation of CD25+ cells via their T cell receptor. This CD25+-mediated suppression seems to involve inhibition of the transcription of interleukin-2, in that it can be abrogated by addition of exogenous IL-2. It is also possible that engagement of cytotoxic T lymphocyte antigen 4 by its ligands CD80 or CD86 on antigen-presenting cells is involved in the induction of suppression. Evidence for this is again based on cell culture systems in which CD4+CD25+ suppression can be reversed by addition of anti-CTLA4 antibody.

It is thought that regulatory T cells might have an important role in preventing autoimmunity. In animal models, depletion of CD25+ cells with anti-CD25 antibody does not lead to the development of autoimmune disease. However, autoimmune diseases induced by CD25– T cells are seen on transfer of CD25– T cells to mice that lack CD25+ cells. Thus, regulatory T cells might inhibit autoimmunity by competing with CD25– cells for space, cytokines or co-stimulatory signals. It has also been noted that immunisation of CD25-depleted mice with the K/T ATPase results in autoimmune gastritis. It is therefore possible that a non-specific inflammatory response could supply a necessary second signal for the activation of CD25– T cells in the absence of CD25+ suppressors.

Manipulation of CD25+ suppressors can be used to produce an enhanced response to tumour antigens used in vaccines. Several studies have shown that the antibody-mediated depletion of CD25+ T cells facilitates the induction of tumour immunity. The combined use of CD25 depletion and CTLA4 blockade was found to be more effective than either approach used separately for the enhancement of immune response to a melanoma vaccine. CD25+ T cell depletion followed by immunisation might also be of use in enhancing immune responses to conventional vaccines for infectious agents, particularly vaccines that are weakly immunogenic, such as HIV vaccines.

Another possible clinical application of suppressor T cell manipulation would be in the treatment of autoimmune diseases. Clearly, enhancement of the number and activity of CD4+CD25+ T cells could be of use in dampening an aggressive autoimmune or allergic process. However, knowledge of the normal physiology and interactions of these elusive cells is less than complete and still requires expansion.

References

Sakaguchi S 2001 Regulatory T cells: key controllers of immunologic self tolerance. Cell 101:455–458

Shevach E M 2002 CD4+ CD25+ suppressor T cells: more questions than answers. Nature Reviews, Immunology 2:389–400

95.   Vaccine development

A. **T**   B. **F**   C. **T**   D. **F**   E. **F**

Several new technologies are under development for the production and delivery of vaccines to a wide range of conditions. Vaccines are being investigated not only for a broad range of infections, including HIV, haemorrhagic fevers, malaria and dengue, but also for autoimmune diseases, including diabetes (with the aim of inducing immune tolerance), for atherosclerosis, neurodegenerative diseases including targeting the production of amyloid in Alzheimer's disease. Tumour- and person-specific vaccines against several malignant diseases, including melanoma, leukaemia and colorectal cancer, are also under investigation and it might also be possible to vaccinate against drugs of addiction, such as cocaine and nicotine.

Most current vaccines are based on either live attenuated viruses or bacteria (e.g. polio, BCG), or killed preparations (e.g. influenza). More recently, acellular, or fragmented vaccines, e.g. for pertussis have been developed. In future, DNA vaccines could well become the norm. The great advantage of DNA vaccines is that a specific antigen can be encoded on DNA, allowing precise targeting of the immune response. This allows the immune response to be targeted to the most antigenic sequence, thus enhancing the effectiveness of the vaccine. DNA can be inserted into viral vectors or it can be inserted into free bacterial plasmids, which are attached to gold beads or a similar substrate before being injected into the host. Unfortunately, aside from some notable successes, e.g. hepatitis B, most trials of DNA vaccines in humans have not produced a sufficiently vigorous immune response to date.

Advances in vaccine delivery are also emerging into clinical practice. A live attenuated influenza vaccine has been tested, which can be delivered via an intranasal spray with excellent efficacy, and promising results have been obtained with a new *Streptococcus pneumoniae* vaccine using polysaccharides conjugated to protein. This conjugate produces a T-cell-dependent immune response, rather than the T-cell-independent response seen with the traditional polysaccharide vaccine. Polysaccharide vaccines tend to produce weak immunity in children below the age of 2; the new conjugated vaccine is expected to circumvent this problem.

Enteric infections can be targeted with oral vaccines, as has been the case with polio for many years. A novel approach to such oral vaccinations is the creation of transgenic plants, e.g. potatoes, expressing antigens. Such an approach has produced a useful immune response to a transgenic enterotoxin subunit. Cutaneous application of cholera or *Escherichia coli* enterotoxins might also be able to stimulate an immune response in the gut mucosa against the toxins responsible for the symptoms of these enteric infections.

Reference

Poland G P, Murray D, Bonilla-Guerrero R 2002 New vaccine development. British Medical Journal 324:1315–1319

CARDIOLOGY
True/False answers

96.   Aldosterone receptor blockade

A. **T**   B. **F**   C. **F**   D. **T**   E. **F**

Aldosterone is the main mineralocorticoid excreted by the adrenal cortex and promotes renal retention of sodium and with it water and loss of potassium. Secretion of aldosterone is stimulated by angiotensin II. Blockade of the aldosterone receptor with spironolactone allows loss of sodium with water. It was previously thought not to provide any benefit to patients with heart failure who were already taking an ACE inhibitor because ACE inhibitors would already have reduced the levels of aldosterone. In addition, the combination was thought to potentially cause serious hyperkalaemia. However, more recent evidence suggests that ACE inhibitors suppress the production of aldosterone only transiently, and that therefore the direct inhibition of the aldosterone receptor might provide additional benefit. Serum potassium has an important role in the regulation of aldosterone production and thus it might become the overriding control in patients treated with ACE inhibitors.

The Randomised Aldactone Evaluation Study (RALES) showed that patients with severe heart failure (NYHA class III or IV) with poor ejection fraction (less than 35%) gained significant benefit by taking low-dose spironolactone (25–50 mg once daily). To be included, all patients had to be already taking an ACE inhibitor, if tolerated, and a loop diuretic. Most patients were also on digoxin, and a minority was taking aspirin (36%) and beta-blockers (10%). The primary endpoint used was all-cause mortality and this showed a significant reduction in the arm treated with spironolactone. This was mainly due to cardiac death, particularly from progressive heart failure and sudden death. The spironolactone-treated group also showed improvement in symptoms and a reduction in hospitalisations from heart failure.

These effects are not thought to be solely due to the effect of aldosterone on the kidneys; significant benefit was seen at the low dose of 25 mg, but little diuretic effect. Aldosterone has been shown to cause myocardial fibrosis, vascular fibrosis and baroreceptor dysfunction, and the benefits of spironolactone might well be in part due to blockade of these effects. Side-effects seen from spironolactone include gynaecomastia and breast pain.

Reference

Pitt B, Zannad F, Remme W J et al (Randomized Aldactone Evaluation Study Investigators) 1999 The effect of spironolactone on morbidity and mortality in patients with severe heart failure. New England Journal of Medicine 341:709–717

---

97.   Cardiac resynchronisation therapy

A. **T**   B. **F**   C. **T**   D. **F**   E. **F**

Patients with severe heart failure have both significant morbidity and mortality. There are high levels of hospitalisation and patients are often very symptomatic with shortness of breath, reduced exercise capacity and tiredness. Drug therapy is clearly the mainstay of treatment for most of these patients but there are some patients who remain symptomatic despite optimal drug treatment.

About 30% of patients with dilated left ventricles and heart failure have intraventricular conduction delay with either left or right bundle branch block. This leads to loss of coordinated ventricular contraction. By a process known as mechanoenergetic uncoupling, it is believed that this dyssynchronous contraction worsens the already impaired use of energy by the heart. It is also known that patients with pathologically wide QRS complexes have a worse outcome than patients with normal QRS duration.

Technology is now available to simultaneously pace both the left and right ventricles at the same time. In addition to the usual two leads positioned in the right atrial appendage and right ventricular apex, a third lead is positioned in the coronary sinus. This has been shown to effectively pace the left ventricular free wall and septum.

Two studies have now shown improvement in symptoms and hospitalisation rates in patients with biventricular pacing systems; both were randomised trials. The first smaller study included only 67 patients with severe heart failure (NYHA class III) and this study was blinded to the patient only. All patients had a pacing system implanted and were randomised to full therapy or fixed rate ventricular (VVI) pacing only. At 3 months, both groups were reprogrammed to cross over. Only 48 patients completed the 6-month study but results were encouraging, with improvement in symptoms and reductions in hospitalisation.

A much larger double-blinded randomised controlled trial has now been published. The MIRACLE study randomised 453 individuals with moderate to severe heart failure (mostly NYHA class III) and wide QRS to active cardiac resynchronisation or medical therapy alone. Most patients were already taking digoxin, diuretics and an ACE inhibitor; over 50% were on beta-blockers. Medications were not altered if possible during the follow-up period. All patients had a device implanted but patients in the control group were left with the pacemaker switched off for 6 months, and no crossover was allowed. This study showed significant improvements in 6-min walk test distances, functional class, quality of life, time on treadmill testing and ejection fraction. There was also a reduction in hospitalisation for heart failure.

No study so far has shown any improvement in survival. Patients with ventricular tachycardia or at high risk of sudden cardiac death should have an implantable cardioverter defibrillator if they meet implantation criteria as biventricular pacing alone has not been shown to reduce sudden cardiac death. Newer systems have been developed and can provide both defibrillation and biventricular pacing; these could be considered in this subgroup of patients.

References

Abraham W T, Fisher W G, Smith A L et al 2002 Cardiac resynchronization in chronic heart failure. New England Journal of Medicine 346:1845–1853

Cazeau S, Leclercq C, Lavergne T et al 2001 Effects of multisite biventricular pacing in patients with heart failure and intraventricular conduction delay. New England Journal of Medicine 344:873–880

98.   Statin therapy

A. **T**   B. **T**   C. **T**   D. **F**   E. **F**

The publication of the Heart Protection Study has altered management strategies for all patients at risk of vascular events. This UK-based study followed-up over 20 000 patients for a mean period of over 5 years. The study was a randomised controlled trial and was analysed with intention-to-treat. The inclusion criteria included age 40–80 years and any of:

- any coronary disease (myocardial infarction, angina, unstable angina, coronary angioplasty, coronary artery bypass surgery)
- any non-coronary artery disease (ischaemic stroke, peripheral arterial disease, peripheral revascularisation with bypass, angioplasty or endarterectomy)
- diabetes
- hypertension (if also male and 65 years old or more).

Blood cholesterol was measured but did not affect inclusion. In this group of high-risk patients, a highly significant reduction in both coronary and non-coronary vascular death was seen. There was no effect on non-vascular death. Importantly, there was no significant difference between the groups for liver impairment, and myopathy and rhabdomyolysis were extremely rare; five patients in the statin group compared to three in the control arm. There were no fatalities due to rhabdomyolysis.

Early studies using statins had suggested associated problems, including increased risk of suicide, worsening of obstructive airways disease and reduction in osteoporosis and fractures. There was no evidence from this study that any of these conditions were associated with statin therapy.

Importantly, the findings from this study seem to remain true for all subgroups, including older people, diabetics and patients with peripheral arterial disease. When subgroup analysis was performed on different levels of LDL cholesterol it was found that patients with LDL cholesterol of 3.0 mmol/L or less still gained significant benefit from statin therapy.

Reference

MRC/BHF 2002 Heart protection study of cholesterol lowering with simvastatin in 20,536 high-risk individuals: a randomised placebo-controlled trial. Lancet 360:7–22

99. Clopidogrel

A. **F**   B. **F**   C. **F**   D. **F**   E. **T**

Clopidogrel is a thienopyridine derivative that blocks the activation of platelets by adenosine diphosphate (ADP). The drug irreversibly binds ADP to the platelet receptor, preventing activation of the GpIIb–IIIa complex. This complex is the major receptor for fibrinogen on platelets and blocking the activation of this receptor prevents platelet aggregation. There is also experimental evidence that clopidogrel not only prevents both arterial and venous thrombosis, but also reduces atherogenesis in several species.

One major study has been published investigating the effects of clopidogrel in patients with acute coronary syndromes. The CURE study (Clopidogrel in Unstable angina to prevent Recurrent Events) was designed to test the benefit of clopidogrel in patients admitted with acute coronary syndromes without ST segment elevation. Over 12 000 patients were randomised to either aspirin with clopidogrel or aspirin with placebo. Endpoints included composite death from cardiovascular causes, non-fatal myocardial infarction and stroke. The study showed that this composite endpoint did show a significant difference between the two groups, with the active arm having fewer events, but there was no significant difference between the groups in death from cardiovascular causes, non-Q-wave or Q wave myocardial infarction, stroke or indeed death from non-cardiovascular causes. Furthermore, there was a significantly higher risk of major bleeding complications in the aspirin with clopidogrel group, although there was no increased risk of haemorrhagic stroke or life-threatening bleeding.

A recent report in the *Drug and Therapeutics Bulletin* summaries this study. It concludes that for every 100 patients with acute coronary syndrome without ST elevation, adding clopidogrel to aspirin will prevent two cardiovascular deaths/non-fatal myocardial infarctions/strokes but will cause major bleeding in one patient. On this basis the authors were unable to recommend routine use of clopidogrel in this patient group.

Furthermore, there is good evidence to suggest that this group of patients should be being treated with glycoprotein IIb/IIIa inhibitors, and there is no evidence to suggest that the addition of clopidogrel to this therapy in addition to aspirin has any benefit. There could be a place for the use of clopidogrel in patients in whom glycoprotein IIb/IIIa inhibitors are contraindicated, although at the present time this use is not licensed.

References

Clopidogrel and acute coronary syndrome. Drug and Therapeutics Bulletin 2002 40:41–42

Yusuf S, Zhao F, Mehta S R 2001 Effects of clopidogrel in addition to aspirin in patients with acute coronary syndromes without ST-segment elevation. New England Journal of Medicine 345:494–502

100.   Asymptomatic aortic stenosis

A. **T**   B. **F**   C. **F**   D. **F**   E. **T**

There is much literature available to confirm that once severe aortic stenosis causes the patient symptoms, the chance of prolonged event-free survival is low, and these patients benefit from valve surgery. Most cardiologists define aortic stenosis as a valve area of < 1.0 cm^2. Alternatively, the peak velocity of blood flow through the aortic valve can be measured by echocardiography. To eject the same volume of blood through a narrow orifice requires the blood to pass through at a higher velocity to maintain the same cardiac output. This flow velocity can be used to estimate the pressure gradient across the valve by use of the Bernoulli equation, which states that:

$$\text{the pressure difference} = 4 \times \text{velocity}^2$$

Some physicians use the peak velocity as an indicator of stenosis severity, and usually in this situation a peak velocity of > 3 m/s is considered significant; > 4 m/s is considered as severe. Pressure gradients are derived from the flow velocity; a peak gradient of > 30 mmHg is usually taken to be significant.

However, the natural history and outcomes of patients without any symptoms have until recently been understudied, with the result that few consistent guidelines have been produced. With the increased availability of echocardiography, more of these patients are being detected, and so guidelines have been drawn up by the European Society of Cardiology.

According to a number of series, the average increase in mean gradient is 7 mmHg per year. Valve area reduces by 0.02 to 0.3 cm^2 per year. Valves narrow more quickly in patients with degenerative disease than in those with congenital bicuspid valves, and other predictors of progression include age, hypertension, smoking and hypercholesterolaemia.

Although a lack of symptoms suggests good outcome with respect to sudden death (< 0.3% per year) there is a high chance of events overall in this group, although some of the studies included in this analysis also included valve surgery itself as an event. One study suggested that event-free survival in patients with aortic flow velocities of < 3 m/s was 84%, whereas those with velocities of > 4 m/s had a 21% chance of event-free survival without surgery at 2 years.

Exercise testing is contraindicated in all symptomatic patients with aortic stenosis. However, there has been recent evidence to suggest that exercising patients who are asymptomatic might not only be relatively safe, but can also provide useful prognostic information that can help guide the decision to refer for surgery. Poor prognostic indicators include:

- symptoms of dyspnoea, angina or syncope
- failure of blood pressure to rise > 20 mmHg, or a fall in blood pressure
- inability to reach 80% predicted level of exercise for sex and age
- ST segment depression of > 2 mm in the absence of causes other than aortic stenosis
- arrhythmias.

Measuring the 'pull back' gradient across the aortic valve at the time of coronary angiography is not necessary in patients with severe aortic stenosis as measured by echocardiography unless the echocardiogram is of inadequate quality or there is a discrepancy between the echocardiographic finding and the clinical picture. Echocardiography can provide highly accurate estimates of valve gradients in the hands of an experienced operator, and attempting to pass a catheter across a stenosed valve carries a risk of complications.

The recent European guidelines suggest that surgery can be considered in patients with severe aortic stenosis compared with their body size (< 0.6 cm/m^2 body surface area) especially if any of the above exercise criteria are met, there is a rapid progression in peak velocity over time, or there is left ventricular dysfunction.

Reference

Recommendations on the management of the asymptomatic patient with valvular heart disease. European Heart Journal 2002 23:1253–1266

101. Exercise training in chronic heart failure

A. **F**   B. **F**   C. **T**   D. **T**   E. **F**

Years ago, exercise was discouraged for patients with chronic heart failure. Although bedresting can certainly help to mobilise oedema in the decompensated phase of the disease, inactivity leads to muscle atrophy and wasting. Although early studies suggested that strenuous exercise can have an adverse effect on ventricular function in heart failure, there is now a large body of evidence showing the beneficial effects of light to moderate exercise training in chronic heart failure.

Patients with chronic heart failure not only have impaired pump function but they suffer from changes to peripheral muscle function. Impaired blood flow, loss of type 1 fibres, lower mitochondrial numbers and early onset of anaerobic metabolism are all features. Muscles in chronic heart failure are easily fatigued and have lower strength on repetitive testing. Other systemic features of chronic heart failure include reduced efficiency of breathing, as well as increased sympathetic drive, increased renin–angiotensin–aldosterone system activity and increased levels of cytokines such as interleukin-6 and tumour necrosis factor. It is still unclear how loss of pump function leads to all of these abnormalities but there is good evidence now that feedback occurs, so that impaired muscle function can increase sympathetic drive and further reduce pump function over the long term.

Moderate exercise training can reverse the pathological changes in peripheral muscles, with consequent improvements in peak oxygen uptake (at least for stamina training) and exercise tolerance. Far from worsening cardiac function, some studies have shown small improvements in left ventricular size and ejection fraction after exercise training. Sympathetic drive and cytokine expression are reduced by exercise and the efficiency of respiration improves. All of these effects translate into improved exercise capacity, reduced symptoms and, in many studies, improved health-related quality of life. Different forms of exercise have different effects; weight training can improve muscle strength without a large effect on peak oxygen uptake, whereas endurance training and interval training improve muscle fatiguability and improve overall stamina.

One of the key unanswered questions is whether exercise training can reduce death and hospitalisation for heart failure. No study has yet been large enough to show this. The benefits of exercise are dependent on continued adherence; benefits are rapidly lost on discontinuing exercise. Exercise training has not been trialled in patients with marked fluid overload; such patients should be treated along standard lines with diuretics and ACE inhibitors to stabilise them prior to commencing a programme of exercise training. Studies to date have also excluded patients with aortic stenosis and a history of primary ventricular fibrillation or sustained ventricular tachycardia; it is therefore not clear whether exercise training can reduce the incidence of ventricular arrhythmias or sudden death.

References

Lloyd-Williams F, Mair F S, Leitner M 2002 Exercise training and heart failure: a systematic review of current evidence. British Journal of General Practice 52:47–55

Recommendations for exercise training in chronic heart failure patients. European Heart Journal 2001 22:125–135

Best-of-5 answers

102. Treatment of ventricular tachycardia

Answer: **E**

Guidelines published recently by NICE clearly lay out the indications for both primary and secondary prophylaxis for treating patients at risk of sudden cardiac death with implantable cardioverter defibrillators.

Sudden cardiac death claims 70 000–90 000 victims in the UK each year; this is over a quarter of all cardiovascular deaths. Most of these are secondary to ventricular arrhythmias – either ventricular tachycardia or ventricular fibrillation. The remaining sudden cardiac deaths are mostly from bradycardias.

Any patient who survives a sudden cardiac event is likely to have further events and is at high risk of death; 15% will have a further event within a year, and many of these will be fatal. The chance of surviving an out-of-hospital cardiac episode in the UK is only about 2%.

Patients who have are recommended to have an implantable cardioverter defibrillator include:

- Secondary prevention:
  - cardiac arrest due to ventricular tachycardia or ventricular fibrillation
  - spontaneous sustained ventricular tachycardia with haemodynamic compromise
  - sustained ventricular tachycardia without compromise but with: ejection fraction < 35% or class I–III NYHA class heart failure.
- Primary prevention – a confirmed history of myocardial infarction and all of:
  - non-sustained ventricular tachycardia on 24-h monitoring
  - inducible ventricular tachycardia on electrophysiological testing
  - ejection fraction < 35%
  - class I–III NYHA class heart failure.
- Any familial condition with high risk of sudden cardiac death, including:
  - long QT syndrome
  - hypertrophic cardiomyopathy
  - Brugada syndrome
  - arrhythmogenic right ventricular dysplasia.

These guidelines are based on evidence from a number of randomised controlled trials following patients postmyocardial infarction randomised to different therapies. To summarise, postinfarct patients benefited from an improved survival with beta-blockers and this improvement was most dramatic in patients with impaired left ventricular function. A number of trials using antiarrhythmic drugs, including flecainide, sotalol and amiodarone have failed to show improved survival in postinfarct patients. Indeed, flecainide and sotalol both caused an increased risk of death. Amiodarone seems to reduce arrhythmias without improving mortality.

The main trials looking at primary prevention using implantable cardioverter defibrillators were the MADIT and MUTT trials. These showed that patients with predefined variables, including poor ejection fraction, non-sustained ventricular tachycardia on monitoring and inducible ventricular tachycardia on stimulation, gained a survival benefit from having a defibrillator implanted.

For patients who have already had a sudden cardiac event and are in the secondary prevention group, a meta-analysis that combined data from three large randomised controlled trials has been performed. This showed that there is a consistent survival benefit in this group of patients with treatment with an implantable defibrillator.

References

Connolly S J, Hallstrom A P, Cappato R et al 2000 Meta-analysis of the implantable cardioverter defibrillator secondary prevention trials. AVID, CASH and CIDS studies. Antiarrhythmics vs implantable defibrillator study. Cardiac Arrest Study Hamburg. Canadian Implantable Defibrillator Study. European Heart Journal 21:2071–2078

Huikuri H V, Castellanos A, Myerburg R J 2001 Sudden death due to cardiac arrhythmias. New England Journal of Medicine 345:1473–1482

103. Drug-eluting stents

Answer: **B**

Ever since coronary angioplasty was introduced, restenosis has always been a problem. The rate of restenosis improved after the introduction of stents but still remains high, with up to 15–20% of patients demonstrating significant in-stent restenosis by 6 months. In-stent stenosis is thought to occur as a result of tissue reaction to the metal stent. This injury causes release of inflammatory mediators, which encourage smooth muscle cell migration and proliferation. This neointimal proliferation causes in-growth of tissue through the struts of the stent and eventually causes narrowing. Most of this reaction occurs within approximately 6 months from the stent implantation, although late stenosis may occur in a minority of cases.

Rapamycin (sirolimus) is a macrolide antifungal agent that was first identified in 1975 on Easter Island, in the South Pacific, when the actinomycete *Streptomyces hygroscopicus* was discovered; this produces the new antibiotic. By chance, rapamycin was also found to have anti-inflammatory, antimigratory and antiproliferative properties.

Originally, it was developed as a drug for use in organ transplant recipients to reduce organ rejection, but as a sideline it was also used to coat a metal stent on the assumption that it might reduce neointimal thickening. A blend of rapamycin and synthetic polymer applied to the stent allows gradual elution of rapamycin over a 30-day period.

The first randomised controlled trial using these coated stents has now been published. The RAVEL study randomised 238 patients with stable angina and single primary coronary stenosis of less than 18 mm long to angioplasty and stenting with either a standard metal stent or the rapamycin-coated stent. The coated stent group had no significant angiographically visible restenosis after a 1-year follow-up. There was no difference in mortality, myocardial infarction or bypass grafting but 27 of the 118 patients randomised to the control group required repeat angioplasty and stenting; none of the coated-stent group did. No episodes of acute thrombosis were seen in either group and both were routinely treated with both aspirin and clopidogrel. A substudy looking at those patients with diabetes found no difference between diabetic and non-diabetic patients in the drug-coated group.

The small total dose of drug and slow release method of administration accounts for the lack of side-effects seen; when administered at higher doses rapamycin can cause hyperlipidaemia and thrombocytopenia. Further data need to be seen to look at longer-term outcomes in more patients using these coated stents, and studies using stents coated with an alternative antiproliferative agent, paclitaxel, are keenly awaited.

Reference

Morice M C, Serruys P W, Sousa J E et al 2002 A randomized comparison of a sirolimus-eluting stent with a standard stent for coronary revascularization. New England Journal of Medicine 346:1773–1780

104. Driving following loss of consciousness

Answer: **D**

The legal basis of fitness to drive comes from the Road Traffic Act of 1988 and subsequent regulations especially the Motor Vehicles Regulations of 1996. The act describes three conditions:

1. A prescribed disability is any condition that renders the patient illegal to drive (e.g. uncontrolled epilepsy).
2. A relevant disability is any condition that renders the driver unsafe to drive (e.g. visual field defects).
3. A prospective disability is any condition that in time might cause one of the above (e.g. diabetes).

It is the duty of licence holders to inform the DVLA if they have any condition that might affect their ability to drive. Ultimately, it is the DVLA who has legal responsibility for this and therefore must be kept informed. Thus it is the responsibility of the doctor to inform patients that they must contact the DVLA if they have a condition that might impair their ability to drive; patients should be told that this is their legal responsiblity. If they cannot understand this, then you should do this directly yourself. Patients refusing to accept the diagnosis should be given advise not to drive and offered a second opinion. If they continue to drive you must try to persuade them to stop, and this might require informing next of kin. Finally, you can inform the DVLA directly, while also informing the patient you are doing this.

   This patient has an unexplained loss of consciousness and, because of the abnormal ECG and frequency of events, is at high risk of reoccurrence. His blackouts are likely to be due to arrhythmia, but other pathology such as aortic valve disease should be excluded. He therefore has a prescribed disability. The patient has a legal obligation to inform the DVLA and he must be told this. If the cause is not identified and treated, the patient cannot drive until he is event free for more than 6 months. If the cause is identified and treated, for example by valve replacement for aortic stenosis, then driving can recommence after 4 weeks. However, there are special rules for defibrillators. Following new implantation, driving cannot occur for at least 6 months presuming that no shock has been delivered. If therapy has been delivered there must not have been any incapacity within the preceding 5 years unless the cause of this has been defined and controlled.

   With respect to heavy goods vehicle licences, driving can resume after 3 months if the cause is identified and treated, or 1 year if not. If the patient has an implantable defibrillator a permanent bar occurs.

Reference

DVLA 2001 At-a-glance guide to the current medical standards of fitness to drive. DVLA, Swansea

105. Vitamin E in arterial disease

Answer: **D**

Two major studies have now been published that finally put to rest the debate about the effects of antioxidants in atherosclerotic arterial disease. LDL cholesterol can be modified by oxidation, which makes it more liable to deposition in arterial walls and to cause atherosclerosis. Prevention of this oxidative process with antioxidants has been shown in animal models to slow the progression of atherosclerotic disease. Vitamin E itself is a potent antioxidant of LDL cholesterol and, in vitro, prolongs resistance of LDL to oxidative damage. Vitamin C is an important antioxidant that, among other effects, can help to repair oxidised vitamin E. Several non-randomised observational studies have suggested a strong link between dietary intake of antioxidants and low levels of cardiovascular disease. For a long time it has been believed that supplementary vitamin E has been of potential benefit in patients at risk of cardiovascular events. A number of small studies did appear to confirm these findings but this was not seen in a number of larger studies looking at the effects of antioxidants in renal disease and cancer. Two of these studies suggested a link between antioxidant therapy and haemorrhagic stroke but this has not been shown since in larger studies. Two well-designed and large studies that looked into the effect of antioxidants in patients at high risk of cardiovascular disease have now been published.

The MRC/BHF Heart Protection Study randomised over 20 500 patients who had coronary disease, other arterial occlusive disease or diabetes to either placebo or a combination of vitamin E, C and beta-carotene with a 5-year follow-up. No difference was found between the groups for all-cause mortality, deaths due to vascular or non-vascular causes. There was no effect on non-fatal or fatal myocardial infarction rate, non-fatal or fatal stroke rate and coronary or non-coronary revascularisation rates. In addition, no effect was found on cancer incidence or hospitalisation for non-cardiovascular causes.

The Heart Outcome Prevention Evaluation (HOPE) study investigators also looked at this subject in detail. As part of this study over 9500 patients were randomised in a two-by-two factorial method to either vitamin E or placebo and either ramipril or matching placebo. Mean follow-up was 4.5 years, and patients were included who had high risk of cardiovascular events either because they already had cardiovascular disease or because they had diabetes with one further addition risk factor. The results from this study mirror the Heart Protection Study data. No differences between the vitamin-E-treated and placebo were found for cardiovascular death, myocardial infarction or stroke. Again, no adverse effects were found in the vitamin-E-treated group.

References

Heart Outcomes Prevention Evaluation (HOPE) Study Investigators 2000 Effects of ramipril on cardiovascular and microvascular outcomes in people with diabetes mellitus: results of the HOPE study and MICRO-HOPE substudy. Lancet 355:253–259

MRC/BHF 2002 Heart protection study of cholesterol lowering with simvastatin in 20,536 high-risk individuals: a randomised placebo-controlled trial. Lancet 360:7–22

106. Genetics of dilated cardiomyopathy

Answer: **A**

Dilated cardiomyopathy is the most common form of cardiomyopathy and is estimated to occur in approximately 15–20 per 100 000 patients. Although treatment with ACE inhibitors, diuretics and beta-blockers has improved outcomes, there is still a poor outlook. An estimated 50% of patients will have died by 5 years from diagnosis.

Most cases are still secondary to viral infection. Adenoviruses and enteroviruses (most commonly coxsackievirus B3 or B4) are the usual culprits. These are mostly self-limiting infections with complete recovery, but sometimes there is persisting infection with subsequent development of dilated cardiomyopathy. Other sporadic causes include alcohol abuse, drug therapy and autoimmune diseases. Autoimmunity is thought to have an important role in the pathogenesis of dilated cardiomyopathy, be it from initial viral insult to genetic causes. Autoantibodies are seen in a significant proportion of all cases. However, it has been discovered that up to 30% of cases have a genetic basis.

Approximately 60% of genetic cases are autosomal dominant. There is a wide variation in penetrance and a number of different gene foci have been identified. Other genetic causes include an autosomal recessive version that is more severe and has a more rapid progression than the dominant version. No gene has yet been identified for this type. Rarely, inheritance is X-linked, on Xp21, associated with a dystrophin gene defect and mitochondrial inheritance. Even within the small group of patients with mitochondrial defects inherited from their mother, there is still further variation. Some of these patients have mitochrondrial deletions whereas others can have one of a number of point mutations. Which point mutation has occurred will dictate which clinical syndrome the patient presents with. The MELAS syndrome (myopathy, encephalopathy, lactic acidosis and stroke-like episodes) has been typed to a mutation of the tRNA leu genes.

Reference

Towbin J A, Bowles N S 2001 Molecular genetics of left ventricular dysfunction. Current Molecular Medicine 1:81–90

RHEUMATOLOGY

True/False answers

107.   Rheumatoid arthritis

A. **F**   B. **F**   C. **T**   D. **F**   E. **T**

Rheumatoid arthritis is a chronic inflammatory arthropathy. The diagnosis is made clinically but the presence of rheumatoid factor substantiates the clinical suspicion. Rheumatoid factor is an IgM antibody that is directed against antigenic determinants on the Fc fragment of IgG. It is present in 75–80% of cases. Seropositive individuals tend to have a more aggressive form of disease and are predisposed to develop the classic seropositive associations for example nodules and lung and cardiac complications.

The differential diagnosis of an acute rheumatoid joint is septic arthritis and it should be noted that infection tends to preferentially settle in a previously damaged joint. In cases where there is doubt, the joint should be aspirated. In either rheumatoid or bacterially infected synovial fluid there is predominance of neutrophils but, in the case of a septic joint, bacteria will be seen on the Gram stain and cultured.

Over the past 2–3 years there have been marked advances in the treatment of rheumatoid arthritis. The new biological agents act to inhibit the activity of TNF-α. Two such agents are on the market at present: etanercept and infliximab. Etanercept is administered subcutaneously whereas infliximab is administered intravenously and is always coadministered with methotrexate. These agents have shown in clinical trials to provide significant symptomatic benefit and halt the progression of joint damage. However, their high cost and incidence of side-effects limit their use. Infliximab therapy costs £10 829 per patient per year and etanercept £8450, as compared with methotrexate, which costs only £30 per patient per annum. The most common side-effect is infection, including some opportunistic infections; reactivation of tuberculosis has been reported. Live vaccines should be avoided during treatment with these agents. The development of anti-double-stranded DNA antibodies, and even of drug-induced lupus-like syndrome is possible. Etanercept can induce CNS demyelinating disorders. TNF-α might be important in the immunological defence against cancer. Theoretically, use of these agents could increase a patient's risk of developing cancer, although so far there is no clinical evidence of this. However, past history of invasive carcinoma is a contraindication to use of these drugs.

Research carried out by several centres over the past few years shows that rheumatoid arthritis patients are at high risk of developing premature atherosclerosis and cardiovascular disease. The mechanism for this is unclear as the incidence of conventional vascular risk factors was similar in the controls to rheumatoid patients. It is thought that chronic inflammation or steroid use may be implicated.

References

Del Rincon I, Williams K, Stern M et al 2001 High incidence of cardiovascular events in rheumatoid arthritis cohort not explained by traditional cardiac risk factors. Arthritis and Rheumatism 44:2737–2745

Etanercept and infliximab for rheumatoid arthritis. Drug and Therapeutics Bulletin 39:49–52

Klippel J H 2000 Biological therapy for rheumatoid arthritis. New England Journal of Medicine 343:1640–1641

Van Doornum S, McColl G, Wicks I P 2002 Accelerated atherosclerosis: an extra-articular feature of rheumatoid arthritis? Arthritis and Rheumatism 46:862–873

108. Systemic lupus erythematosus (SLE)

A. **F**   B. **F**   C. **F**   D. **F**   E. **T**

Systemic lupus erythematousus (SLE) usually presents between the ages 16 and 55 years, but it can occur at almost any age. It is more common and severe in Asians and black Americans but seldom occurs in black Africans. It is ten times more common in females than males. The incidence of SLE has more than tripled over the past four decades. Using the 1982 American College of Rheumatology criteria, the adjusted incidence of SLE was 5·56 per 100 000 during 1980–92, compared with only 1·51 per 100 000 during 1950–79.

The diagnostic criteria state that four of the following must be present:

• malar rash
• discoid rash
• photosensitivity
• oral ulcers
• arthritis
• serositis
• renal disease
• neurological disorder
• haematological disorder
• positive autoantibodies
• antinuclear antibody.

Therefore, individuals who are seronegative (negative antinuclear antibody) can still meet the diagnostic criteria for the disease. Discoid lupus is generally confined to the skin and only very rarely progresses to systemic disease.

The 10-year survival rate is 75–85%, with more than 90% of patients surviving longer than 5 years. Mortality has a bimodal distribution; early deaths are usually due to active disease, whereas atherosclerosis is a leading cause of late (5–10 years) deaths. In a study of women with SLE aged between 35 and 44 years of age, it was found that they had a 52-fold higher risk of having a myocardial infarction than matched women from the Framingham cohort. The reason for premature atherosclerosis in lupus patients is not known as yet. It is almost certainly multifactorial. Steroids are known to propagate atherosclerosis. It might therefore be due to steroid use, disease activity or both. What is known, however, is that hydroxychloroquine has a beneficial effect on serum cholesterol and there is suggestion that patients should not, wherever possible, be treated with steroid without the coprescription of hydroxychloroquine.

References

Hall F, Walport M 1998 Systemic lupus erythematosis. Medicine 26:5–11

Manzi S, Meilhn E N, Rairie J E et al 1997 Age specific incidence rates of myocardial infarction and angina in women with SLE: comparison with the Framingham study. American Journal of Epidemiology 145:408–415

Rahman P, Gladman D D, Urowitz M B et al 1999 The cholesterol lowering effect of antimalarial drugs is enhanced in patients with lupus taking corticosteroid drugs. Journal of Rheumatology 26(2):325–330

109. Myositis

A. **F**   B. **F**   C. **T**   D. **T**   E. **T**

This man has dermatomyositis. Dermatomyositis is an idiopathic inflammatory myopathy with characteristic cutaneous manifestations. These cutaneous features include malar erythema, poikiloderma in a photosensitive distribution, violaceous erythema on the extensor surfaces, and periungual and cuticular changes. Skin lesions of dermatomyositis can precede the development of myopathy and might persist well after the control of the myositis. Myopathy primarily affects proximal muscles, is generally symmetrical, and is slowly progressive over a period of weeks to months.

Dermatomyositis is a multisystem disorder. Arthralgias or arthritis occur in a quarter of patients. Oesophageal disease, which presents with dysphagia, occurs in 15–50% of patients. Pulmonary disease occurs in 15–30% of patients. This can be interstitial pneumonitis but might also be a complication of muscle disease (e.g. hypoventilation or aspiration in patients with dysphagia) or as a result of treatment (i.e. opportunistic infection or drug-induced hypersentivity pneumonitis). Both oesophageal and pulmonary involvement are associated with a poor prognosis. Cardiac involvement occurs in 50% of patients. Symptomatic cardiac involvement is also associated with a poor prognosis. Calcinosis of skin or muscle is unusual in adults but occurs in up to 40% of children.

Large studies report the rate of malignant disease in dermatomyositis to be 20–25%; the association is strongest for those aged over 50 years. Malignancy can come to light before, after or during the myositis, which can follow the course of malignant disease (paraneoplastic course) or its own course independent of the treatment of malignant disease. Gynaecological malignancy, particularly ovarian carcinoma, is overrepresented in patients with dermatomyositis. Concern about immunosuppression predisposing patients to an increased risk of cancer has not been proven.

The cause of dermatomyositis is unknown. In a few patients, the cutaneous manifestations are caused, or exacerbated, by drugs. This has been reported for hydroxycarbamide (hydroxyurea), quinidine, non-steroidal anti-inflammatory drugs, penicillamine and statins.

The diagnosis of dermatomyositis should be suspected in patients with compatible cutaneous findings. With muscle involvement enzymatic testing shows an increase in creatinine kinase, aldolase, lactate dehydrogenase or alanine aminotransferase. Creatine kinase is the most specific and widely available test and it is useful to assess response to treatment. Additional tests, including electromyography, muscle biopsy, ultrasonography or magnetic resonance imaging, can be done for patients in whom other tests have been inconclusive. Antinuclear antibody is commonly positive. Antibodies to Jo-1 are predictive of pulmonary involvement but rarely seen in patients with dermatomyositis. Antibodies to Mi-2 are found in about 25% of patients. This test is specific but not sensitive.

The severity of the myositis frequently correlates with enzyme concentrations and degree of weakness. Patients should be assessed for oesophageal, pulmonary and cardiac involvement. Investigations for malignant disease should be done in all adult patients with dermatomyositis. The type of investigations depends on the patient's age and sex. Assessment of malignant disease is repeated if new symptoms arise, or each year for the first 3 years after diagnosis because overrepresentation of cancer seems to normalise after 3 years.

The mainstay therapy for dermatomyositis is systemic corticosteroids. Traditionally, 0·5–1·0 mg/kg bodyweight prednisolone is given as initial therapy. The treatment should continue for at least 1 month after myositis has become clinically and enzymatically inactive, thereafter the dose is slowly tapered. About 25% of patients will not respond to corticosteroids and 25–50% will develop substantial steroid-related side-effects. Early intervention with steroid-sparing agents (immunosuppressants) appears to be effective in inducing or maintaining a remission. Between 50 and 75% of patients treated with an immunosuppressant will respond with an increase in strength, a decrease in enzyme concentrations, or a decrease in corticosteroid dose. However, no double-blind, placebo-controlled studies show the effectiveness of any of these agents.

Patients who do not respond to these immunosuppressants might respond to pulse methylprednisolone or combination immunosuppressive therapy. High-dose intravenous immunoglobulin has been shown to be beneficial in refractory dermatomyositis. Cutaneous disease in patients with dermatomyositis often does not respond to corticosteroids or immunosuppressive drugs; however, hydroxychloroquine is effective in about 80% of patients.

References

Bohan A, Peter J B 2000 Polymyositis and dermatomyositis. New England Journal of Medicine 292:344–347, 403–407

Callen J P 2000 Dermatomyositis. Lancet 355:53–57

Dalakas M C, Illa I, Dambrosia J M et al 1993 A controlled trial of high-dose intravenous immune globulin infusions as treatment for dermatomyositis. New England Journal of Medicine 329:1993–2000

Siguregeirsson B, Lindelöf B, Edhag O, Allander E 1992 Risk of cancer in patients with dermatomyositis or polymyositis. New England Journal of Medicine 325:363–367

110. Non-steroidal anti-inflammatory drugs (NSAIDs)

A. **T**   B. **F**   C. **F**   D. **F**   E. **F**

Non-steroidal anti-inflammatory drugs (NSAIDs) are among the most widely prescribed drugs worldwide. The discovery that NSAIDs such as aspirin exert their actions primarily by inhibiting the production of prostaglandins was made in 1971. Cyclo-oxygenase (COX), the key enzyme catalysing the biosynthesis of prostaglandins, was purified in 1976 and cloned in 1988. A second COX gene was discovered in

1991. We now know that the two genes express two similar but distinct isoforms of the enzyme – COX I and COX II.

The two known COX isoforms are similar in size, substrate specificity and kinetics, but vary in their expression and distribution. COX I is present in most cells throughout the body and catalyses the formation of prostaglandins involved in physiological function. In the stomach, COX I catalyses the synthesis of PGE_2 and PGI_2, which have cytoprotective actions and play an important role in maintaining the integrity of the gastroduodenal mucosa; it is also responsible for maintaining renal function. COX II is an inducible isoform that is found mainly in inflammatory and immune cells as well as in the kidney. Proinflammatory cytokines and growth factors induce COX II and it is responsible for the generation of the hyperalgesic and proinflammatory prostaglandins at the site of inflammation.

It is estimated that 25% of patients using NSAIDs experience some kind of side-effect and about 5% develop serious health consequences (e.g. massive gastrointestinal bleed, acute renal failure). All currently available NSAIDs inhibit both COX I and COX II to varying degrees. Studies support the theory that the undesirable side-effects such as gastric erosion and renal dysfunction are due to the inhibition of COX I, whereas the antiinflammatory (therapeutic) effects are due to the inhibition of COX II. Selectivity of the conventional NSAIDs for COX I and COX II vary greatly. Some NSAIDs are relatively COX I selective, some are essentially non-selective, whereas others are relatively COX II selective. Inhibitory effects of NSAIDs on gastric PGE_2 synthesis correlate with COX I selectivity. However, even COX-II-selective NSAIDs can have sufficient anti-COX I activity to cause inhibition of gastric PGE synthesis and therefore predispose to mucosal damage.

Guidelines on the use of four COX-II-selective drugs for the treatment of osteoarthritis and rheumatoid arthritis in England and Wales were issued by NICE in July 2001. Celecoxib, etodolac, rofecoxib and meloxicam are not recommended for routine (regular) use in patients with rheumatoid arthritis or osteoarthritis. They should be used instead of standard NSAIDs only in those who are at 'high risk' of developing serious gastrointestinal problems. High-risk patients include those age 65 or over, those already taking other medicines that can cause gastrointestinal problems and those with existing gastrointestinal problems. The risk of gastrointestinal problems is particularly increased in patients with a previous history of gastroduodenal ulcer, gastrointestinal bleeding or gastroduodenal perforation. The use of even a COX-II-selective drug should be considered especially carefully in this situation. All NSAIDs can cause side-effects and they should be prescribed only when there is a demonstrable clinical need and for diseases for which they are licensed. Long-term use of these products should be avoided unless the person taking the drug is monitored and is checked to see if these medicines are still required.

Patients who have cardiovascular disease as well as osteoarthritis or rheumatoid arthritis usually take low-dose aspirin and this can increase the risk of gastrointestinal problems. Prescribing COX-II-selective agents instead of standard NSAIDs in this situation is therefore not justified. All NSAIDs should be avoided. In the past, proton pump inhibitors have been prescribed with COX-II-selective inhibitors with the aim of further reducing potential gastrointestinal problems. However, there is no evidence to support the prescription of these drugs with COX-II-selective inhibitors and therefore NICE does not recommend this practice.

There have been recent suggestions that COX-II-selective NSAIDs are associated with an increased cardiovascular risk but further studies have shown this is more likely due to the standard NSAIDs (in particular naproxen) having a greater antiplatelet effect, therefore perhaps making them cardioprotective.

References

Bombardier C, Laine L, Reicin A et al 2000 Comparison of upper gastrointestinal toxicity of rofecoxib and naproxen in patients with rheumatoid arthritis. New England Journal of Medicine 343:1520–1528

NICE 2001 Guidance on COX II inhibitors for osteoarthritis and rheumatoid arthritis (press release 025). Issued 26 July 2001

NSAIDs and COX-2 inhibitors. Internet On-line Medical Monograph Series 1999 9(3). Online. Available: webcampus.med.mcphu.edu/cme/medicine/med_study.html

Silversteine F, Faich G, Goldsteine J et al 2000 Gastrointestinal toxicity with celecoxib vs non-steroidal anti-inflammatory drugs for osteoarthritis and rheumatoid arthritis: The CLASS study. Journal of the American Medical Association 284:1247–1255

Best-of-5 answers

111.   Glucosamine

Answer: **A**

Osteoarthritis is a major cause of disability and is among the most frequent forms of musculoskeletal disorders. The goal of pharmacological treatment is usually to control symptoms of the disease, pain and limitation of function. This is traditionally accomplished by the use of analgesic agents or NSAIDs. Drugs for the treatment of osteoarthritis can be classified as symptom modifying or structure modifying. Structure-modifying drugs can alter the joint structure favourably and thus actually interfere with the progression of the disease.

Glucosamine sulfate is the sulfate derivative of the natural aminomonosaccharide glucosamine. Glucosamine is a normal constituent of glycosaminoglycans in cartilage matrix and synovial fluid. Crystalline glucosamine sulfate is a pure substance that is synthesised from chitin and in which glucosamine, sulfate, chloride and sodium ions are present in stoichiometric ratios of 2:1:2:2. This product is approved as a prescription treatment for osteoarthritis in many countries in Europe and elsewhere. A number of GPs in the UK prescribe glucosamine, and it is listed in the *Drug Tariff*.

A Belgian group carried out a randomised, double-blind, placebo-controlled trial, in which 212 patients with knee osteoarthritis were randomly assigned 1500 mg oral glucosamine sulfate or placebo once daily for 3 years. The 106 patients on placebo had a progressive joint-space narrowing, with a mean joint-space loss after 3 years of 0·31 mm. There was no significant joint-space loss in the 106 patients on glucosamine sulfate. Visual analogue scores of symptoms worsened slightly in patients on placebo compared with the improvement after treatment with glucosamine sulfate. There were no differences in safety or reasons for early withdrawal between the treatment and placebo groups. The authors did not find glucose homeostasis to be impaired in any one in the treatment group, although glucosamine is known to increase insulin resistance in animal studies and should therefore be used with caution in diabetics.

There is no evidence that glucosamine has any disease-modifying effect in rheumatoid arthritis.

Reference

Reginster J Y, Deroisy R, Rovati L et al 2001 Long-term effects of glucosamine sulphate on osteoarthritis progression: a randomised, placebo-controlled clinical trial. Lancet 357:251–256

112. Ankylosing spondylitis

Answer: **C**

This man has ankylosing spondylitis; the prevalence of ankylosing spondylitis is in the region of 1% and the ratio of affected males to females is 2.5:1. Males tend to get more severe spinal disease whereas females tend to have peripheral joint involvement more often. Peripheral joint involvement occurs in 20–40% of cases and more commonly affects the lower than upper limb joints. HLA-B27 is found in 95%; only around 45% of HLA-B27 positive patients will develop iritis.

The classic finding in ankylosing spondylitis is sacroiliitis and this is graded radiologically from 0 to 4, 0 being normal and 4 fused. Squaring of the inferior and superior margins of the vertebrae occurs with eventual fusion to form the classic 'bamboo spine'.

The mainstay of treatment is to relieve pain, reduce inflammation and maintain normal posture and function. This is achieved by the use of NSAID, regular physiotherapy and hydrotherapy. The so-called 'question mark' posture is very uncommon in those who carry out regular spinal strengthening exercises.

There is no evidence that sulfasalazine improves spinal mobility but a 3-year study published in 1993 showed that sulfasalazine does improve outcome for peripheral joint involvement. Disease progression is monitored by the Schober's test (which measures degree of spinal flexion), wall to tragus length and chest expansion. It is important to note that ankylosis (fusion) can occur at the site of articulation of the rib with the spine.

Enthesopathy (inflammation at site of tendinous insertion) and tendinitis are both common in ankylosing spondylitis. Often a steroid injection can be helpful but never in the Achilles tendon, as tendon rupture is a likely complication.

The other complications of ankylosing spondylitis are pulmonary fibrosis, aortic valve incompetence and pericarditis.

References

Calin A 1998 Ankylosing spondylitis. In: Maddison P J, Isenberg D A, Woo P, Glass D N (eds) Oxford textbook of rheumatology (vol 2). Oxford University Press, Oxford p 681–690

Kirwin J, Edwards A, Huitfeldt B et al 1993 The course of established ankylosing spondylitis and the effects of sulphasalazine over 3 years. British Journal of Rheumatology 32:729–733

113. Gout

Answer: **C**

Gout is the constellation of clinical features that result from the deposition of monosodium urate monohydrate or uric acid. These features include acute arthritis, tenosynovitis, bursitis or cellulitis, tophaceous deposits, renal disease and urolithiasis. It is often thought to be relatively rare but is in fact underdiagnosed; several British and American surveys have estimated the prevalence of gout to be 2.6–8.4 per 1000 overall in adults, with the prevalence increasing with age to rates of 24 per 1000 in men and 16 per 1000 in women aged 65–74. In fact, it is the most common cause of inflammatory arthropathy in men over the age of 40.

Hyperuricaemia is a common but not obligatory feature. It is important to realise that the serum urate concentration can be high, normal or even low during an acute attack. Idiopathic hyperuricaemia occurs more often than clinical gout. The main predisposing factors for gout in men are family history, obesity, excessive alcohol intake, high purine diet, and raised triglyceride concentrations. Patients can be broadly classified as overproducers or undersecretors of urate. In most cases of gout, decreased urinary excretion of urate is the most common metabolic abnormality. This can be due to genetic factors but is usually the result of drugs that reduce renal urate clearance. This is a particular problem in elderly people, who are often taking thiazide diuretics and low-dose aspirin, and have concomitant impaired renal function. Low-dose aspirin blocks urate secretion in renal tubule thus increasing serum concentrations, whereas high-dose aspirin blocks urate reabsorbtion thus increasing excretion.

NSAIDs are the first line of therapy in the treatment of acute gout and should be given in full doses unless there is a history of a peptic ulcer, a background of renal impairment and hypertension, or cardiac failure. Unfortunately, many of the patients who develop acute gout have these contraindications. Clearly, this patient has dyspepsia and a history of alcohol excess and therefore NSAIDs should be avoided. Colchicine given orally or intravenously is an alternative, but is often poorly tolerated by older people. It tends to cause nausea, vomiting and diarrhoea (which can be bloody) and treatment is often limited by these side-effects. Intra-articular steroids and systemic steroids are useful in older patients with impaired renal function.

An acute attack of gout can take up to 7 days to settle and in the acute phase the patient might have leucocytosis and a fever. The most important differential diagnosis of gout is septic arthritis and therefore whenever possible the joint should be aspirated and fluid sent for crystal analysis as well as Gram stain and culture. This is particularly important where steroid is to be used. In acute gout one would expect to see needle-shaped negatively birefringent crystals under polarised light as compared to pseudo-gout where the crystals are brick-shaped and positively birefringent.

Long-term prophylaxis in gout should be with allopurinol but this drug should not be started until 1 month after an acute episode, as it can precipitate an acute attack in the early stages of treatment. A useful alternative in urate undersecretors, provided renal function is normal and there is no history of urate stones, is benzbromarone, a powerful uricosuric agent. Diuretic need should be assessed and alcohol consumption should be reduced if this has been excessive. Recurrent attacks of gout occurring despite what seems to be adequate prophylactic therapy are almost always associated with continued alcohol abuse and poor compliance with treatment, especially in men.

References

Nuki G 1998 Gout. Medicine 26:54

Sturrock R D 2000 Gout, easy to misdiagnose. British Medical Journal 320:132–133

114. Temporal arteritis

Answer: **D**

Temporal arteritis originates from a generalised vasculopathy affecting medium and large arteries. New-onset headache in any patient older than 50 years should prompt consideration of this diagnosis. Early recognition and treatment remain critical to prevent monocular or binocular blindness. Visual impairment results from inflammation of branches of the ophthalmic artery, particularly the posterior ciliary artery, leading to ischaemic optic neuritis. Additionally, the central retinal artery might be affected. Visual loss can affect as many as 50% of patients who are untreated. Temporal arteritis occurs more frequently in patients of northern European descent and rarely in patients of African or Asians descent. Women develop temporal arteritis 4–6 times more frequently than men. Temporal arteritis rarely occurs in patients younger than 50 years; the mean age of onset is 70 years. The incidence is higher, almost 1%, in patients over 80. Confusion still surrounds the terminology used to classify this vasculitis. Temporal arteritis is a commonly employed term, because inflammation often affects the temporal artery, causing headache in the temporal area. Findings from biopsy of the superficial temporal artery assist in establishing the diagnosis. Giant cell arteritis, an alternative name for this disorder, describes the pathological appearance of affected vessels infiltrated by lymphocytes, plasma cells and multinucleated giant cells. Patchy or segmental changes occur in medium and large arteries of the head and neck and can extend into the carotid arteries and aorta.

Headache, the most universal symptom, is present in more than 85% of patients with temporal arteritis. It tends to be new or changed in character from a previous headache pattern, yet few features distinguish a headache caused by temporal arteritis from those arising from other aetiologies. Jaw claudication is especially prominent when patient is chewing or talking and occurs in 65% of patients with temporal arteritis. Constitutional symptoms including anorexia, weight loss, fever, malaise, fatigue or depression can occur. Palpation of the affected artery can reveal exquisite tenderness, warmth and a lack of palpable pulsation. Inflamed arteries can be dilated and thickened, allowing vessels to be rolled between the fingers and skull.

An ESR should be done on suspicion of temporal arteritis. Most patients with temporal arteritis have an ESR of greater than 80 mm/h but approximately 10% of patients have an ESR less than 30 mm/h. ESR can serve as a useful guide to disease activity. Full blood count might reveal leucocytosis, mild anaemia or thrombocytosis. Definitive diagnosis relies on a temporal artery biopsy but treatment should not be delayed until this is done. False-negative biopsies can occur because the disease tends to be segmental in nature and steroid therapy can affect results. However, inflammatory changes usually persist for 2–4 weeks after initiation of treatment. It should be noted that the 1990 American College of Rheumatology criteria for classification of giant cell arteritis states that three of a possible five items must be present. This means that a patient could have a negative biopsy but still fulfill the diagnostic criteria (Table 114.1).

Treatment consists of high-dose prednisolone (40–60 mg/day). Intravenous steroids can be considered if visual deficit is established. Symptoms should begin to resolve within 1–3 days. Duration of maintenance therapy is usually 1–2 years, depending on the patient's response. Methotrexate or azathioprine can act as steroid-sparing agents. NSAIDs provide supplemental pain relief but do not prevent progressive vasculitis that can lead to blindness. Generally, temporal arteritis appears as a self-limited condition lasting up to 2 years.

Reference

Egland A G 2000 Temporal arteritis. *eMedicine Journal* 2(10). Online. Available: www.emedicine.com

Table 114.1   1990 American College of Rheumatology criteria for classification of giant cell arteritis

Three of the following five should be present:
Development of symptoms in patients older than 50 years
Temporal artery tenderness on palpation
New onset of headache or localized head pain
Decreased pulsations not related to arteriosclerosis of cervical arteries
Erythrocyte sedimentation rate (ESR) greater than 50

115.   Pseudogout

Answer: **D**

Pseudogout is the most common cause of acute monoarthritis in elderly people; it is more common in females. Acute attacks of pseudogout are due to shedding of pyrophosphate crystals from articular cartilage. Factors that can precipitate such shedding of crystals include trauma, surgery (especially parathyroidectomy), institution of thyroxine replacement therapy or intercurrent illness. The joints that are most likely to be affected are the knee, wrist and shoulder.

The patient will present with systemic features of fever, malaise or confusion sufficient to suspect sepsis. Aspiration of joint fluid is mandatory. Confirmation requires the demonstration of crystals 1–10 μm long, rhomboidal, with weak positive birefringence under compensated polarised light. Crystals are usually short and stubby, often much smaller than urate crystals. It should be noted that crystals are often difficult to find in the synovial fluid, which can lead to diagnostic uncertainty; centrifuging the sample can increase detection.

Pyrophosphate arthropathy can also present as a chronic arthropathy. This form is common in elderly females. The knees are the most commonly affected joint, followed by wrists and shoulders. Synovitis can be marked. The clinical and radiological appearance of affected joints resembles that of osteoarthritis. Chondrocalcinosis (radiological calcification of articular cartilage) is the classic radiological finding in this condition but does need not be present to make the diagnosis.

Treatment can be local or systemic. Local steroid injection into the affected joint is useful, once sepsis has been excluded. NSAIDs are often helpful during an acute attack, as is colchicine. There is no prophylactic agent available.

References

Nuki G 1998 Crystal arthropathies: calcium pyrophosphate dihydrate (CPPD) deposition. In: Maddison P J, Isenberg D A, Woo P, Glass D N (eds) Oxford textbook of rheumatology (vol 2). Oxford University Press, Oxford p 997–1001

Snaith M L 1995 ABC of rheumatology: gout, hyperuricaemia, and crystal arthritis. British Medical Journal 310:521–524

116.   Reactive arthritis

Answer: **E**

Reactive arthritis is an aseptic arthritis that develops after an infection elsewhere in the body. The classic triad of arthritis, urethritis and conjunctivitis – Reiter's syndrome – is a distinct variety of reactive arthritis. Many microorganisms can induce reactive arthritis. The condition is most commonly associated with urogenital or enteric infections with *Chlamydia trachomatis*, *Yersinia enterocolitica*, *Salmonella*, *Shigella* and *Campylobacter*. In about one-quarter of cases the triggering organism remains unknown.

Between 60 and 90% of patients with postvenereal or postenteric reactive arthritis are positive for HLA-B27. The arthritis usually develops within 4 weeks of the primary infection; it is typically oligoarticular and asymmetric. Painful joints and muscle and tendon insertions are common. Extra-articular manifestations occur in 10–50% of cases and include mucocutaneous symptoms, ocular inflammation, urethritis, nephritis and carditis. The average duration of the arthritis is 4–5 months and 15–30% develop chronic arthritis or sacroiliitis. The presence of HLA-B27 predicts prolonged and more severe disease.

Research over the past 10 years has increased understanding of the relation between host and microbial factors. Persistently high plasma concentrations of antibodies, mainly IgA, directed against lipopolysaccharides and also outer membrane proteins, have been found in serum from patients with reactive arthritis triggered by *Yersinia* and *Salmonella*. Both lipopolysaccharide and outer membrane protein antigens from *Salmonella*, *Shigella* and *Yersinia* have been found in synovial tissue from patients with reactive arthritis, indicating an inflammatory process that might be driven by continuous antigen stimulation. Chlamydial inclusion bodies and chlamydial DNA have also been found in synovial specimens. The relation between HLA-B27 and bacteria in the pathogenesis of reactive arthritis remains unclear. It is possible that there is immunological cross-reactivity between HLA-B27 and microbial antigens, or HLA-B27 might act as a receptor for bacterial proteins, resulting in a foreign complex subjected to immune attack.

All patients with acute monoarthrits should have the joint aspirated and the contents sent for culture because the most important differential diagnosis is septic arthritis. Theoretically, this young man could have a urinary tract infection with septic arthritis. The other possibility would be gonoccocal arthritis but the onset of symptoms tends to be more acute, and it is far more common in females.

The treatment of reactive arthritis is with NSAIDs and intra-articular injections of steroid. Joint sepsis must be excluded before considering local steroid injection. The place of antibiotics in reactive arthritis is still controversial. In retrospective studies, no difference in preventing arthritis was found between patients who were given antibiotics and those who were not. This suggests that the events causing reactive arthritis take place early during the infection. However, relapses of postvenereal arthritis in patients with Reiter's syndrome have been shown to be reduced when the urethritis is treated with antibiotics.

References

Miller M L 1998 Pyogenic arthritis in adults. In: Maddison P J, Isenberg D A, Woo P, Glass D N (eds) Oxford textbook of rheumatology (vol 2). Oxford University Press, Oxford p 529–538

Svenungsson B 1994 Reactive arthritis. British Medical Journal 308:671–672

EPIDEMIOLOGY
True/False answers

117. Confounding

A. **T**   B. **F**   C. **T**   D. **T**   E. **T**

A confounding factor is defined as a factor associated with the risk of a disease in subjects unexposed to the exposure of interest (i.e. not affected by either the exposure or disease) and that is associated with the exposure in the population from which cases arise. For example, if a researcher wanted to determine whether drinking coffee increased the risk for lung cancer, it would be important to control for confounding by smoking. Smoking is associated with a risk of lung cancer regardless of coffee intake and it is reasonable to believe that those who drink more coffee might smoke more. Hence a study that does not control for confounding by smoking could demonstrate an association between coffee drinking and lung cancer that is attributable entirely to the heavier smoking habit of some coffee drinkers.

There are a number of methods to control for confounding factors. Some methods involve designing a study in a particular way and some methods make use of specific statistical analytic techniques. Each method has potential advantages and disadvantages, and can often be used in combination.

Three of these methods involve how a study is designed: randomisation, restriction and matching (matching also requires specific analysis):

- *Randomisation* has the potential to control for confounding more completely than perhaps any other method, but can be used only for interventional studies. With this technique, subjects are allocated exposure status (e.g. an intervention group and a placebo group) at random. The great strength of randomisation is that if the sample size is sufficient, both known and unknown confounding factors are controlled for. All the other methods can only be used for known or suspected confounding factors. Randomisation confers upon interventional studies the ability to produce the highest quality of epidemiological evidence.

- *Restriction* involves limiting the participants of the study to those not exposed to the confounding factor in question. For example, if an investigator wished to explore the association of coffee drinking and lung cancer and control for potential confounding by smoking, the study could be restricted to non-smokers. Restriction has the advantages of being straightforward and convenient but has several significant limitations. First, the results cannot be generalised to include those excluded from the study. In our hypothetical study of coffee drinking and lung cancer, the inability to generalise the result to include smokers would almost certainly severely limit the clinical relevance. Second, to use restriction as a method of confounding control, particularly for more than one factor, might create difficulties for recruitment, because so many potential subjects will need to be excluded. Finally, and perhaps most importantly, restriction prevents the investigator from exploring how the association between the exposure and outcome in question varies according to the level of the confounding factor.

- *Matching* is a more complicated process that involves features of both the design and the analysis of a study. It is most typically employed in case control studies, although it can also be used in other analytical study types. Like restriction, matching requires that the confounding factors to be controlled for are identified in advance. However, instead of restricting all subjects to the same level of the confounding factor, matching ensures that the potential confounding factors are distributed in exactly the same manner between the cases and controls. This is achieved by selecting a control subject with the same levels of exposure in each of the confounding factors in question. Such matching of cases and controls can be time consuming and expensive and requires special analysis. Like restriction, matching does not permit the analysis of how exposure and outcome vary according to the level of the confounding factor. However, matching can be very useful in certain circumstances, including when the number of available cases is small or the when the exposures of interest are particularly complex.

There are two methods for controlling for potential confounding factors using analytic techniques: stratification and multivariate analysis:

- *Stratification* seeks to control confounding by assessing the relationship between the exposure and outcome of interest within strata of the confounding factor. Using a study of coffee drinking (exposure), lung cancer (outcome) and smoking (confounder) once again as an example, cases and controls would be separated into strata depending on their smoking history, for example non-smokers, < 10 pack years, 10–20 pack years and > 20 pack years. The odds ratio calculated within each stratum would provide an estimate for that stratum of the risk of lung cancer from coffee drinking relatively unconfounded by smoking. The odds ratios from each stratum can then be combined to produce a single estimate for the relationship after control for confounding. One of the most common techniques of calculating this single pooled estimate is called the Mantel–Haenzel method. Although stratification can be performed relatively easily and quickly, it can struggle to deal with several confounding factors at the same time.

• *Multivariate analysis* involves the construction of a mathematical model that best describes the relationship between various exposures and an outcome. The choice of the mathematical model depends on many issues and assumptions. Multiple regression is used most commonly to simultaneously control for multiple factors. Different forms of multivariate analysis commonly encountered in medicine include logistic regression (where the outcome of interest is binary variable, e.g. myocardial infarction versus no myocardial infarction) and proportional hazards modelling/Cox regression (where the outcome of interest is the time to an event). Used appropriately, multivariate analysis is a powerful tool for the control of multiple confounding factors in analytical studies, but caution must be exercised to ensure that investigators understand their data rather than performing endless regression modelling until a *P* value < 0.05 results.

References

Hennekens C H, Buring J E, Mayrent S L 1987 Epidemiology in medicine, 1st edn. Little Brown, Boston

Last J M 1995 A dictionary of epidemiology, 3rd edn. Oxford University Press, New York

118. Observational studies

A. **F**   B. **T**   C. **F**   D. **F**   E. **T**

Epidemiological studies are often subdivided into observational studies and intervention studies (clinical trials). Although intervention studies have the potential to produce the highest quality of evidence, not all questions can be examined by this type of design.

Correlational studies, sometimes called ecological studies, examine the relationship between a disease-related characteristic of an entire population (e.g. deaths from coronary heart disease per 100 000) and an exposure of interest, such as cigarettes sold per capita. The results of this type of study are expressed by a correlation coefficient, which quantifies the extent to which there is a linear relationship between exposure and disease. Correlational studies can often be performed relatively quickly and inexpensively but are limited in their ability to link exposure with disease in particular individuals and by the inability to control for confounding factors.

A cross-sectional survey examines the relationship between disease and exposure in a population at one point in time. Unlike a correlational study, data is collected from each individual in that population (or a representative sample). A cross-sectional survey can be used to calculate the prevalence of a disease or condition and allows limited hypothesis testing of causality if the exposure is one that is likely to remain unchanged with time, for example sex or race. Cross-sectional studies are generally faster and less expensive to perform than prospective studies, but because prevalent and not incident cases are used the data will always reflect issues that influence survival or disease duration, as well as aetiology.

In case-control studies, subjects are selected for inclusion on the basis of whether they have a disease or condition and the proportions of these groups that have a history of exposure to a characteristic of interest are compared. The results of a case-control study are typically expressed as an odds ratio. The strengths of a case-control study are the ability to examine multiple potential causes of rare diseases relatively quickly and cheaply. However, a case-control study can be particularly prone to bias compared with other study designs (especially selection bias and recall bias) and in some situations the temporal relationship between exposure and disease might be difficult to establish. Further limitations include an inability to assess rare exposures for a disease or to calculate incidence rates of a disease.

By contrast, cohort studies are well suited to the study of rare exposures and allow the measurement of the incidence of a disease. In this type of study subjects are selected on the basis of the presence or absence of a particular exposure and the subsequent incidence of the disease in question is compared in the two groups. Cohort studies can be performed prospectively or retrospectively. Prospective cohort studies minimises the potential for bias in the ascertainment of exposure but are more expensive and time consuming than retrospective cohort studies.

References

Hennekens C H, Buring J E, Mayrent S L 1987 Epidemiology in medicine, 1st edn. Little Brown, Boston

Last J M 1995 A dictionary of epidemiology, 3rd edn. Oxford University Press, New York

Best-of-5 answers

119. **Homocysteine and ischaemic heart disease**

Answer: **C**

The ongoing assessment of homocysteine as a risk factor for ischaemic heart disease is an excellent example of how an understanding of the importance of confounding factors and the relative strengths and weaknesses of observational studies should alter one's degree of belief in the study results. It also demonstrates the value of well-performed systematic reviews and meta-analyses.

The great majority of studies examining the relationship between homocysteine and ischaemic heart disease outcomes, particularly initially, were cross-sectional or case-control studies. Prospective studies have only been performed more recently. Unlike the cross-sectional and case-control studies, the prospective studies have suggested that homocysteine is either not a risk factor for ischaemic heart disease or is only a weak risk factor. These conclusions are well discussed in a number of recent systematic reviews and meta-analyses. In a recent meta-analysis, Ford et al (2002) included 57 publications and reported the following odds ratios by study type for the risk of ischaemic heart disease for a 5 μmol/L increase in homocysteine: cohort studies 1.06 (95% CI 0.99–.13), nested case-control studies 1.23 (95% CI 1.07–1.41), case-control studies 1.70 (95% CI 1.50–1.93). This suggests that the more robust the study design, the weaker the association between homocysteine level and ischaemic heart disease.

There are several reasons for the apparent discrepancy between the results of the different types of observational studies. First, it has been shown that there is probably a significant publication bias among the cross-sectional and case-control studies, suggesting that at least some negative studies were not published. There does not appear to be evidence for a publication bias among prospective studies. Second, the quality of control of confounding factors is higher among prospective studies than among many of the cross-sectional and case-control studies. Even within the case-control studies there is a gradient of result according to the degree of control for confounding, that is, the more confounding factors that are assessed adequately, the lower the estimate of the association between homocysteine and ischaemic heart disease. Finally, prospective studies are better able to demonstrate a temporal link between an exposure and an outcome, and the association demonstrated in cross-sectional and case-control studies might be due to pre-existing vascular disease of which homocysteine may be a surrogate marker.

In conclusion, the best current epidemiological evidence in humans suggests that homocysteine is probably not a strong risk factor for ischaemic heart disease, if at all. Folate has been shown to lower homocysteine levels but has not yet been demonstrated to have an impact on ischaemic heart disease outcomes. The role of folate supplementation for patients with ischaemic heart disease is even less clear now that the association of homocysteine and risk of ischaemic heart disease appears less certain, and cannot be recommended currently.

References

Christen W G, Ajani U A, Glynn R J et al 2000 Blood levels of homocysteine and increased risk of cardiovascular disease: causal or casual? Archives of Internal Medicine 160:422–434

Cleophas T J, Hornstra N, van Hoogstraten B et al 2000 Homocysteine, a risk factor for coronary artery disease or not? A meta-analysis. American Journal of Cardiology 86:1005–1009

Ford E S, Smith S J, Stroup D F et al 2002 Homocysteine and cardiovascular disease: a systematic review of the evidence with special emphasis on case-control studies and nested case-control studies. International Journal of Epidemiology 31:59–70

NEUROLOGY
True/False answers

120.   Paraneoplastic syndromes

A. **F**   B. **T**   C. **T**   D. **F**   E. **T**

Paraneoplastic syndromes account for about 1% of the effects of cancer on the nervous system. These remote effects of tumours are thought to be antibody mediated and an increasing number of antibodies is associated with these syndromes. Paraneoplastic antibodies can either be the direct cause of the neurological syndrome (usually directed against a receptor or ion channel) or are associated with the syndrome and are usually directed against intracellular components of central neurons.

Lambert–Eaton myasthenic syndrome is a paraneoplastic syndrome associated with small cell lung cancer in which the antibody is directed against presynaptic voltage-gated calcium channels in the peripheral nerve terminal. This syndrome can also occur as an autoimmune disease (50% of cases). The characteristic symptoms include fatigability, limb girdle weakness, an incremental response to repetitive electrical stimulation on EMG and in about half of cases autonomic symptoms such as dry mouth and impotence. As antibodies against voltage-gated calcium channels are the direct cause of the symptoms, removing the antibody with immune therapy such as plasma exchange improves symptoms. Of course, the underlying tumour also needs treatment.

Myasthenia gravis is an autoimmune disease with antibodies directed against acetylcholine receptor antibodies in about 85% of cases. It has recently been shown that in 10% of antibody-negative cases there is an antibody against a muscle-specific kinase (anti-MuSK antibodies). This kinase is thought to be important in maintaining the acetylcholine receptor complex. Thymomas are associated with myasthenia gravis in 10–15% of cases and are mainly epithelial rather than lymphocytic in origin; about 10% of thymomas are malignant. Thymic hyperplasia is seen in about 50% of patients with myasthenia gravis, particularly in patients under 45 years of age. The treatment for thymic hyperplasia or thymoma is thymic resection. The main antibodies associated with central nervous system paraneoplastic syndromes are anti-Hu, anti-Yo and anti-Ri. Increasing numbers of other antibodies are being determined but these were the first discovered and the clinical syndromes are best described. Anti-Hu antibodies are associated with small cell lung cancer. The clinical syndrome is varied but includes sensory (often painful) neuropathies, cerebellar syndromes and encephalomyelitis. Anti-Yo antibodies are associated with ovarian, breast and other gynaecological cancers and are primarily associated with a cerebellar syndrome. Anti-Ri antibodies are associated with small cell cancer and retinal degeneration.

References

Dalmau J O, Posner J B 1999 Paraneoplastic syndromes. Archives of Neurology 56:405–408

Vincent A, Palace J, Hilton-Jones D 2001 Myasthenia gravis. Lancet 357:2122–2128

121. Inflammatory neuropathies

A. **T**   B. **F**   C. **F**   D. **T**   E. **F**

Guillain–Barré syndrome is an acute inflammatory demyelinating polyneuropathy. The pathogenesis is thought to be an autoimmune disease triggered by a preceding infection. Antibodies are thought to be produced in response to acute infection and cross-react with gangliosides in the peripheral nervous system. Gangliosides are glycolipids that are present on cell membranes. Although the antibodies against gangliosides, such as anti-GM1, are thought to be pathogenic, there has, as yet, been no proof of pathogenesis with passive transfer to animal models. Recent studies have indicated that there is a correlation between clinical features and antiganglioside antibodies. Anti-GM1 antibodies are thought to be more common in the motor variants of Guillain–Barré syndrome and anti-GQ1b are present in about 90% of cases of Miller–Fisher variant, which presents with ophthalmoplegia, areflexia and ataxia. Interestingly, the GQ1b ganglioside is particularly represented in the ocular nerves perhaps accounting for the prominent ocular symptomatology.

The mainstay of treatment for Guillain–Barré syndrome is supportive care, with good nursing care of pressure areas, intensive respiratory/autonomic monitoring and care. However, some major studies have shown a benefit of plasma exchange whereas others have shown that intravenous immunoglobulin has equivalent benefit and reduced side-effects. The largest trial published (the PSGBS trial) confirmed that plasma exchange or intravenous immunoglobulin are equivalent but that there is no benefit from combining treatment. Either of these treatments is indicated for patients within the first 2 weeks of onset with bulbar weakness, respiratory dysfunction or the inability to walk without assistance. Treatment is probably indicated for milder weakness earlier in the course. No benefit from steroids has been shown in major studies.

Chronic inflammatory demyelinating polyneuropathy occurs in males twice as often as in females. The average age of onset is 50, although it can occur at any age. Most presentations are with a slowly progressive onset over 2 months (to distinguish it from Guillain–Barré syndrome), however, 30% (and in particular younger subjects) present with a relapsing–remitting form. The symptoms are similar to Guillain–Barré syndrome, with motor symptoms being more prominent than sensory symptoms, distal and proximal weakness and distal sensory loss with absent or reduced tendon reflexes in 90%. The diagnosis is confirmed with nerve conduction studies showing slow conduction velocities and conduction block. Examination of the cerebrospinal fluid (CSF) demonstrates a high protein level. Nerve biopsy shows demyelination and remyelination, which can resemble onion bulbs. First-line treatment is with corticosteriods, starting at 60–100 mg a day and reducing according to clinical effect. Intravenous immunoglobulin and plasma exchange are also efficacious in the short term. Other immunosuppressants, such as ciclosporin, azathioprine, methotrexate and cyclophosphamide, have been used in more refractory cases. Although there is thought to be an immune-mediated mechanism causing chronic inflammatory demyelinating polyneuropathy, few antibodies to gangliosides have been found.

Besides neuropathies associated with malignant monoclonal gammopathies, such as multiple myeloma or POEMS, neuropathies are also associated with monoclonal gammopathies of undetermined significance. Between 8 and 37% of patients with monoclonal gammopathies of undetermined significance will have a neuropathy and the most common abnormality is an IgM paraprotein and not an IgG paraprotein, which is more common in cases without a neuropathy. About half of the IgM paraproteins associated with neuropathy have the paraprotein directed against myelin-associated glycoprotein, that is, the paraprotein is an antimyelin-associated glycoprotein antibody. Myelin-associated glycoprotein is a member of the immunoglobulin superfamily and is an adhesion molecule; its precise role and how antibodies against it cause neuropathy is not clear. It is found in the central nervous system and peripheral nervous system and is present in myelinating Schwann cells. Neuropathies associated with monoclonal gammopathies result in a predominant distal sensory neuropathy. There is a clinical response to immune therapies in a proportion of patients. About half of patients with a neuropathy associated with IgM monoclonal gammopathy of undetermined significance syndrome respond to steroids, plasma exchange, cytotoxic agents such as cyclophosphamide or intravenous immunoglobulin.

References

Ad hoc Subcommittee of the American Academy of Neurology AIDS Task Force 1991 Research criteria for diagnosis of chronic inflammatory demyelinating polyneuropathy (CIDP). Neurology 41:617–618

Nobile-Orazio E, Carpo M 2001 Neuropathy and monoclonal gammopathy. Current Opinion in Neurology 14:615–620

Plasma Exchange/Sandoglobulin Guillain–Barré Syndrome Trial Group 1997 A randomised trial of plasma exchange, intravenous immunoglobulin, and combined treatments in Guillain–Barré syndrome. Lancet 349:225–230

Van der Meche F G, Schmitz P I for the Dutch Guillain–Barré Study Group 1992 A randomised trial comparing intravenous immune globulin and plasma exchange in Guillain–Barré syndrome. New England Journal of Medicine 326:1123–1129

122. Subarachnoid haemorrhage

A. **F**   B. **F**   C. **F**   D. **T**   E. **T**

Subarachnoid haemorrhage is responsible for about 5% of all cerebrovascular events with an incidence of about 15–25 per 100 000. Case fatality is about 50% with a third of patients becoming dependent postsubarachnoid haemorrhage. The main risk factors are as for other stroke disorders with most patients presenting under the age of 60. Genetic causes of subarachnoid haemorrhage, such as polycystic kidney disease, are rare. The classic presenting feature is a sudden explosive headache. Most patients with this history do not have a subarachnoid haemorrhage but all need investigating to exclude a subarachnoid haemorrhage, particularly as rebleeds are common if untreated, even in the mildest initial bleeds. All patients require a CT scan, which shows subarachnoid blood in about 95% of cases. If the CT scan is negative then a lumbar puncture needs to be performed at least 12 h after the onset of headache. The delay is necessary to guard against the uncertainty of a traumatic tap. Xanthochromia, or the yellowing of the supernatant suggests the breakdown products of blood and this can be confirmed on spectrophotometry. Thus red cells in the CSF are not diagnostic for subarachnoid haemorrhage and the presence of xanthochromia 12 h after the event needs to be determined before the diagnosis is made.

The most common cause of a subarachnoid haemorrhage is aneursymal rupture in about 85% of cases, with perimesencephalic haemorrhage in 10% and rarer causes in 5%. Thus all cases need further imaging, usually catheter angiography to exclude an aneurysm, which needs surgical or radiological treatment. There are few controlled trials comparing the benefits of early (< 3 days) or delayed (10–12 days) surgery, but once the aneurysm is occluded there is no more risk of rebleeding. This is the only mechanism to reduce rebleeding.

The main complications after subarachnoid haemorrhage are obstructive hydrocephalus, due to blood in the ventricular system, and delayed cerebral ischaemia or vasospasm. Any deterioration in conscious level warrants a CT scan to exclude hydrocephalus, which would require surgical intervention. Therapies shown to reduce delayed cerebral ischaemia include nimodipine (60 mg 4-hourly), avoiding antihypertensives and maintaining good hydration with intravenous fluids.

Reference

Van Gijn J, Rinhel G J 2001 Subarachnoid haemorrhage: diagnosis, causes and management. Brain 124:249–278

123. Epileptic seizures

A. **F**   B. **F**   C. **T**   D. **T**   E. **T**

Seizures can be classified into generalised seizure disorders (such as absence seizures, myoclonic seizures and tonic–clonic seizures) and partial seizure disorders, which are subclassified into complex partial seizures (in which consciousness is impaired) and simple partial seizures. Partial seizures can also evolve into generalised tonic–clonic convulsions. This patient describes a typical complex partial seizure with secondary generalisation to a tonic-clonic episode.

It is increasingly difficult to generalise regarding starting epilepsy treatment as more epilepsy syndromes with distinct prognoses become characterised. The patient should be treated when the clinician thinks the patient will probably have another seizure without treatment. In a patient with a single generalised unprovoked tonic–clonic seizure, the risk of a further seizure is 20–70% and so treatment is normally deferred until a second seizure has occurred. The type of seizure, EEG abnormalities and underlying cause affect the risk of developing further seizures. For example, patients with a structural brain lesion or EEG abnormalities are more likely to have further seizures and starting treatment after a single seizure might be appropriate.

The clinical manifestations of partial seizures depend on the area of the brain involved in the seizure and can be motor, sensory or an experiential phenomenon such as déjà vu. If consciousness is also impaired, or there is an abnormal response to the environment, seizures are described as complex partial and often involve the temporal lobes. All seizures with the suggestion of focal onset, even if they go on to generalise, need further investigation with neuroimaging (preferably MRI). The most common findings are trauma, brain tumours, vascular disease and congenital malformations. Interictal EEG abnormalities are seen in about 35–40% of patients with clinically determined epilepsy after a single examination. Multiple EEG examination or sleep-deprived EEG examination can increase the yield to 60%.

Before starting anticonvulsants in women of child-bearing age it is vital to counsel regarding the risk of fetal abnormalities. The risk increases with the number of anticonvulsants and the dose of anticonvulsants but the risk of major fetal abnormalities on one anticonvulsant is three times (6%) the general population risk (2%). Sodium valproate is particularly implicated, with 10% of children born to mothers on this drug having minor cognitive abnormalities. Recently, lamotrigine has shown similar rates to other anticonvulsants. The advice to women on anticonvulsants wanting to try and conceive is to reduce polypharmacy, reduce the dose of drug to the minimal effective dose and take folic acid prior to conception.

References

Canger R, Battino D, Canevini M P et al 1999 Malformations in offspring of women with epilepsy: a prospective study. Epilepsia 40:1231–1236

Reiff-Eldridge R, Heffner C R, Ephross S A et al 2000 Monitoring pregnancy outcomes after prenatal drug exposure through prospective pregnancy registries: a pharmaceutical company commitment. American Journal of Obstetrics and Gynecology 182:159–163

124. Genetics of neurological disease

A. **F**   B. **T**   C. **F**   D. **T**   E. **T**

Our genetic understanding of a multitude of neurological disorders is expanding rapidly. Charcot–Marie–Tooth disease, also known as peroneal muscular atrophy, is the most common inherited neuropathy. The modern name for this disorder is hereditary motor sensory neuropathy (HMSN), of which there are two common types. HMSN 1 refers to a demyelinating neuropathy and HMSN 2 is an axonal neuropathy. HMSN 1 is an autosomal disorder with duplication or point mutations in the *PMP-22* gene (peripheral myelin protein 22). The PMP protein is thought to be important in compacting myelin around axons. Interestingly, another condition affecting peripheral nerves – hereditary neuropathy with liability to pressure palsies – is caused by a deletion of the same gene. Other mutations have been found in other myelin proteins (e.g. myelin protein zero (Po)), that cause variants of HMSN.

The neurological diseases associated with triplet repeats are: myotonic dystrophy (myotonic dystrophy protein kinase gene), fragile X, Huntington's disease (huntingtin gene), X-linked spinobulbar muscular atrophy (androgen receptor gene), dentatorubral-pallido-luysian atrophy, spinocerebellar ataxias (especially SCA-1; ataxin-1 gene) and Friedreich's ataxia (frataxin gene).

The dystrophin gene is mutated in both Duchenne and Becker muscular dystrophies, now increasingly called dystrophinopathies. Dystrophin is a large subsarcolemmal protein in skeletal and cardiac muscle that is thought to be structurally important in linking the intracellular cytoskeleton and extracellular matrix, and has a probable functional role in differentiation of muscle fibres and organisation of the postsynaptic membrane. The gene is located on the X chromosome (Xp21). Duchenne muscular dystrophy presents with progressive proximal weakness around the ages 6–11; there is calf hypertrophy, which is due to muscle fibrosis. There can be an associated cardiomyopathy and intellectual impairment. Becker muscular dystrophy presents similarly with a progressive proximal myopathy but has a milder and more variable clinical picture.

Mitochondral DNA is a double-stranded circular molecule encoding for 37 genes (13 peptides in the mitochondrial respiratory-chain complex). There are between two and ten copies in each mitochondrion and over 1000 in each cell. The inheritance is maternal. The normal situation is for homoplasmy, with all copies of the mitochondrial DNA being identical, but single cells can contain different mitochondrial DNA populations in different mitochondria (heteroplasmy). This produces tissue variation with the highest levels seen in postmitotic tissues such as neurons, skeletal and cardiac muscle and endocrine tissue. The presence of heteroplasmy with pathogenic mitochondrial mutations is thought to account for differing susceptibilities of different tissues to the effects of these mutations.

Alzheimer's disease is divided into familial and sporadic forms. Three genes have been linked to early onset familial Alzheimer's disease: the amyloid precursor protein gene on chromosome 21, presenilin 1 (chromosome 14) and presenilin 2 (chromosome 1). All these mutations are thought to affect amyloid metabolism supporting the amyloid hypothesis of pathogenesis in Alzheimer's disease. The amyloid hypothesis suggests that accumulation of beta-amyloid, by overproduction or failure of breakdown, leads to amyloid deposition, causing amyloid plaques, and leading to neurofibrillary tangles and cell death.

In Down syndrome there is overexpression of the amyloid precursor protein gene (trisomy 21),which leads to diffuse amyloid deposits in the brains of patients around 15 years old and Alzheimer changes are visible in all brains by the age of 40. In sporadic older cases there is an association between the inheritance of the apoprotein E allele E4 and Alzheimer's disease.

Von Hippel–Lindau syndrome is a dominantly inherited condition that includes haemangioblastoma of the cerebellum and retina, with renal and pancreatic cysts and carcinomas and phaeochromocytomas. The gene is located on the short arm of chromosome 3 and is a tumour suppressor gene that is inactivated in von Hippel–Lindau syndrome and most sporadic renal carcinomas.

References

Lindblad K, Schalling M 1999 Expanded repeat sequences and disease. Seminars in Neurology 19(3):289–299

Berger P, Young P, Suter U 2002 Molecular cell biology of Charcot–Marie–Tooth disease. Neurogenetics 4:1–15

Best-of-5 answers

125.   Multiple sclerosis

Answer: **A**

Multiple sclerosis is a common inflammatory disease of the central nervous system in which immunocompetent cells destroy myelin. The clinical patterns of disease fall into several types: relapsing remitting, secondary progressive and primary progressive. Relapsing remitting multiple sclerosis is the most common presentation of disease, with a subacute onset of neurological symptoms in a 20–40-year-old patient. After years of intermittent relapses these patients tend to develop neurological disability and signs between relapses and are then said to have become secondarily progressive. There have been studies suggesting that the time to disability is dependent on the relapse rate in the early years of the disease. Primary progressive multiple sclerosis has an insidious onset, is more common in older people and accounts for about 10% of multiple sclerosis patients.

Treatments concentrate on immune modulation, with steroids being used for acute attacks of demyelination to resolve symptoms more quickly. There is no evidence that steroids reduce the disability associated with later disease. Immunosuppressants such as azathioprine and methotrexate have been used in some cases to try and modify the course of the disease, but there have been few prospective randomised control trials and no benefit has been shown so far.

In the last few years there have been several large-scale randomised control trials of beta interferon therapy in patients with relapsing remitting and secondary progressive multiple sclerosis. In the three trials investigating relapsing remitting patients, all of the studies restricted entry to patients who were ambulant and who were having more than two relapses a year, and found a significant reduction in the frequency and severity of relapses of about 30%. Thus the recommendations are that patients fulfilling these criteria should have access to beta interferon (Association of British Neurologists 2001). This now happens in the NHS.

The studies in secondary progressive disease have not been so clear-cut; no effects on disease progression have been shown but there does appear to be a reduction in the rate of relapses. Beta interferon is not recommended in progressive multiple sclerosis at present. Similar results and recommendations result from studies using glatiramer, a compound comprised of four amino acids that was developed to suppress experimental allergic encephalomyelitis in guinea pigs. Its mode of action in human multiple sclerosis is not known.

References

Association of British Neurologists 2001 Guidelines for the use of beta interferon and glatiramer acetate in multiple sclerosis. January 2001

IFNB Multiple Sclerosis Study Group 1993 Interferon beta-1b is effective in relapsing-remitting multiple sclerosis. Neurology 43:655–661

Jacobs L D, Cookfair D L, Rudick R A et al 1996 Intramuscular interferon beta-1a for disease progression in relapsing multiple sclerosis. Annals of Neurology 39:285–294

PRISMS Study Group 1998 Randomised double-blind placebo controlled study of interferon-1a in relapsing/remitting multiple sclerosis. Lancet 352:1498–1504

126. Emergency neurology

Answer: **D**

A sudden onset cerebellar syndrome requires urgent investigation with imaging of the head to diagnose or exclude a cerebellar haematoma. A cerebellar haemorrhage can be lethal through compression of the brainstem and surgical evacuation is the appropriate treatment, so a prompt diagnosis is critical. Hydrocephalus is a complication. The onset is usually acute with a sudden occipital headache, vomiting and ataxia. A decline in conscious level is an ominous sign and indicates the need for urgent decompression.

An internuclear ophthalmoplegia implies pathology in the medial longitudinal fasiculus in the midbrain. The most common cause for bilateral lesions is multiple sclerosis and for unilateral lesions is a vascular event. A sudden onset foot drop could be due to a central event (such as a stroke) or might be peripheral in origin. The most likely cause is compression of the common peroneal nerve at the head of the fibula, and the differential includes an L4 or L5 radicular lesion. The most likely cause of an isolated seventh nerve palsy is a Bell's palsy (i.e. idiopathic). The treatment is with high-dose steroids and aciclovir (to treat herpes zoster as a potential cause). If there are any unusual features at onset, or an atypical course, further investigation is warranted. A painful complete third nerve palsy warrants urgent investigation to exclude an aneurysm of the posterior communicating artery. The onset is usually acute with severe pain and the pupil is almost always affected (dilated and fixed to light). An incomplete third nerve palsy with pupil sparing is most likely due to medical causes of nerve infarction (such as diabetes) as the more peripheral papillary fibres are spared.

Reference

Moore A 2000 What to refer to a neurosurgeon. Medicine 28:82–84

127. Variant Creutzfeldt–Jakob disease

Answer: **B**

Prion diseases are a group of conditions that until recently included Creutzfeldt–Jakob disease (CJD), Gerstmann–Straussler–Scheinker disease and kuru. These can be divided into hereditary, sporadic or acquired forms.

More recently, a variant of classic CJD has been described. First reported in 1996, more than 100 cases have now been reported and the number of cases seems set to rise. The features seen in this variant condition are quite distinct from those seen in the sporadic or acquired classic pattern of disease. The patients tend to be younger, with a median age of only 26 years, and there is no history of recent neurosurgery or family history of the condition. Median survival is 13.0 months. At presentation 15% patients had neurological signs only, 22% had a combination of neurological and psychological features and the rest had only psychological features at presentation. However, it is not usually long before neurological features occur. Over half of the first 100 patients had at least one neurological feature within 2 months of presentation.

Common early psychological features include dysphonia, withdrawal, anxiety, irritability and insomnia as well as loss of interest. Less common early features included behavioural change, panic attacks and suicidal ideation. Late psychiatric features are highly variable and include bizarre behaviour, paranoid ideation, confabulation, impaired recognition, impaired comprehension and change in eating preferences.

There does not appear to be any common early neurological signs although uncommon presentations include loss of consciousness, a predisposition to dropping things, headaches and excess sweating. Most of the neurological features tend to occur late in the course of the disease. Most common features include hyperreflexia, impaired coordination, myoclonus, incontinence, and eye signs. Many other features can also be seen, again tending to occur later on.

From this it can be seen that initial recognition of the disease can be difficult. Referral leading to diagnosis was often to psychiatrists or neurologists in these early patients, but also general physicians, paediatricians and others.

Suspicion of variant CJD should lead to referral to a neurological centre. Diagnosis is initially made clinically. The EEG shows no typical appearance, unlike classic CJD. Approximately half of these patients test positive for 14-3-3 immunoassay and 70% demonstrate bilateral pulvinar high signal on MRI. All patients are homozygous for methionine at codon 129 of the prion protein gene.

References

Collinge J 1999 Variant Creutzfeldt–Jakob disease. Lancet 354:317–323

Spencer M D, Knight R S, Will R G 2002 First hundred cases of variant Creutzfeldt–Jakob disease: retrospective case note review of early psychiatric and neurological features. British Medical Journal 324:1479–1482

Will R G, Zeidler M, Stewart G E et al 2000 Diagnosis of new variant Creutzfeldt–Jakob disease. Annals of Neurology 47:575–582

128. Parkinson's disease

Answer: **E**

Although the introduction of levodopa preparations has revolutionised the management of Parkinson's disease, in recent years there has been increasing concern regarding the long-term motor complications of treatment and the potential neurotoxicity of levodopa. Motor complications include dyskinesias, dystonia and response fluctuations. These complications affect 10% of patients with each year of levodopa treatment such that after 5 years 50% of patients will suffer them. This risk is higher in patients with disease onset below the age of 40, with 100% suffering complications after 6 years of treatment. Attempts to reduce the onset of motor complications include delaying treatment as long as possible (i.e. until functionally disabled) and starting treatment at this stage with a dopamine agonist.

Dopamine agonists were initially introduced as adjuvants to levodopa in late stage disease. Trials with dopamine agonists such as bromocriptine, pergolide, pramipexole and ropinirole have demonstrated a delay in the onset of motor complications. This was not seen with combination treatment with levodopa and an agonist. However, there were more adverse events, necessitating withdrawal of therapy and possibly reducing efficacy with agonist monotherapy. This appears to be a class effect of these drugs but there are limited studies comparing different agonists. Additionally, the trials used predominantly younger patients with Parkinson's disease so it is difficult to generalise these results to an elderly population. Current acceptable practice with newly diagnosed patients would therefore be to delay treatment until functionally disabled and then to start either a dopamine agonist alone in younger patients (under 65 years) and to try and delay the initiation of levodopa treatment; in older patients it would be acceptable to start levodopa initially and consider adding an agonist when/if motor complications develop.

A large trial (PD MED) is currently underway in the UK in which early disease patients are randomised to levodopa, dopamine agonist or selegiline and followed for a minimum of 5 years, which will hopefully help to clarify these management issues.

References

Clarke C 2000 Medical management of Parkinson's disease. Journal of Neurology, Neurosurgery and Psychiatry 72(suppl 1):122–127

Parkinson Study Group 2000 Pramipexole verus levodopa as initial treatment for Parkinson's disease. Journal of the Americal Medical Association 284:1931–1938

Rascol O, Brooks D, Korczyn A et al 2000 A five year study of the incidence of dyskinesia in patients with early Parkinson's disease who were treated with ropinirole or levodopa. New England Journal of Medicine 342:1484–1491

129. Reversible causes of dementia

Answer: **A**

This clinical scenario gives the characteristic features of normal pressure hydrocephalus. Normal pressure hydrocephalus is characterised by urinary incontinence, gait apraxia and cognitive decline. A previous history of meningitis, head injury or subarachnoid haemorrhage is sometimes obtained. The dementia has subcortical features such as reduced attention and psychomotor slowing, similar to a vascular (or multi-infarct) dementia picture. The imaging demonstrates enlargement of the cerebral ventricles. It can be difficult to distinguish on imaging from the atrophy associated with Alzheimer's disease or vascular dementia. Intracranial pressure monitoring is now undertaken prior to shunt insertion to help determine who would benefit from neurosurgical intervention. Removing 40–50 ml of CSF and observing any clinical improvement has also been used to predict who would benefit from a ventriculoperitoneal shunt. Reviews have suggested that about 30% of patients shunted show significant improvements, with a 6% risk of complications. Patients with a short duration of dementia, gait disturbance before cognitive disturbance, a history of a potential secondary cause and a lack of dysphasia have the best prognosis.

Although the majority of patients with progressive loss of memory and intellectual abilities have an irreversible dementing disorder, it is important to remember to search for treatable causes. Chronic subdural haematomas present with headache, drowsiness and bilateral pyramidal signs. The history of head injury might be forgotten or trivial but good results are obtainable from draining subdural haematomas, provided that the conscious level is not severely impaired. Brain tumours, especially frontal tumours, can mimic dementing illnesses and can occasionally be treatable, as in the case of meningioma.

Pseudodementia, caused by depressive illness, is increasingly recognised, especially in older people. It can be very difficult to distinguish without a trial of antidepressants. A number of systemic organic diseases can also mimic dementia, including hypothyroidism, hyper- or hypocortisolaemia, vitamin deficiency (e.g. B_{12}), cerebral vasculitis and syphilis. Alcohol must also not be forgotten; although the damage might be irreversible, vitamin supplementation can improve cognitive function in Wernicke's disease and sobering up might allow the patient to make the most of the residual cognitive function.

References

Galton C, Hodges J 1999 The spectrum of dementia and its treatment. Journal of the Royal College of Physicians, London 33:234–239

Hebb A, Cusimano M 2001 Idiopathic normal pressure hydrocephalus: a systemic review of diagnosis and outcome. Neurosurgery 49:1166–1184

HAEMATOLOGY

True/False answers

130.   Blood transfusion

A. **F**   B. **T**   C. **F**   D. **T**   E. **T**

Blood transfusion can be lifesaving in emergencies and can improve symptoms and quality of life in some chronic anaemic states, but it is associated with a range of side-effects and adverse outcomes. The Serious Hazards of Transfusion (SHOT) audit, an ongoing audit of all transfusion activity in the UK, suggests that serious errors in giving blood occur at a rate of 1 per 16 000 units transfused; 1 in 500 000 units is contaminated with bacteria and 1 in 100 000 to 1 in 400 000 contains hepatitis B, but only one in 3 million leads to hepatitis C infection, the result of a new RNA test for hepatitis C.

There is a theoretical risk of vCJD transmission via blood transfusion; B lymphocytes might facilitate the transmission of this agent. However, no cases of vCJD have been shown to have occurred due to blood transfusion as yet. No screening test for vCJD that is applicable to blood has been developed, although a number of companies are working on this. A leucodepletion process is carried out on all blood to be used for red cell transfusion in the UK; this may might reduce the chance of vCJD transmission and reduces the risk of cytomegalovirus transmission. Pooled plasma from UK citizens cannot be used for production of blood fractions such as albumin. In the US and Canada, people who have lived in the UK between 1980 and 1996 cannot give blood because of the theoretical risk of vCJD contamination.

Apart from the risks of acute haemolytic reactions (1 in 250 000 to 1 in 1 million) and infection, blood transfusion appears to cause a degree of immune suppression. This might explain why patients with colorectal cancer who undergo transfusion have a worse outcome than those who avoid transfusion.

Liver transplant often demands a very large amount of transfused blood, with the attendant problems of possible infection, transfusion reactions, hypocalcaemia and clotting derangements. Aprotinin is a proteolytic enzyme that degrades plasmin and kallikrein, and thus inhibits the fibrinolytic side of clotting haemostasis. A randomised trial of aprotinin in liver transplantation showed that aprotinin reduced the blood loss by up to 60%, and reduced the transfusion requirement by up to 37%. There was no difference in mortality or thromboembolic events at 30 days.

References

Porte R J, Molenaar I Q, Begliomini B et al 2000 Aprotinin and transfusion requirements in orthotopic liver transplantation: a multicentre randomised double-blind study. Lancet 355:1303–1309

Regan F, Taylor C 2002 Recent developments: blood transfusion medicine. British Medical Journal 325:143–147

131. Haemolytic–uraemic syndrome/thrombotic thrombocytopenic purpura

A. T   B. F   C. F   D. F   E. T

Haemolytic–uraemic syndrome (HUS) and thrombotic thrombocytopenic purpura (TTP) form a spectrum of conditions. Intravascular thrombosis with widespread organ damage, haemolysis, microangiopathy and renal impairment occur. In children, HUS has a relatively benign prognosis – with renal support therapy, the mortality rate is 3–5% and most, but not all children regain dialysis independence. In the elderly, the condition is usually lethal – the mortality rate is > 85%.

HUS is most commonly caused by shigatoxin-producing enterobacteria – usually *Escherichia coli* 0157:H7; between 3 and 15% of such infections lead to HUS. Shigatoxins bind to a family of glycosphingolipid receptors found on red blood cells and on capillaries in the brain and glomeruli. The toxin is endocytosed after binding and causes ribosomal inactivation leading to cell death. This disruption of the endothelium leads to microangiopathy and capillary thrombus formation.

Although antibiotic therapy to kill the culprit bacteria would appear to be a logical way of reducing the amount of shigatoxin produced, it is not at all clear that this is the case in practice. Most data currently available is based on retrospective case series; the only large prospective study (71 patients) of *E. coli* 0157:H7 infection showed that early antibiotic therapy was associated with a much greater chance of developing HUS. Certainly, in vitro experiments suggest that subtherapeutic concentrations of antibiotics can increase the release of shigatoxin by *E. coli* 0157:H7.

Not all cases of HUS are due to infection, however. Some familial cases have been found to be associated with defective or deficient complement factor H, a regulatory protein that can bind to, and promote the breakdown of, the activated C3b complement component. It thus acts as a brake on runaway complement cascade activation, which can cause significant bystander tissue damage and further complement cascade activation.

TTP is thought to be an autoimmune condition, mediated by IgG autoantibodies directed against a protease that cleaves von Willebrand factor. Von Willebrand factor is then free to form multimeric complexes, which bind and activate platelets, leading to microthrombus formation. Several drugs have been implicated in the development of TTP, including penicillin, rifampicin, cytotoxics, risperidone, aciclovir, quinolones and, most recently, clopidogrel. The condition is extremely rare, however, and proving a definite causal link might well be an elusive goal.

References

Hankey G J 2000 Clopidogrel and thrombotic thrombocytopenic purpura. Lancet 356:269–270

Taylor C M 2001 Complement factor H and the haemolytic uraemic syndrome. Lancet 358:1200–1202

Todd W T A 2001 Prospects for the prevention of haemolytic–uraemic syndrome. Lancet 359:1636–1638

132. Deep venous thrombosis

A. **T**   B. **T**   C. **F**   D. **F**   E. **T**

Deep venous thrombosis is a very common and, at the time of writing, newsworthy condition. The standard risk factors include advancing age, malignancy, obesity, previous thromboembolic disease, family history of thromboembolic disease, surgery (especially hip, knee or pelvic), limb paresis, intravenous drug abuse, pregnancy, immobility, including plaster casts and serious illness, and known hypercoagulable states.

The oral contraceptive pill has been known to increase the risk of deep venous thrombosis for many years but recent research has suggested that so-called 'third-generation' contraceptives containing gestodene or desogestrel confer a greater risk of deep venous thrombosis than 'second-generation' contraceptives containing levonorgestrel. A meta-analysis of 13 such studies suggested that third-generation contraceptives confer 1.7 times the risk of deep venous thrombosis of second-generation contraceptives.

Another focus of media attention has been on deep venous thrombosis (and sudden death) following long-haul air flights. Despite the furore that several recent cases have generated, the evidence for an increased risk from long-haul flights is mixed. Some studies have failed to find an increased risk whereas others have suggested a prevalence of up to 10% for asymptomatic deep venous thrombosis after flying. At least one trial has shown a marked reduction in asymptomatic deep venous thrombosis after flying by using compression stockings.

Clinical examination is notoriously unreliable for making the diagnosis of deep venous thrombosis, although the use of clinical scoring systems can give an estimate of the likelihood of a swollen leg being due to deep venous thrombosis. D-dimers are a highly sensitive test for deep venous thrombosis; a negative D-dimer test has 98% negative predictive value. D-dimers are not specific for deep venous thrombosis, however; they are raised in sepsis, myocardial infarction and inflammatory conditions. Venography and ultrasonography remain the best tests for positively identifying deep venous thrombosis.

The incidence of deep venous thrombosis after hip or knee surgery approaches 80% in the absence of any prophylactic therapy. Prophylactic subcutaneous heparin is usually given until discharge from hospital but a recent meta-analysis has shown that extended duration prophylaxis (30–40 days) can further reduce the incidence of symptomatic and asymptomatic deep venous thrombosis in this patient group. There was a small increased risk of minor bleeds but no difference in major bleeding episodes between the groups.

A somewhat surprising new risk factor for deep venous thrombosis has been identified recently – the use of antipsychotic agents. A case-control study suggested that the odds of developing deep venous thrombosis in those taking antipsychotics was seven times that of the control group. It is unclear why this should be; all classes of antipsychotic were implicated, although low potency agents appeared to have a higher risk.

References

Eikelboom J W, Quinlan D J, Douketis J D 2001 Extended-duration prophylaxis against venous thrombosis after total hip or knee replacement: a meta-analysis of the randomised trials. Lancet 358:9–15

Kemmeren J M, Algra A, Grobbee D E 2001 Third generation oral contraceptives and risk of venous thrombosis: meta-analysis. British Medical Journal 323:1–9

Scurr J H, Machin S J, Bailey-King S et al 2001 Frequency and prevention of symptomless deep-vein thrombosis in long-haul flights: a randomised trial. Lancet 357:1485–1489

Zornberg G L, Jick H 2000 Antipsychotic drug use and risk of first-time idiopathic venous thromboembolism: a case-control study. Lancet 356:1219–1223

Best-of-5 answers

133. Thalassaemias

Answer: **D**

The genetic basis of the thalassaemias is now well understood; hundreds of insertion and deletion mutations affecting single bases or large chunks of DNA have been described. These lead to reduced or absent production of beta-globin (beta thalassaemia) or alpha-globin (alpha thalassaemia). Reduced production leads to the formation of unstable and inefficient homotetramers, with consequent reduced oxygen-carrying ability, membrane damage, short red cell life, anaemia and splenomegaly. Ineffective bone marrow also hypertrophies, leading to skeletal malformation.

Thalassaemia can be detected via chorionic villus sampling early in pregnancy, allowing a decision about abortion to be made if the disease is likely to be very severe or lead to stillbirth. Patients who are heterozygous for beta thalassaemia display an elevated HbA2 concentration, along with microcytic, hypochromic red cells; such patients are thus easily identified and can undergo prenatal counselling.

Some new treatments for thalassaemia are now available. Blood transfusion plus regular desferrioxamine infusions allow the bone marrow to be switched off, preventing skeletal malformation; the desferrioxamine chelates iron and stops progressive iron overload, which can culminate in cirrhosis, diabetes, hypogonadism and cardiomyopathy. Desferrioxamine infusions have been associated with retinal nerve damage, sensorineural hearing loss, *Yersinia* spp. infections, vertebral disc calcification, hepatic and renal impairment. Deferiprone is an orally active iron chelator; although it appears to be effective at stopping tissue iron deposition in at least some patients with thalassaemia, and can improve compliance and quality of life, there are concerns that: (1) it might not be as effective as desferrioxamine; and (2) side-effects might be more troublesome than those of desferrioxamine. It can cause hepatic fibrosis, arthritis and neutropaenia, which can be severe in some cases. Thrombocytopaenia does not appear to be a significant side-effect.

Bone marrow transplantation is an effective treatment for thalassaemia if an HLA-matched sibling donor is available. It is more effective if carried out early in life. Splenomegaly, especially if accompanied by increasing requirements for blood transfusion, is still an indication for splenectomy. Vaccination against capsulated bacteria (e.g. pneumococcus, meningococcus and *Haemophilus influenzae*) is required after splenectomy.

References

Giardina P J, Grady R W 2001 Chelation therapy in beta-thalassaemia: an optimistic update. Seminars in Hematology 38:360–366

Merson L, Olivier N 2002 Orally active iron chelators. Blood Reviews 16:127–134

Weatherall D J, Provan A B 2000 Red cells I: inherited anaemias. Lancet 355:1169–1175

134. Stem cell transplantation

Answer: **D**

Stem cell transplantation is now a well-established therapy for a number of haematological conditions, including acute and chronic myeloid leukaemia, myelodysplasia, refractory aplastic anaemia and thalassaemia. It is also used in lymphoma, myeloma and some solid tumours such as neuroblastoma. Interest is currently focused on exploring the range of solid tumour types for which this therapy might be useful, and on exploring its role in treating autoimmune conditions (e.g. systemic sclerosis), metabolic derangements, sickle-cell anaemia, amyloidosis and osteopetrosis.

Therapy consists of three phases. First, material is procured for transplant. This can come from an allogeneic source (sibling blood or bone marrow, umbilical cord blood, or unrelated donor blood or bone marrow), or from the patient (autologous blood or bone marrow). Peripheral blood stem cells are harvested by using growth factors to mobilise stem cells into the circulation, then taking blood, separating out the stem cells and returning the blood. Autologous blood and bone marrow donations are usually 'cleaned up' to remove as many malignant cells as possible.

Second, conditioning is performed. This entails high-dose chemotherapy together with whole body irradiation to destroy the bone marrow and any malignant cells that are present. Third, the transplant material is reintroduced and allowed to form new bone marrow. This third phase can take several weeks, during which close supportive care is needed to maintain haemoglobin levels, combat infection and guard against haemmorhage due to the lack of platelets.

Autologous transplantation has the advantage of being an exact tissue match, thus graft versus host reactions do not occur. Engraftment is slower with autologous transplantation, both for peripheral blood and for bone marrow transplants, but the mortality rate from the transplant is lower than with allogeneic transplants. The disadvantages are that no graft versus tumour response can occur and that, despite cleaning up of the donation, malignant cells can sometimes be reintroduced along with the stem cells.

Allogeneic transplants are effective but carry a substantial treatment-related mortality, often due to graft versus host disease. Sibling donations have a better outcome than those from unrelated donors. Peripheral stem cell transplants appear to engraft more quickly than bone marrow transplants, both for allogeneic and autologous grafts. Another source of stem cells is neonatal umbilical cord blood; this is rich in stem cells and has a lower rate of graft versus host disease than with adult allogeneic donor cells. The volumes of blood and overall number of available stem cells are small, however, and cord blood is thus usually reserved for use in children.

Cytomegalovirus-negative donors are preferred for transplantation, as the rate of cytomegalovirus infection in recipients is much lower. However, recent data suggests that in recipients who are HLA-A2 positive, stem cell transplants from cytomegalovirus-positive donors lead to an improved outcome in leukaemia. This is thought to be because of a graft versus leukaemia effect; cytotoxic T cells in the donor, which are active against cytomegalovirus infection, appear to recognise an epitope on the HLA-A2 molecule, allowing the donor cells to kill host cells, including leukaemia cells. Such graft versus tumour effects are currently under intense scrutiny; a lesser degree of myeloablation might be necessary if such graft versus tumour effects are capable of mopping up the remaining tumour cells. Reduced myeloablative therapy may be better tolerated, leading to better outcomes.

References

Lennard A L, Jackson G H 2000 Stem cell transplantation. British Medical Journal 321:433–437

Nachbaur D, Bonatti H, Oberaigner W et al 2001 Survival after bone marrow transplantation from cytomegalovirus seropositive sibling donors. Lancet 358:1157–1159

Powles R, Mehta J, Kulkani S et al 2000 Allogeneic blood and bone-marrow stem-cell transplantation in haematological malignant diseases: a randomised trial. Lancet 355:1231–1237

MOLECULAR BIOLOGY

True/False answers

135.   Biofilms

A. **F**   B. **T**   C. **F**   D. **T**   E. **F**

When bacteria adhere to surfaces such as plastic, metal or damaged tissue (e.g. bone), they can form a biofilm – a layer of bacteria encased in protein and polysaccharides. Bacteria in such a biofilm behave very differently to those floating freely in body fluids. Access to nutrients is often a limiting factor, and bacteria within a biofilm often slow their metabolism dramatically, with a consequent reduction in their doubling time. Such bacteria are intrinsically resistant to many antibiotics that target metabolic or cell-division processes with bacteria. Some bacterial cells take this process to extremes, forming spore-like structures with minimal metabolic activity, which are very resistant to antibiotic attack. Furthermore, biofilms can retard the diffusion of antibiotics, allowing resistance enzymes such as beta lactamases to destroy antibiotics before they accumulate to lethal levels.

Similarly, biofilms impede the free diffusion of metabolic waste products. The deeper layers of a biofilm can be highly acidic and anaerobic, conditions favouring the growth of other species of bacteria, as well as inhibiting the action of some antibiotics. Thus although a biofilm often starts with a single species of bacterium, for example, *Pseudomonas aeruginosa* or *Staphylococcus aureus*, most established biofilms are polymicrobial, with different species taking advantage of the microenvironments to be found in the biofilm. Cooperative interactions can occur not only between individual bacterial cells of the same species but also between species, helping to stabilise the biofilm environment.

Biofilms are notoriously difficult to remove with antimicrobial therapy; such therapy often damps down signs of infection by killing free-floating bacterial cells but signs of infection return on stopping the antibiotics. Combination therapy can prove more effective in a few situations but it is usually necessary to remove the damaged tissue (e.g. osteomyelitis) or the prosthetic substrate (e.g. prosthetic heart valve, prosthetic hip joint).

Reference

Stewart P S, Costerton J W 2001 Antibiotic resistance of bacteria in biofilms. Lancet 358:135–138

136. Apoptosis

A. F   B. T   C. T   D. T   E. T

Apoptosis is a form of programmed cell death that is central to the understanding of embryological morphogenesis, the pathogenesis of cancer, autoimmune disease, HIV infection and perhaps even neurodegenerative diseases, including Alzheimer's disease. Apoptosis can be triggered by cell–cell interactions or by cellular damage from radiation, cytotoxic drugs or withdrawal of growth factors.

Two pathways exist to trigger the apoptotic cascade. The extrinsic pathway is triggered by receptor–ligand interactions at the cell surface; there are several so-call 'death receptors', including Fas, TNF-receptor 1 and the TRAIL (TNF-related apoptosis-inducing ligand) receptors. These receptors trigger a proteolytic cascade involving the caspase family of enzymes, which ends in the activation of 'executioner caspases' – the enzymes that digest chromatin and induce cell fragmentation. The second pathway is the intrinsic pathway. Damage to mitochondria by a variety of stimuli leads to release of cytochrome c, which combines with several other proteins to form a complex know as the apoptosome. This complex then triggers the caspase cascade.

As would be expected, such a process is subject to multiple controls at different points. The tumour suppressor gene p53 is capable not only of causing cell-cycle arrest but can also trigger expression of 'death receptors' at the cell surface, Other inhibitors, for example the FLIP protein, can prevent the activated death receptor from triggering the caspase cascade; still others (bcl-2) can trigger apoptosis via the intrinsic pathway; a process that is inhibited by the BAX protein. A series of caspase inhibitors has also been discovered.

There is evidence that dysregulation of apoptosis is a feature of many disease states. Many cancers have mutations of genes involved in apoptosis (e.g. p53, bcl-2), suggesting that such cancers manage to avoid the normal triggers for apoptosis in order to proliferate. Some cancers, however, have increased rates of apoptosis – their proliferative rate appears to exceed the rate at which apoptosis can be induced. An interesting phenomenon known as tumour cell counterattack has also been described, whereby tumour cells express the Fas ligand on their surface. Any cytotoxic lymphocyte making contact with such a tumour cell will have its own apoptotic programme triggered by the Fas ligand, thus destroying the tumour-cell-specific lymphocyte response.

HIV infection leads to excessive apoptosis in the T helper cell population; many cells that die are not directly infected with HIV but die as a bystander effect. The mechanisms are unclear, but transfer of HIV-Tat protein to bystander cells might play a role in sensitising bystander cells to apoptosis. Autoimmune conditions such as SLE and autoimmune thyroid disease show evidence of deranged apoptosis; it could be that a failure of apoptosis occurs, thus autoreactive immune cells are not deleted effectively. Such cells are thus left free to attack the body's own tissues. Neurological death often occurs via similar mechanisms to apoptosis; cell death in the area of penumbral ischaemia in acute stroke, as well as cell death in Huntingdon's chorea and Alzheimer's disease all occur via an apoptosis-like pathway. It remains to be seen whether manipulation of the apoptotic pathway will translate into clinical benefit in this wide range of disease processes.

References

Eichhorst S T, Kramner P H 2001 Derangement of apoptosis in cancer. Lancet 358:345–346

Haslett C, Savill J 2001 Why is apoptosis important? British Medical Journal 322:1499–1500

Renehan A G, Booth C, Potten C S 2001 What is apoptosis, and why is it important? British Medical Journal 322:1536–1538

Sjostrom J, Bergh J 2001 How apoptosis is regulated, and what goes wrong in cancer. British Medical Journal 322:1538–1539

137.   Oxidative phosphorylation

A. **T**   B. **T**   C. **T**   D. **T**   E. **T**

The oxidative phosphorylation pathway is a major energy generating metabolic pathway contained within the mitochondria. Five complexes (I–V), which are located on the inner mitochondrial membrane, act to pass electrons down the chain. This energy source is used to pump hydrogen ions across the membrane and the resultant electrochemical transmembrane gradient drives an ATPase in complex V that produces ATP.

Defects of the oxidative phosphorylation pathway can be primary (due to an intrinsic defect of the pathway constituents) or secondary, for example due to toxins (e.g. cyanide). There are 83 proteins involved in the pathway, 13 of which are encoded by mitochondrial DNA; the other 70 are coded for by nuclear DNA. Diseases such as MELAS (myoclonus, epilepsy, lactic acidosis and stroke-like episodes), chronic progressive external ophthalmoplegia and MERRF (myoclonic epilepsy with ragged red fibres) are encoded on mitochondrial DNA, and are thus maternally inherited. Other diseases, such as Friedreich's ataxia and Huntington's chorea, involve nuclear encoded proteins. Frataxin, the attected gene product in Friedreich's ataxia, appears to be involved in iron handling within mitochondria. Frataxin defects lead to iron accumulation and to severe deficiencies of complexes I, II and III.

Many mitochondrial diseases affect the muscles and brain; a reflection of the dependence that these organs have on the oxidative phosphorylation pathway. Many of these diseases have a highly variable distribution in terms of severity and organs affected. This could reflect the fact that mitochondria appear to segregate to different organs and tissues early on in embryogenesis; a mutation in one mitochondrion at this stage might therefore affect only a certain subset of tissues.

Several other well-known neurodegenerative diseases display abnormalities of the pathway, including Parkinson's disease, Alzheimer's disease and Wilson's disease. Whether such abnormalities are a non-specific response to cellular damage from other pathogenic processes, or whether they are in fact causative, remains to be elucidated.

References

Leonard J V, Schapira A H V 2000a Mitochondrial respiratory chain disorders I: mitochondrial DNA defects. Lancet 355:299–304

Leonard J V, Schapira A H V 2000b Mitochondrial respiratory chain disorders II: neurodegenerative disorders and nuclear gene defects. Lancet 355:389–394

138. Selenium

A. **F**   B. **T**   C. **T**   D. **T**   E. **F**

Selenium is an essential trace element with a number of important roles in maintaining health. It forms a complex with cysteine (selenocysteine) in a number of enzymes; over thirty such enzymes have been discovered so far. Examples of enzymes include several types of glutathione peroxidases, which act as antioxidants and protect cellular contents from oxidative damage. Iodothyronine deiodinases also contain selenium; these enzymes convert thyroxine to triiodothyronine. Several selenium-containing proteins have also been found in sperm and appear to be important for sperm motility and protection of sperm during development.

A number of health problems have been associated with low selenium levels; Keshan disease (a cardiomyopathy) and Kashin–Beck disease (arthritis) occur in areas of China with very low selenium levels in the soil. Selenium deficiency also appears to lead to loss of immune function, both cell-mediated and humoral, and is correlated with reduced male fertility and increased rates of miscarriage. Low mood also correlates with selenium deficiency, as do subtle perturbations of the triiodothyronine:thyroxine ratio.

Viral illness can alter the measured selenium level; this might account for the lower levels of selenium seen in HIV infection, but low selenium levels also appear to change the natural history of some viral infections. Low selenium levels resulting in impaired immune function might allow viral infections to escape from immune control, but animal models have also suggested that low selenium levels can lead to an increase in viral virulence.

The relationship between selenium and cardiovascular disease is controversial. Selenium is known to have antioxidant properties, probably mediated by its role in the reaction centre of glutathione peroxidase enzymes. In patients with coronary artery disease, selenium levels correlate inversely with platelet aggregability – a reflection of the effects of selenium on the balance of arachidonic acid metabolites. Prospective studies examining the incidence of cardiovascular disease in relation to selenium levels have mostly failed to show an association between cardiovascular disease and selenium, however.

Selenium supplementation has been tried as a therapy in a number of conditions. It appears to improve mood in depressed individuals with low selenium levels and can improve sperm motility and fertility in subfertile men. Selenium has been shown to reduce pain and exacerbations of chronic pancreatitis. There is weak evidence that selenium might be able to reduce the incidence of hepatocellular cancer in hepatitis-B-positive patients, and perhaps reduce mortality in patients with a history of cancer who are deficient in selenium. No data is yet available regarding the effect of selenium supplementation on cardiovascular disease.

Reference

Rayman M P 2000 The importance of selenium to human health. Lancet 356:233–241

139. Angiogenesis

A. **T**   B. **T**   C. **F**   D. **T**   E. **F**

Angiogenesis is a complex phenomenon, controlled by several growth factors and inhibitors. Therapeutic interest in angiogenesis has been stimulated by two groups of diseases. Ischaemic conditions, such as coronary artery disease, stroke and peripheral vascular disease, could benefit from the administration of angiogenic factors to grow new vessels and hence improve blood supply. Tumour growth, on the other hand, depends on new vessel growth accompanying the growth of the tumour. Antiangiogenic factors could therefore be expected to halt tumour growth or confine tumours to very small sizes.

Many substances have been shown to have angiogenic activity, including vascular endothelial growth factor, fibroblast growth factor, tumour necrosis factor, interleukin-8, the transforming growth factors, angiogenin, proliferin, hepatocyte growth factor and platelet-derived growth factor. Both leptin and thyroxine have also been shown to have angiogenic effects. Of these substances, attention has concentrated on vascular endothelial growth factor and fibroblast growth factor. Vascular endothelial growth factor is released in response to stimuli such as exercise and hypoxia. It binds to receptors on endothelial cells, stimulating mitogenesis and migration of endothelial cells to form new endothelial channels. Formation of the extracellular matrix and recruitment of smooth muscle cells then occurs to form new blood vessels.

Fibroblast growth factor, especially FGF-2, has more widespread effects. It too is released in response to hypoxia; it binds to a variety of cells including endothelial cells, fibroblasts and smooth muscle cells, causing proliferation and migration. It acts as a vasodilating agent and also stimulates endothelial cells to produce matrix metalloproteinases, which facilitate cell movement and cell matrix remodelling. Fibroblast growth factor and vascular endothelial growth factor are under study in intractable angina as well as in peripheral vascular disease; the recent TRAFFIC study showed that fibroblast growth factor infusion for peripheral vascular disease can improve walking distance.

The effects of angiogenic factors are balanced by naturally occurring antiangiogenic substances. These include interferon alpha, angiostatin, platelet factor 4, tissue inhibitors of metalloproteinases, thrombospondin and pigment-epithelium-derived factor. A number of trials of such substances (e.g. angiostatin) are underway to establish whether antiangiogenic factors can cause regression of tumours or prevent the growth of metastases.

References

Donnelly R, Yeung J M 2002 Therapeutic angiogenesis: a step forward in intermittent claudication. Lancet 359:2048–2050

Henry T D 1999 Therapeutic angiogenesis. British Medical Journal 318:1536–1539

Lederman R J, Mendelsohn F O, Anderson R D et al 2002 Therapeutic angiogenesis with recombinant fibroblast growth factor-2 for intermittent claudication (the TRAFFIC study): a randomised trial. Lancet 359:2053–2058

140. Mechanisms of bone turnover

A. **T**   B. **T**   C. **T**   D. **T**   E. **T**

Bone turnover relies on a balance between the activity of osteoclasts and osteoblasts. Both types of cell work together in small units of bone turnover, with osteoclasts first resorbing an area of bone and then osteoblasts laying down new bone after a delay. Bone loss (leading eventually to osteoporosis) occurs when osteoclastic activity exceeds osteoblastic activity. This can be due to increased osteoclast activity or lifespan, reduced osteoblast activity or lifespan, or both phenomena working together. In the postmenopausal period, osteoblast lifespan appears to fall, probably as a result of lower estrogen levels.

Osteoblasts not only form new bone, they are responsible for triggering the formation and activity of osteoclasts. Factors such as parathyroid hormone, estrogen and vitamin D act upon osteoblasts, which in turn produce the receptor activator of nuclear factor κ ligand (RANK ligand). This molecule, similar in structure to the soluble tumour necrosis factor receptor, acts on precursor cells in bone to produce osteoclasts. The precursor cells are also under the control of osteoblasts via osteoblast production of macrophage colony stimulating factor, which encourages the precursor cells to proliferate. Osteoblasts also influence stromal cells and osteoclast activity via cytokines, including interleukin-6. Further regulation is provided by osteoprotegerin, which inhibits osteoclast formation.

Estrogen is well known to influence bone mineral density, as witnessed by the accelerated loss of bone after the menopause and in low estrogen states (e.g. primary ovarian failure). Estrogen is an important determinant of bone loss in older men as well as women; low free estradiol levels correlate with low bone mineral density in older men. Androgens also play a role, however; they promote bone formation to counter the increased resorption seen in low estrogen states.

Most of the variance in peak bone mass in younger adults appears to be genetic rather than environmental, as suggested by twin studies. Despite this, the genes that underlie this variance have proved elusive; most of the obvious candidates such as genes involved in calcium homeostasis, vitamin D metabolism, collagen and collagen synthesis and cellular activation factors can explain only a very small amount of the observed genetic variance. Furthermore, no genetic loci have been shown to predict fracture rates or response to therapies such as calcium, vitamin D or bisphosphonates as yet.

Reference

Seeman E 2002 Pathogenesis of bone fragility in women and men. Lancet 359:1841–1850

141. Biology of the senses

A. **T**   B. **T**   C. **T**   D. **F**   E. **F**

Recent research has extended the receptor paradigm to a number of special sensory inputs. Cold stimuli activate an excitatory ion channel (cold and menthol receptor, CMR1), a member of the transient receptor potential family of ion channels. The CMR1 channel is an excitatory calcium-conducting channel found on small trigeminal nerve endings, and can be activated by menthol as well as by cold stimuli. Related transient receptor potential family members, the vanilloid receptors, detect heat. Vanilloid receptor 1 is activated by temperatures above 43°C, and also by capsaicin, the active ingredient in chilli powder. The related VRL-1 channel is activated by temperatures above 52°C but not by capsaicin.

Controversy surrounds the existence of human pheromones, despite the widespread availability of so-called pheromone preparations now available to help boost the wearer's sexual attractiveness. Although no substance has been found in humans that would serve as a putative pheromone, recent work has led to the detection of analogues of known mammalian pheromone receptors in the human genome. One receptor sequence, *V1RL1* is of particular interest, and mRNA expression from this gene has been found to be confined to the nasal mucosa. It remains to be seen if specific agonists of this receptor display pheromone-like effects.

The four primary tastes – sweet, salt, sour and bitter – have not as yet been associated with specific receptors. A fifth taste – referred to in Japanese as 'umami' and describing a meaty, filling taste – has recently been associated with a truncated version of the glutamate receptor mGluR4. The truncated receptor is found in the taste buds and is much less sensitive to glutamate than normal glutamate receptors. The function of the receptor might be to signal the presence of foods with a high protein content, such as meat – its existence also explains the effectiveness of monosodium glutamate as a flavour enhancer.

References

Chaudhari N, Landin A M, Roper S D 2000 A metabotropic glutamate receptor variant functions as a taste receptor. Nature Neuroscience 3:113–119

McKemy D, Neuhausser W M, Julius D 2002 Identification of a cold receptor reveals a general role for TRP channels in thermosensation. Nature 416:52–58

Morris K 2000 Candidate receptor turns on human pheromone debate. Lancet 356:835

142. Channelopathies

A. **T**   B. **F**   C. **T**   D. **F**   E. **F**

'Channelopathy' is an umbrella term that refers to any disorder affecting electrically active membrane channels. Such disorders can affect the function of nerve and muscle, both skeletal and cardiac. Channelopathies can be congenital (due to mutated genes) or acquired, due to drugs, antibodies, toxins or the effects of pathological processes such as inflammation on the expression and action of channels.

Several cardiac diseases are now known to be due to disorders of channel function. Congenital long QT syndromes are known to be due to mutations in the SCN5A sodium channel, causing increased sodium flux, or to potassium channel mutations (e.g. KCNQ1, KCNE1), which lead to a loss of potassium channel function. Acquired long QT syndromes can be produced by the action of a variety of drugs; e.g. amiodarone and dofetilide block the action of the inward-rectifying potassium channel.

Heart failure is notorious for the high incidence of malignant ventricular arrhythmias associated with the condition; it is noteworthy that downregulation of potassium channels is a prominent feature of heart failure. Computer modelling has demonstrated that this downregulation, resulting in QT prolongation, can produce afterdepolarisations leading to ventricular tachycardia. The downregulation in potassium channels might be another example of an adaptive response that has long-term deleterious effects; in the short term, potassium channel downregulation would be expected to increase the depolarisation voltage, thus enhancing calcium influx and improving excitation-contraction coupling, hence improving myocyte contractility.

The Brugada syndrome is an uncommon congenital condition characterised by sudden death or ventricular fibrillation in structurally normal hearts. It often affects young adults and is most common in patients of South East Asian origin. The resting ECG shows characteristic 'coved' ST elevation in leads V1 to V3, together with a partial right bundle branch block. The syndrome has been linked to loss-of-function mutations of the SCN5A fast sodium channel.

The familial periodic paralyses are examples of inherited channelopathies affecting skeletal muscle. Hyperkalaemic periodic paralysis is due to mutations of the alpha 1 subunit of the skeletal muscle sodium channel; hypokalaemic periodic paralysis is due to mutations of the alpha 1 subunit of a skeletal muscle calcium channel – not a potassium channel.

Disordered function and distribution of sodium channels on neurons has been noted in multiple sclerosis, e.g. in the Purkinje cells of the cerebellum. This acquired channelopathy might explain the reversible loss of neuronal function seen in relapsing multiple sclerosis, but is not thought to be the primary pathological process. Rather, the channelopathy is thought to occur secondary to inflammation, or possibly even to antibodies directed against channels. Demyelination remains the hallmark of multiple sclerosis pathology, but the channelopathy does appear to contribute to the loss of neuronal function.

References

Marban E 2002 Cardiac channelopathies. Nature 415:213–218

Rose M R 1998 Neurological channelopathies. British Medical Journal 316:1104–1105

Waxman S G 2001 Acquired channelopathies in nerve injury and MS. Neurology 56:1621–1627

143.   Antimicrobial peptides

A. **F**   B. **T**   C. **T**   D. **T**   E. **F**

Over 500 naturally occurring peptides have now been discovered to possess antimicrobial activity. Most are very small, often only a few dozen amino acids in length, and most have an 'amphipathic' configuration, that is, there are well separated hydrophobic and cationic areas. Such peptides have been found in all members of the animal kingdom, including in humans.

The mechanism of action of such peptides is still under intense scrutiny but many of them appear to exploit a fundamental difference between eukaryotic and prokaryotic cell membranes. Negatively charged phospholipids are present on the outer and inner leaflets of bacterial membranes, whereas the outer leaflet of eukaryotic cell membranes is usually neutral in charge. This allows antimicrobial peptides to bind preferentially to the outer leaflet of bacterial cell membranes. Several mechanisms that could result in bacterial cell death have been postulated, including pore formation, destabilisation of membranes or energy gradients, or translocation of the peptides into the bacterial cytoplasm. The intracellular target (if any) of such peptides is unclear at present.

In humans, antimicrobial peptides, such as defensins and buforin, are found on most epithelial surfaces. In the gut, excess quantities of histone A2 are produced and secreted by gut epithelial cells; the histone is then cleaved in the gut lumen by pepsin to buforin, a powerful antimicrobial peptide. The ionic environment in which the peptides act appears to have an important influence on their activity; the disruption caused to the ionic milieu of the lung by cystic fibrosis leads to reduced activity of defensins secreted by the lung epithelium. This might contribute to the susceptibility to bacterial infection seen in cystic fibrosis.

Antimicrobial peptides are integrated into the overall function of the immune system; proinflammatory cytokines such as interleukin-1 induce epithelial surfaces to produce antimicrobial peptides and antimicrobial peptides released by neutrophils and epithelial cells act as chemoattractive agents for T lymphocytes. A variety of antimicrobial peptides are being trialled for use as anti-infectives in topical, systemic or catheter-associated form, but none have been approved for routine use as yet.

Reference

Zasloff M 2002 Antimicrobial peptides of multicellular organisms. Nature 415:389–395

144. Molecular biology of hypoxia

A. **F**   B. **T**   C. **F**   D. **T**   E. **F**

Hypoxia is known to trigger a series of adaptive responses in eukaryotic cells, including the stimulation of erythropoiesis and angiogenesis, the production of cellular growth and mitotic factors, a switch to glycolytic energy production, alterations in ion and substrate transport and changes in cell–matrix interactions. An understanding of the mechanisms underlying these changes is important not only in ischaemic diseases such as myocardial infarction, but also in cancer biology, as large areas of many solid tumours exist under hypoxic conditions.

Recent work has shown that many of the above changes are mediated by hypoxia-inducible factor, a two-component protein system that binds to promoter areas present on many genes – the hypoxic response element. Hypoxia-inducible factor is synthesised continuosly but, in the presence of oxygen, proline residues on hypoxia-inducible factor are hydroxylated. This process allows the protein to be tagged with ubiquitin, the modified protein is then bound by the von Hippel–Lindau protein, which targets the modified hypoxia-inducible factor to the proteasome for destruction. Under hypoxic conditions this process of protein tagging and destruction does not occur, leading to increased levels of hypoxia-inducible factor.

Hypoxia-inducible factor can activate a large series of genes, including the erythropoietin gene, growth factors including IGF-1, matrix factors such as collagen, angiogenic factors such as vascular endothelial growth factor, and metabolic machinery, such as glucose transporters and glycolytic enzymes. Thus, hypoxia-inducing factor appears to be central to the hypoxic cellular response. Erythropoietin is responsible for the enhanced erythropoietic response to hypoxia but does not appear to directly mediate other aspects of the hypoxic response; the production of erythropoietin is under the control of hypoxia-inducible factor. The role of oxygen as the trigger for the hypoxic response has been shown by studying the effects of growing cells under different levels of hypoxia; also by the fact that cyanide, which depletes ATP but does not change oxygen levels, does not cause an increase in erythropoietin levels.

Von Hippel–Lindau protein is a tumour suppressor gene that is inactivated in a variety of cancers, including renal cell carcinoma. As noted above, it plays an important role in regulating the hypoxic response; whether failure to destroy hypoxia-inducible factor, with consequent widespread gene upregulation can explain all of the tumourigenic effects of von Hippel–Lindau protein remains to be seen.

Reference

Maxwell P H 2002 Oxygen homeostasis and cancer: insights from a rare disease. Clinical Medicine 2:356–362

145. Hypocretin/orexin

A. **F**   B. **F**   C. **T**   D. **T**   E. **F**

Hypocretins (also known as orexins) are a recently discovered pair of small neuropeptides. They bind to two forms of hypocretin receptor, which are G-protein-coupled transmembrane receptors. Hypocretins appear to act as excitatory neurotransmitters; the cell bodies of neurons that release hypocretins are found only in the dorsolateral hypothalamus in humans. From there, the neurons project to the locus ceruleus, amygdala, nucleus tractus solitarus, reticular formation, thalamus and basal ganglia.

The hypocretin sytem has been implicated in two major disease areas so far – narcolepsy and obesity. Levels of hypocretin in the cerebrospinal fluid are usually remarkably uniform across a wide range of age and sex within the human population, but most patients with narcolepsy have undetectable or suppressed levels of hypocretin. Postmortem brain studies show that most sufferers of narcolepsy have lost over 90% of their hypocretin-secreting neurons. It is not clear how or why these neurons are destroyed; gliosis is present in some but not all patients. It has been postulated that the few narcolepsy patients with normal hypocretin levels might have resistance to the effects of hypocretin. Hypocretin or hypocretin receptor mutations appear to be a very rare cause of narcolepsy.

Hypocretins have also been implicated in appetite and weight regulation, a not unsurprising finding given the site of hypocretin neurons in the hypothalamus. Animal studies suggest that hypocretin stimulates appetite and weight gain, although the situation appears rather different in humans. Given the fact that hypocretin levels in narcolepsy are reduced, low body mass indices would be expected in narcolepsy. This is not the case, however; body mass index is elevated in most narcolepsy sufferers, and the prevalence of diabetes is higher than in control populations. Further work is underway to examine the effect of hypocretins and hypocretin receptor blockers in humans.

References

Ebrahim I O, Howard R S, Kopelman M D et al 2002 The hypocretin/orexin system. Journal of the Royal Society of Medicine 95:227–230

Schuld A, Hebebrand J, Geller F, Pollmacher T 2000 Increased body-mass index in patients with narcolepsy. Lancet 355:1274–1275

Taheri S, Zeitzer J M, Mignot E 2002 The role of hypocretins (orexins) in sleep regulation and narcolepsy. Annual Review of Neuroscience 25:283–313

ONCOLOGY
True/False answers

146. Therapy for malignant gliomas

A. **F**   B. **T**   C. **F**   D. **T**   E. **F**

Malignant gliomas have a very poor prognosis; the 2-year survival from diagnosis for patients with high-grade lesions is only 5–10%. Malignant gliomas are difficult to treat because their infiltrating nature makes surgical excision virtually impossible, and the blood–brain barrier prevents good tissue penetration by most cytotoxic agents.

A recent meta-analysis showed that adding chemotherapy in the form of nitrosoureas to surgery plus radiotherapy confers a small survival advantage; the 1-year survival rate rose from 40% to 46%.

Currently, chemotherapeutic interest centres around temozolomide, a DNA methylating agent with good penetration of the blood–brain barrier. Objective radiographic changes were seen in 35% of patients receiving temozolomide, and a randomised controlled trial of temozolomide versus procarbazine demonstrated a small but significant improvement in median survival. However, progression-free survival at 6 months was still only 21% in the temozolomide group. Temozolomide was well tolerated, with few side-effects, and led to improvements in health-related quality of life scores.

Cognitive function often declines in patients with low-grade malignant gliomas; a recent analysis suggests that although the majority of this decline is attributable to the presence of the tumour, radiotherapy can affect memory function if administered in fractions above 2 Gy. Antiepileptic medications were associated with problems in attention and executive function.

Radiotherapy can be carried out using a gamma knife, which is not, in fact, a knife and cannot be used for biopsy. It is a highly focused source of gamma rays, which can be used to apply radiation to a cerebral tumour or metastasis in a precise, targeted manner. Investigations are ongoing to ascertain whether the technique provides additional survival, function or quality of life advantages over conventional therapy.

References

Batchelor T 2000 Temozolomide for malignant brain tumours. Lancet 355:1115–1116

Glioma Meta-analysis (GMT) Group 2002 Chemotherapy in adult high-grade glioma: a systematic review and meta-analysis of individual patient data from 12 randomised trials. Lancet 359:1011–1018

Klein M, Heimans J J, Aaronson N K et al 2002 Effect of radiotherapy and other treatment-related factors on mid-term to long-term cognitive sequelae in low-grade gliomas: a comparative study. Lancet 360:1361–1368

147.   Estrogen and breast cancer

A. **F**   B. **T**   C. **F**   D. **F**   E. **F**

Estrogen has long been known to play an important role in breast cancer – one of the earliest treatments for breast cancer failing to respond to local surgery was bilateral oophorectomy. Estrogen receptors are present on many breast cancers and estrogen is a powerful mitogen and growth promoter for many breast tumours. Cumulative exposure to estrogen correlates with risk of breast cancer, hence early menarche, late menopause and late first pregnancy all increase the risk of breast cancer. High estradiol levels in postmenopausal women also correlate with an increased risk and bone mineral density (a crude correlate of lifetime estrogen exposure) is inversely correlated with the risk of developing breast cancer.

The biosynthetic pathway for estrogen is complex and several genetic polymorphisms have been found to confer increased risk of breast cancer. These include 17α-hydroxylase and aromatase enzymes; mutant varieties that lead to high circulating estrogen concentrations are associated with breast cancer development. Conversely, alterations in the degradation pathways for estrogen, e.g. cytochrome P450 1A1 and catechol-O-methyltransferase can also confer increased risk. In the case of catechol-O-methyl transferase, mutations with low activity predispose to breast cancer, as more estrogen is metabolised by an alternative pathway that produces carcinogenic intermediates.

Rates of breast cancer are low in parts of the world that ingest a large amount of soya. Soya is known to be a rich source of phytestrogens, which have complex effects, being both agonists and antagonists at estrogen receptors. It is unclear whether these antiestrogenic effects can explain the observed dietary link, or whether other factors are responsible, the high intake of soya being nothing more than a bystander effect.

Anastrozole is a specific aromatase inhibitor, which reduces circulating estrogen levels by 97–99%. It has shown at least equivalent efficacy to tamoxifen (and superior efficacy in some trials) as a treatment for metastatic breast cancer and trials are ongoing regarding its role in adjuvant therapy. No data exist as yet to show that it can reduce the incidence of first occurrence breast cancer in high-risk individuals.

Hormone replacement therapy has been known to carry a small increased risk of breast cancer for some time; the recent Women's Health Initiative (WHI) trial confirmed a relative risk of 1.26 versus placebo – a result of borderline significance. This trial also suggested that the cardioprotective effects of hormone replacement therapy were not present – in fact the risk of both coronary heart disease and stroke were increased in the treatment arm. This clearly has implications for the risk:benefit balance in using hormone replacement therapy, and many women are re-evaluating their decision to take hormone replacement therapy in the light of these trial results. Despite this, the absolute increase in breast cancer seen in the WHI trial is small – 8 cases per 10 000 person-years.

References

Clemons M, Goss P 2001 Estrogen and the risk of breast cancer. New England Journal of Medicine 344:276–285

Lonning P E 2001 Aromatase inhibitors and inactivators in breast cancer. British Medical Journal 323:880–881

Writing group for the Women's Health Initiative (WHI) investigators 2002 Risks and benefits of estrogen plus progestin in health postmenopausal women. Journal of the American Medical Association 288:321–333

148. Hypercalcaemia of malignancy

A. **T**   B. **T**   C. **F**   D. **F**   E. **F**

Hypercalcaemia in malignancy can be a paraneoplastic condition, usually mediated by circulating parathyroid hormone-related peptide (PTHrP), or it can be due to bony metastases, as is almost certainly the case in this woman. Recent studies have elucidated the molecular mechanisms underlying the activity of bony metastases in more detail and it has become apparent that PTHrP is a key player in bony metastases from breast cancer and other cancers producing osteolytic lesions. It is released by tumour cells and acts on osteoblasts to stimulate production of RANKL and downregulate osteoprotegerin production. These changes lead to osteoclast overactivity and consequent bone resorption.

Calcium is released as a result of osteoclast overactivity but rather than this leading to increased excretion of calcium by the kidneys, the increased circulating levels of PTHrP in fact encourage tubular reabsoprtion of calcium by the kidneys, exacerbating the hypercalcaemia. Growth factors such as transforming growth factor beta and IGF-1 are released by overactive osteoclasts and these factors, together with elevated extracellular calcium, act to stimulate further tumour mitogenesis and growth, thus setting up a vicious cycle. In breast cancer cells, transforming growth factor beta drives production of PTHrP by the tumour cells, creating a vicious cycle of osteolysis.

It has been known for many years that bisphosphonates inhibit osteoclast activity and this is the principal mechanism by which they reduce elevated calcium levels. They appear to have cytotoxic effects against other cell types including osteoblasts, macrophages and tumour cells; however, bisphosphonates can interrupt cellular energy production and can induce apoptosis. These effects might underlie the improved survival noted in some trials of bisphosphonate therapy.

Osteoprotegerin is not yet available as a calcium-lowering therapy in humans; trials are awaited. There are powerful theoretical reasons for thinking that it will be highly effective. Endothelin antagonists have not been trialled as a therapy for hypercalcaemia in humans as yet; molecular studies show that endothelin and factors such as fibroblast growth factor and platelet-derived growth factor are important in the establishment of osteoblastic bone metastases (e.g. from prostate cancer), thus inhibitors of endothelin might be found to have a place in the treatment or prevention of osteoblastic metastatic disease.

References

Body J J 2000 Current and future directions in medical therapy – hypercalcaemia. Cancer 88:3054–3058

Diel I J, Solomayer E F, Bastert G 2000 Bisphosphonates and the prevention of metastasis. Cancer 88:3080–3088

Mundy G R 2002 Metastasis to bone: causes, consequence and therapeutic opportunities. Nature Reviews. Cancer 2:584–593

Best-of-5 answers

149. Non-small cell lung cancer

Answer: **D**

The place of chemotherapy in non-small cell lung cancer has undergone something of a reappraisal over the last few years. Previous teaching was that non-small cell lung cancer responds better to radiotherapy, and that small cell lung cancer is much more sensitive to chemotherapy (although it almost always becomes resistant later). Recent trials using newer agents such as the taxanes, irinotecan and gemcitabine have shown modest tumour responses that nevertheless translate into overall survival benefits and progression-free periods for stage III and stage IV (metastatic) disease. Chemotherapy also appears to enhance the efficacy of radiotherapy for non-small cell lung cancer when used as induction therapy for stage III disease.

There is currently no clear evidence that adjuvant chemotherapy improves survival after surgical resection, although some studies have shown a survival advantage for stage II/III resected disease, others have not shown any benefit of adjuvant chemotherapy as compared to adjuvant radiation alone. Neoadjuvant chemotherapy has been shown to improve survival in patients with locally advanced lymph node disease (N2 disease); trials are underway examining the role of neoadjuvant chemotherapy for early stage lung cancer prior to surgical resection.

Chest X-ray screening has not proven to be sufficiently sensitive as a screening test to detect lung cancer at an early stage, even when combined with sputum cytology. Furthermore, the ambiguity associated with shadowing on a chest X-ray often requires further imaging and investigation to interpret, thus specificity of the test is low. It is therefore little surprise that trials in the 1960s and 1970s failed to show any benefit on survival from chest X-ray screening.

Low-dose CT scanning of the chest has generated much interest as a screening tool in recent years following the publication of the ELCAP study. This showed that low-dose CT of the chest was both sensitive and specific at detecting malignant chest lesions in the context of population screening. The sample size and follow-up in this study was insufficient to show a reduction in mortality from screening but several very large population screening studies are now underway, with follow-up periods of 5–6 years. These studies should hopefully tell us whether CT screening is an effective tool for reducing lung cancer mortality.

References

Baas P 2002 Inductive and adjuvant treatment strategies for localzed nonsmall cell lung cancer in operable and inoperable patients. Current Opinion in Oncology 14:180–184

Hoffman P C, Mauer A M, Vokes E E 2000 Lung cancer. Lancet 355:479–485

Van Klaveren J D, Pedersen J H, de Koning H J et al 2001 Lung cancer screening by low-dose spiral computed tomography. European Respiratory Journal 18:857–866

150. Second malignancy after chemotherapy and radiotherapy

Answer: **E**

A number of malignancies have become curable over the past 30 years, at least in a high proportion of affected patients. These include childhood leukaemia, Hodgkin's disease and testicular cancer – all of which affect comparatively young patients. Therapy for all of these conditions is based on aggressive radiotherapy and chemotherapy regimes.

The long-term survival of these patients has brought with it the problem of long-term side-effects of their anticancer therapy, namely second malignancies. Haematological malignancies, e.g. acute myeloid leukaemia, appear to be related to some forms of chemotherapy, and radiotherapy has been linked to solid tumours, e.g. lung cancer in the case of Hodgkin's disease and primary brain tumours in the case of children undergoing intensive cranial irradiation for acute lymphoblastic leukaemia. Testicular cancer radiotherapy has been linked to stomach and bladder tumours.

The risk of leukaemia after alkylating chemotherapy appears to be highest in the decade after treatment but the risks of radiation exposure do not appear to plateau; they continue to rise with time. Risk increases with increasing total radiation dose received. Combination chemoradiotherapy is associated with a greater risk of second malignancy and wide-field radiotherapy is also associated with a greater risk. The genetic makeup of the patient appears to play a part as well; patients with hereditary retinoblastoma receiving radiation therapy are at a much greater risk of developing bone cancer. There appears to be no effect of sex on the incidence of second malignancies, but patients whose primary malignancy presented later on in life are at reduced risk of a second malignancy compared with those who presented early in life.

Awareness of the risk of second malignancies has stimulated efforts to use milder treatment protocols, for example abandoning the use of cranial irradiation, using smaller radiation fields and reducing the number of cycles of chemotherapy. It is to be hoped that more precisely targeted therapy (e.g. monoclonal antibody therapy) will also reduce the carcinogenic risk of cancer therapy in the future.

References

Dong C, Hemminki K 2001 Second primary neoplasms among 53,159 haematolymphoproliferative malignancy patients in Sweden, 1958–1996: a search for common mechanisms. British Journal of Cancer 85:997–1005

Ng A K, Bernardo P, Weller E et al 2002 Second malignancy after Hodgkin disease treated with radiation therapy with or without chemotherapy: long-term risks and risk factors. Blood 100:1989–1996

Relling M V, Rubnitz J E, Rivera G K et al 1999 High incidence of secondary brain tumours after radiotherapy and antimetabolites. Lancet 354:34–39

Robison L L 1996 Second primary cancers after childhood cancers. British Medical Journal 312:861–862

References

ENDOCRINOLOGY

Atkinson M A, Eisenbarth G S 2001 Type 1 diabetes: new perspectives on disease pathogenesis and treatment. Lancet 358:221–229

Barker D J P 1997 Intrauterine programming of coronary heart disease and stroke. Acta Paediatrica (suppl):178–182

Barker D J P, Forsen T, Uutela A et al 2001 Size at birth and resilience to effects of poor living conditions in adult life: longitudinal study. British Medical Journal 323:1273–1276

Bertagna X 2001 Cushing's syndrome. Medicine 29:16–19

Betterele C, Greggio N A, Volpato M 1998 Clinical review 93. Autoimmune polyglandular syndrome type 1. Journal of Clinical Endocrinology and Metabolism 83:1049–1055

Boscaro M, Barzon L, Fallo F et al 2001 Cushing's syndrome. Lancet 357:783–791

Dayan C M 2001 Interpretation of thyroid function tests. Lancet 357:619–624

Dornholst A 2001 Insulinotropic meglitinide analogues. Lancet 358:1709–1716

Duncan E, Wass J A H 1999 Investigation protocol: Acromegaly and its investigation. Clinical Endocrinology 50:285–293

Eriksson J, Forsen T, Tuomilehto J et al 2001 Early growth and coronary heart disease in later life: longitudinal study. British Medical Journal 322:949–953

Feher MD 2002 Diabetes and hypertension. Medicine 30:30–32

Heart Outcome Prevention Evaluation (HOPE) study investigators 2000 Effects of ramipril on cardiovascular and microvascular outcomes in people with diabetes mellitus. Results of the HOPE study and MICRO-HOPE substudy. Lancet 355:246–259

Inzucchi S E 2002 Oral antihyperglycemic therapy for type 2 diabetes. Journal of the Americal Medical Association 287:360–372

James W P T, Astrup A, Finer N et al 2000 Effect of sibutramine on weight maintenance after weight loss: a randomised trial. Lancet 356:2119–2125

Julius S, Majahalme S, Palatini P 2001 Antihypertensive treatment of patients with diabetes and hypertension. American Journal of Hypertension 14:310S–316S

Lindholm L, Ibsen H, Dahlof B et al 2002 Cardiovascular morbidity and mortality in patients with diabetes in the Losartan Intervention for Endpoint reduction in hypertension study (LIFE): a randomised trial against atenolol. Lancet 359:1004–1010

Morris A D, Boyle D I R, McMahon A D et al 1997 Adherence to insulin treatment, glycaemic control, and ketoacidosis in insulin-dependent diabetes mellitus. Lancet 350:1505–1510

Myhre A G, Halonen M, Eskelin P et al 2001 Autoimmune polyendocrinopathy syndrome type 1 (APS 1) in Norway. Clinical Endocrinology 54:211–217

NICE 2000 Full guidance on rosiglitazone for type 2 diabetes mellitus. Technology appraisal guidance No 9. Online. Available: www.nice.org.uk/article.asp?a=1189

NICE 2001 Full guidance on the use of orlistat for the treatment of obesity in adults Technology appraisal guidance No 22. Online. Available: www.nice.org.uk/article.asp?a=1189

NICE 2001 Full guidance on the use of pioglitazone for type 2 diabetes mellitus Technology appraisal guidance No 21. Online. Available: www.nice.org.uk/article.asp?a=1189

NICE 2001 Full guidance on the use of sibutramine for the treatment of obesity in adults. Technology appraisal guidance No 31. Online. Available: www.nice.org.uk/article.asp?a=1189

Obermayer-Straub P, Manns M P 1998 Autoimmune polyglandular syndromes. Ballière's Clinical Gastroenterology 12:293–315

Parle J V, Masionneuve P, Sheppard M C et al 2001 Preduction of all-cause and cardiovascular mortality in elderly people from one low serum thyrotropin result: a 10-year cohort study. Lancet 358:861–865

Pearce S H S, Cheetham T D 2001 Autoimmune polyendocrinopathy syndrome type 1: treat with kid gloves. Clinical Endocrinology 54:433–435

Pickup J, Keen H 2002 Continuous subcutaneous insulin infusion at 25 years. Diabetes Care 25(3):593–598

Robinson R 2001 The fetal origins of adult disease. British Medical Journal 322:375–376

Schoonjans K, Auwerx J 2000 Thiazolidinediones: an update. Lancet 355:1008–1010

Shapiro A M J, Lakey J R T, Ryan E A et al 2000 Islet transplantation in seven patients with type 1 diabetes mellitus using a glucocorticoid-free immunosuppressive regimen. New England Journal of Medicine 343:230–238

Trainer P J, Drake W M, Katznelson L et al 2000 Treatment of acromegaly with the growth hormone-receptor antagonist pegvisomant. New England Journal of Medicine 342:1171–1177

Van der Lely A J, Hutson R K, Trainer P J et al 2001 Long-term treatment of acromegaly with pegvisomant, a growth hormone receptor antagonist. Lancet 358:1754–1759

Wardle C A, Fraser W D, Squire C R 2001 Pitfalls in the use of thyrotropin concentration as a first-line thyroid-function test. Lancet 357:1013–1014

RESPIRATORY

British Thoracic Society (BTS) Standards of Care Committee 1997 Suspected acute pulmonary embolism: a practical approach. Thorax 52(suppl 4):S1–S24

British Thoracic Society (BTS) and Society of Cardiothoracic Surgeons of Great Britain and Ireland Working Party 2001 Guidelines on the selection of patients with lung cancer for surgery. Thorax 56:89–108

British Thoracic Society (BTS) Standards of Care Committee 2002 Non-invasive ventilation in acute respiratory failure. Thorax 57:192–211

BTS Guidelines for the management of community acquired pneumonia in adults. Thorax 2001; 56(suppl 4):IV1–64

Burge P S, Calverley P M, Jones P W et al 2000 Randomised, double blind, placebo controlled study of fluticasone propionate in patients with moderate to severe chronic obstructive pulmonary disease: the ISOLDE trial. British Medical Journal 320:1297–1303

Compton C H, Gubb J, Nieman R et al 2001 Cilomilast, a selective phosphodiesterase-4 inhibitor for treatment of patients with chronic obstructive pulmonary disease: a randomised, dose-ranging study. Lancet 358:265–270

Drazen J M, Israel E, O'Byrne P M 1999 Treatment of asthma with drugs modifying the leukotriene pathway. New England Journal of Medicine 340:197–206

Frew A J, Plummeridge M J 2001 Alternative agents in asthma. Journal of Allergy and Clinical Immunology 108:3–10

Gross G, Thompson P J, Chervinsky P, Van den Burgt J 1999 Hydrofluoroalkane-134a beclomethasone dipropionate, 400 μg, is as effective as chlorofluorocarbon beclomethasone dipropionate, 800 μg, for the treatment of moderate asthma. Chest 115:343–351

Hoeper M M, Schwarze M, Ehlerding S et al 2000 Long-term treatment of primary pulmonary hypertension with aerosolized iloprost, a prostacyclin analogue. New England Journal of Medicine 342:1866–1870

Hoffman P C, Mauer A M, Vokes E E 2000 Lung cancer. Lancet 355:479–485

Jenkinson C, Davies R J, Mullins R, Stradling J R 1999 Comparison of therapeutic and subtherapeutic nasal continuous positive airway pressure for obstructive sleep apnoea: a randomised prospective parallel trial. Lancet 353:2100–2105

Joint Tuberculosis Committee of the British Thoracic Society 1998 Chemotherapy and management of tuberculosis in the United Kingdom: recommendations 1998. Thorax 53:536–548

Joint Tuberculosis Committee of the British Thoracic Society 2000 Control and prevention of tuberculosis in the United Kingdom: code of practice 2000. Thorax 55:887–901

Jorenby D E, Leischow S J, Nides M A et al 1999 A controlled trial of sustained-release bupropion, a nicotine patch, or both for smoking cessation. New England Journal of Medicine 340:685–691

Kemmeren J M, Algra A, Grobbee D E 2001 Third generation oral contraceptives and risk of venous thrombosis: meta-analysis. British Medical Journal 323:131–134

Leff J A, Busse W W, Pearlman D et al 1998 Montelukast, a leukotriene-receptor antagonist, for the treatment of mild asthma and exercise-induced bronchoconstriction. New England Journal of Medicine 339:147–152

Lipworth B J, White P S 2000 Allergic inflammation in the unified airway: start with the nose. Thorax 55:878–881

Lorut C, Ghossains M, Horellou M H et al 2000 A noninvasive diagnostic strategy including spiral computed tomography in patients with suspected pulmonary embolism. American Journal of Respiration and Critical Care Medicine 162:1413–1418

O'Byrne P M, Barnes P J, Rodriguez-Roisin R et al 2001 Low dose inhaled budesonide and formoterol in mild persistent asthma: the OPTIMA randomized trial. American Journal of Respiration and Critical Care Medicine 164:1392–1397

Pieterman R M, van Putten J W, Meuzelaar J J et al 2000 Preoperative staging of non-small-cell lung cancer with positron-emission tomography. New England Journal of Medicine 343:254–261

Plant P K, Owen J L, Elliott M W 2000 Early use of non-invasive ventilation for acute exacerbations of chronic obstructive pulmonary disease on general respiratory wards: a multicentre randomised controlled trial. Lancet 355:1931–1935

Poole P J, Black P N 2001 Oral mucolytic drugs for exacerbations of chronic obstructive pulmonary disease: systematic review. British Medical Journal 322:1271–1274

Recommendations on the management of pulmonary hypertension in clinical practice. Heart 2001; 86(suppl 1):I1–13

Rubin L J, Badesch D B, Barst R J et al 2002 Bosentan therapy for pulmonary arterial hypertension. New England Journal of Medicine 346:896–903

Sahn S A 1998 Use of fibrinolytic agents in the management of complicated parapneumonic effusions and empyemas. Thorax 53(suppl 2):S65–S72

Shrewsbury S, Pyke S, Britton M 2000 Meta-analysis of increased dose of inhaled steroid or addition of salmeterol in symptomatic asthma (MIASMA). British Medical Journal 320:1368–1373

Stradling J R, Pepperell J C, Davies R J 2001 Sleep apnoea and hypertension: proof at last? Thorax 56(suppl 2):ii45–ii49

Subcommittee of the Joint Tuberculosis Committee of the British Thoracic Society 2000 Management of opportunist mycobacterial infections: Joint Tuberculosis Committee Guidelines 1999. Thorax 55:210–218

The COPD Guidelines Group of the Standards of Care Committee of the BTS 1997 BTS guidelines for the management of chronic obstructive pulmonary disease. Thorax 52(suppl 5):S1–S28

Wood K E 2002 Major pulmonary embolism: review of a pathophysiologic approach to the golden hour of hemodynamically significant pulmonary embolism. Chest 121:877–905

DERMATOLOGY

Bindslev-Jensen C 1998 ABC of allergies: food allergy. British Medical Journal 316:1299–1302

Braun M, Lowitt M H 2001 Pruritus. Advances in Dermatology 17:1–27

Chaudhari U, Romano P, Mulcahy, LD et al 2001 Efficacy and safety of Infliximab monotherapy for plaque-type psoriasis: a randomised trial. Lancet 357:1842–1847

Ellis C N 1991 Cyclosporine for plaque type psoriasis; results of a multidose double blind trial. New England Journal of Medicine 324:277–284

Ferranger T, Miller F 2002 Cutaneous manifestations of diabetes mellitus. Dermatology Clinics 20:483–492

Gutgesell C, Heise S, Seubert S et al. 2001 Double blind placebo controlled trial of house dust avoidance measures in adult patients with atopic dermatitis. British Journal of Dermatology 145:70–74

Jull A, Waters J, Arroll B 2002 Pentoxifylline for treatment of venous leg ulcers: a systematic review. Lancet 359:1550–1554

Lanigan S W 2000 Lasers in dermatology. Medicine 28:16–18

Lebwohl M 2001 Treatment of psoriasis. Part 2. Systemic therapies. Journal of the American Academy of Dermatology 45:649–661

Marcil I, Stern R S 2001 Squamous-cell cancer of the skin in patients given PUVA and ciclosporin: nested cohort crossover study. Lancet 358:1042–1045

Nelson E A, Cullum N, Jones J 2001 Clinical evidence, 5th edn. BMJ Publishing, London, p 1366–1375

Owen C M, Telfer N R 2000 Skin cancer. Medicine 28:39–43

Roenigk H H 1998 Methotrexate in psoriasis: consensus conference. Journal of the American Academy of Dermatology 38(3):478–485

Schmelz M 2002 Itch: mediators and mechanism. Journal of Dermatological Science 28:91–96

CLINICAL PHARMACOLOGY

Amfebutamone/bupropion for smoking cessation: new preparation. Nicotine replacement therapy is safer. Prescrire International 2001 10:163–167

Anderson T J 1999 Assessment and treatment of endothelial dysfunction in humans. Journal of the American College of Cardiologists 34:631–638

Auerbach A D, Goldman L 2002 Beta-blockers and reduction of cardiac events in noncardiac surgery: scientific review. Journal of the American Medical Association 287:1435–1444

Benzaquen B S, Cohen V, Eisenberg M J 2001 Effects of cocaine on the coronary arteries. American Heart Journal 142:402–410

Boaz M, Smetana S, Weinstein T et al 2000 Secondary prevention with antioxidants of cardiovascular disease in endstage renal disease (SPACE): randomised placebo-controlled trial. Lancet 356:1213–1218

Brenner B M, Cooper M E, de Zeeuw D et al 2001 Effects of losartan on renal and cardiovascular outcomes in patients with type 2 diabetes and nephropathy. New England Journal of Medicine 345:861–969

Brown B G, Zhao X Q, Chait A et al 2001 Simvastatin and niacin, antioxidant vitamins, or the combination for the prevention of coronary disease. New England Journal of Medicine 345:1583–1592

Bupropion to aid smoking cessation. Drug and Therapeutics Bulletin 2000 38: 73–75

Dackis C A, O'Brien C P 2001 Cocaine dependence: a disease of the brain's reward centers. Journal of Substance Abuse and Treatment 21:111–117

Dahlof B, Devereux R B, Kjeldsen S E et al 2002 Cardiovascular morbidity and mortality in the Losartan Intervention For Endpoint reduction in hypertension study (LIFE): a randomised trial against atenolol. Lancet 359:995–1003

Dumont L, Mardirosoff C, Tramer M R 2000 Efficacy and harm of pharmacological prevention of acute mountain sickness: quantitative systematic review. British Medical Journal 321:267–272

Fattinger K, Benowitz N L, Jones R T, Verotta D 2000 Nasal mucosal versus gastrointestinal absorption of nasally administered cocaine. European Journal of Clinical Pharmacology 56:305–310

Frei B 1999 On the role of vitamin C and other antioxidants in atherogenesis and vascular dysfunction. Proceedings of the Society for Experimental Biology and Medicine 222:196–204

Fried S K, Ricci M R, Russell C D, Laferrere B 2000 Regulation of leptin production in humans. Journal of Nutrition 130:3127S–3131S

Fugh-Berman A 2000 Herb–drug interactions. Lancet 355:134–138

Ghoshal U C, Chaudhuri S, Pal B B et al 2001 Randomized controlled trial of intrasphincteric botulinum toxin A injection versus balloon dilatation in treatment of achalasia cardia. Diseases of the Esophagus 14:227–231

Gokce N, Keaney J F, Hunter L M et al 2002 Risk stratification for postoperative cardiovascular events via noninvasive assessment of endothelial function: a prospective study. Circulation 105:1567–1572

Gruppo Italiano per lo Studio della Sopravvivenza nell'Infarto miocardico 1999 Dietary supplementation with n-3 polyunsaturated fatty acids and vitamin E after myocardial infarction: results of the GISSI-Prevenzione trial. Lancet 354:447–455

He F J, MacGregor G A 2001 Fortnightly review: beneficial effects of potassium. British Medical Journal 323:497–501

Heart Outcomes Prevention Evaluation Study Investigators 2000 Effects of ramipril on cardiovascular and microvascular outcomes in people with diabetes mellitus: results of the HOPE study and MICRO-HOPE substudy. Lancet 355:253–259

Heintzen M P, Strauer B E 1994 Peripheral vascular effects of beta-blockers. European Heart Journal 15(suppl C):2–7

Heitzer T, Schlinzig T, Krohn K et al 2001 Endothelial dysfunction, oxidative stress, and risk of cardiovascular events in patients with coronary artery disease. Circulation 104:2673–2678

Hickey M S, Calsbeek D J 2001 Plasma leptin and exercise: recent findings. Sports Medicine 31:583–589

Hohenhaus E, Niroomand F, Goerre S et al 1994 Nifedipine does not prevent acute mountain sickness. American Journal of Respiratory and Critical Care Medicine 150:857–860

Holm K J, Spencer C M 2000 Bupropion: a review of its use in the management of smoking cessation. Drugs 59:1007–1024

Hurlimann D, Enseleit F, Noll G, Luscher T F, Ruschitzka F 2002 Endothelin antagonists and heart failure. Current Hypertension Reports 4:85–92

Influence of pravastatin and plasma lipids on clinical events in the West of Scotland Coronary Prevention Study (WOSCOPS). Circulation 1998 97:1440–1445

Kennedy J M, van Rij A M, Spears G F et al 2000 Polypharmacy in a general surgical unit and consequences of drug withdrawal. British Journal of Clinical Pharmacology 49:353–362

Krum H 1998 Effect of endothelin 1 on endothelium derived vascular responsiveness in man. Clinical Science 95:151–156

Le Bars P L, Kastelan J 2000 Efficacy and safety of a Ginkgo biloba extract. Public Health and Nutrition 3:495–499

Mantzoros C S 1999 The role of leptin in human obesity and disease: a review of current evidence. Annals of Internal Medicine 130:671–680

Medline Plus health information (National Library of Medicine) medical encyclopedia. Online. Available: www.nlm.nih.gov/medlineplus

Mogensen C E, Neldam S, Tikkanen I et al 2000 Randomised controlled trial of dual blockade of renin–angiotensin system in patients with hypertension, microalbuminuria, and non-insulin dependent diabetes: the candesartan and lisinopril microalbuminuria (CALM) study. British Medical Journal 321:1440–1444

Munchau A, Bhatia K P 2000 Uses of botulinum toxin injection in medicine today. British Medical Journal 320:161–165

Parving H H, Lehnert H, Brochner-Mortensen J et al 2001 The effect of irbesartan on the development of diabetic nephropathy in patients with type 2 diabetes. New England Journal of Medicine 345:870–878.

Pitt B, Zannad F, Remme W J et al 1999 The effect of spironolactone on morbidity and mortality in patients with severe heart failure. Randomized Aldactone Evaluation Study Investigators. New England Journal of Medicine 341:709–717

Rubin L J, Badesch D B, Barst R J et al 2002 Bosentan therapy for pulmonary arterial hypertension. New England Journal of Medicine 346:896–903

Schachinger V, Britten M B, Zeiher A M 2000 Prognostic impact of coronary vasodilator dysfunction on adverse long-term outcome of coronary heart disease. Circulation 101:1899–1906

Schiffrin E L 2001 Role of endothelin-1 in hypertension and vascular disease. American Journal of Hypertension 14:83S–89S

Schwartz G G, Olsson A G, Ezekowitz M D et al 2001 Effects of atorvastatin on early recurrent ischemic events in acute coronary syndromes: the MIRACL study: a randomized controlled trial. Journal of the American Medical Association 285:1711–1718

Smith J C, Kacker A, Anand V K 2002 Midline nasal and hard palate destruction in cocaine abusers and cocaine's role in rhinologic practice. Ear Nose and Throat Journal 81:172–177

Steiner M, Li W 2001 Aged garlic extract, a modulator of cardiovascular risk factors: a dose-finding study on the effects of age on platelet functions. Journal of Nutrition 131:980S–984S

Tam S W, Worcel M, Wyllie M 2001 Yohimbine: a clinical review. Pharmacology and Therapeutics 91:215–243

Teter C J, Guthrie S K 2001 A comprehensive review of MDMA and GHB: two common club drugs. Pharmacotherapy 21:1486–1513

Tramer M R, Carroll D, Campbell F A et al 2001 Cannabinoids for control of chemotherapy induced nausea and vomiting: quantitative systematic review. British Medical Journal 323:16–21

van Nieuwenhoven M A, Kovacs E M, Brummer R J et al 2001 The effect of different dosages of guar gum on gastric emptying and small intestinal transit of a consumed semisolid meal. Journal of the American College of Nutrition 20:87–91

Vaughan C J, Delanty N 2000 Hypertensive emergencies. Lancet 356:411–417

Wollina U, Karamfilov T, Konrad H 2002 High-dose botulinum toxin type A therapy for axillary hyperhidrosis markedly prolongs the relapse-free interval. Journal of the Americal Academy of Dermatology 46:536–540

Yusuf S, Zhao F, Mehta S R et al 2001 Effects of clopidogrel in addition to aspirin in patients with acute coronary syndromes without ST-segment elevation. New England Journal of Medicine 345:494–502

PSYCHIATRY

Adnet P, Lestavel P, Krivosic-Horber R 2000 Neuroleptic malignant syndrome. British Journal of Anaesthesia 85:129–135

Allison D, Mentore J, Heo M et al 2000 Review: most antipsychotic drugs are associated with weight gain. Evidence Based Medicine 3:58

Britton J, Jarvis J 2000 Buproprion: a new treatment for smokers. British Medical Journal 321:65–66

Cattell H 2000 Suicide in the elderly. Advances in Psychiatric Treatment 6:102–108

Clark C, Buchwald D, MacIntyre A et al 2002 Chronic fatigue syndrome: a step towards agreement. Lancet 359:97–98

Cookson J 2001 Use of antipsychotic drugs and lithium in mania. British Journal of Psychiatry 178(suppl 41):148–156

Dunner D 2000 Optimizing lithium treatment. Journal of Clinical Psychiatry 61(suppl 9):76–80

Ernst E 1999 Second thoughts about safety of St John's wort. Lancet 354:2014–2015

Gelder M, Mayou R, Cowen P et al 2000 Cognitive impairment syndromes with specific psychological dysfunctions. Oxford Textbook of Psychiatry, 3rd edn. Oxford University Press, Oxford, p 314–316, 449–450

Gillman P 1999 The serotonin syndrome and its treatment. Journal of Psychopharmacology 13:100–109

Green I, Patel JK, Goisman RM 2000 Weight gain from novel antipsychotic drugs: need for action. General Hospital Psychiatry 22:224–235

Hasan S, Buckley P 1998 Novel antipsychotics and the neuroleptic malignant syndrome; a review and critique. American Journal of Psychiatry 155:1113–1136

Hypericum depression study group 2002 The effect of *Hypericum perforatum* (St John's wort) in major depressive disorder. Journal of the American Medical Association 287:1807–1814

Jobst K, Wheatley D 2000 Safety of St John's wort (*Hypericum perforatum*). Lancet 355:575–576

Lancaster T 2000 Effectiveness of interventions to help people stop smoking: findings from the Cochrane Library. British Medical Journal 321:355–357

Lingford-Hughes A, Potokar J, Nutt D 2002 Treating anxiety complicated by substance misuse. Advances in Psychiatric Treatment 8:107–716

Luty J 2002 Nicotine addiction and smoking cessation treatments. Advances in Psychiatric Treatment 8:42–48

Mason B 2001 Treatment of alcohol-dependent out-patients with acamprosate: A clinical review. Journal of Clinical Psychiatry 62(suppl 20):42–47

McKeith I 2002 Dementia with Lewy bodies. British Journal of Psychiatry 180:144–147

Meager D 2001 Delirium: optimizing management. British Medical Journal 322:144–149

Meager D 2001 Delirium: the role of psychiatry. Advances in Psychiatric Treatment 7:433–443

Niaura R, Abrams D 2001 Stopping smoking: a hazard for people with a history of major depression? Lancet 357:1900–1901

Peet M 2002 Essential fatty acids: theoretical aspects and treatment implications for schizophrenia and depression. Advances in Psychiatric Treatment 8:223–229

Powell P, Bentall R, Nye F, Edwards R 2001 Randomized controlled trial of patient education to encourage graded exercise in chronic fatigue syndrome. British Medical Journal 322:387–389

Raistrick D 2000 Management of alcohol detoxification. Advances in Psychiatric Treatment 6:348–354

Reid S, Chalder T, Cleare A et al 2000 Extracts from clinical evidence: chronic fatigue. British Medical Journal 320:292–296

Snowden J, Neary D, Mann D 2002 Frontotemporal dementia. British Journal of Psychiatry 180:140–143

Stewart R 2002 Vascular dementia: a diagnosis running out of time. British Journal of Psychiatry 180:152–155

World Health Organization 1998 Pocket guide to the ICD-10 classification of mental and behavioural disorders. Churchill Livingstone, London, p 131–137

MISCELLANEOUS ANSWERS

Age-related Eye Disease Study Group 2001 A randomised, placebo-controlled clinical trial of high-dose supplementation with vitamins C and E, beta carotene, and zinc for age-related macular degeneration and vision loss. Archives of Ophthalmology 119:1417–1436

Arya O P 1996 Tropical STDs. Medicine 24:18–21

Bartalena L, Marcocci C, Bogazzi F et al 1998 Relation between therapy for hyperthyroidism and the course of Graves' ophthalmopathy. New England Journal of Medicine 338:73–78

Denniston A, Dodson P, Reuser T 2002 Diagnosis and management of thyroid eye disease. Hospital Medicine 63:152–157

DVLA 2001 At-a-glance guide to current medical standards of fitness to drive. Drivers Medical Unit, DVLA, Swansea, p 2–31

Fielder A R, Bentley C, Moseley M J 1999 Recent advances: ophthalmology. British Medical Journal 318:717–720

Hall N F, Gale C L, Syddall H et al 2001 Risk of macular degeneration in users of statins: cross sectional study. British Medical Journal 323:375–376

Hughes G, Fenton K A 2001 Epidemiology of STIs: UK. Medicine 29:1–2

Mabey D 2001 Epidemiology of STIs: worldwide. Medicine 29:3–5

Taylor H R, Tikellis G, Robman L D et al 2002 Vitamin E supplementation and macular degeneration: randomised controlled trial. British Medical Journal 325:11–14

Wong T Y 2001 Effect of increasing age on cataract surgery outcomes in very elderly patients. British Medical Journal 322:1104–1106

INFECTIOUS DISEASES

Barlow G D, Nathwani D, Davey P 2001 Appropriate antimicrobial prescribing. Report on a joint symposium between the Royal College of Physicians,

Edinburgh and the Royal Pharmaceutical Society of Great Britain. Proceedings of the Royal College of Physicians, Edinburgh 31:310–316

Begg N, Cartwright K A V, Cohen J et al 1999 Consensus statement on diagnosis, investigation, treatment and prevention of acute bacterial meningitis in immunocompetent adults. Journal of Infection 39:1–15

Bernard G R, Vincent J-L, Laterre P-F et al 2001 Efficacy and safety of recombinant human activated protein C for severe sepsis. New England Journal of Medicine 344:699–709

British Medical Association, Royal Pharmaceutical Society of Great Britain 2001 *Helicobacter pylori* infection. British National Formulary, September 42:37

Cassell G H 1998 Infectious causes of chronic inflammatory diseases and cancer. Emerging Infectious Diseases 4:475–487

Farr B M, Salgado C D, Karchmer T B, Sherertz R J 2001 Can antibiotic-resistant nosocomial infections be controlled? Lancet, Infectious Diseases 1:38–45

Friedland J 1998 Cytokines in infectious diseases. Journal of the Royal College of Physicians, London 32:195–198

Gubareva L V, Kaiser L, Hayden F G 2000 Influenza virus neuraminidase inhibitors. Lancet 355:827–835

Guzmán M G, Goustavo K 2001 Dengue: an update. Lancet Infectious Diseases 2:33–42

Jeljaszewicz J 1996 The epidemiology of the systemic inflammatory response syndrome. Current Opinion in Infectious Disease 9:261–264

Lanciotti R S, Roehrig J T, Deubal V et al 1999 West Nile virus confirmed as cause of an encephalitis outbreak in the New York region. Science 286:2333–2337

Lorber B 1996 Are all diseases infectious? Annals of Internal Medicine 125:844–851

Members of the American College of Chest Physicians/Society of Critical Care Medicine Consensus Conference Committee 1992 Members of the American College of Chest Physicians/Society of Critical Care Medicine consensus conference: definitions of sepsis and organ failure and guidelines for the use of innovative therapies in sepsis. Critical Care Medicine 20:864–874

Monath T P 2001 Yellow fever: an update. Lancet Infectious Diseases 1:11–20

Morgan-Capner P, Crowcroft N S, on behalf of the PHLS Joint Working Party of the Advisory Committees of Virology and Vaccines and Immunisation 2002 Guidelines on the management of, and exposure to, rash illness in pregnancy (including consideration of relevant antibody screening programmes in pregnancy). Communicable Disease and Public Health 5:59–71

Nadelman R B, Wormser G P 1998 Lyme borreliosis. Lancet 352:557–565

Nathwani D, Maclean A, Conway S, Carrington D 1998 Varicella infection in pregnancy and the newborn. Journal of Infection 36:59–71

Oliveira E C, Marik P E, Colice G 2001 Influenza pneumonia: a descriptive study. Chest 119:1717–1723

Public Health Laboratory Service. Information available online: www.phls.co.uk

Raoult D, Foucault C, Brouqui P 2001 Infections in the homeless. Lancet, Infectious Diseases 1:77–84

Salgado C D, Farr B M, Hall K K, Hayden F G 2002 Influenza in the acute hospital setting. Lancet Infectious Diseases 2:145–155

Scottish Centre for Infection and Environmental Health. Information available online: www.show.scot.nhs.uk/scieh

Standing Medical Advisory Committee Sub-Group on Antimicrobial Resistance 1998 The path of least resistance. Department of Health, London

Stuart J M, Gilmore A B, Ross A et al 2001 Preventing secondary meningococcal disease in health care workers: recommendations of a working group of the PHLS Meningococcus Forum. Communicable Disease and Public Health 4:102–105

Swartz M N 2001 Recognition and management of anthrax – an update. New England Journal of Medicine 345: 1621–1626

WHO 2000 Overcoming antimicrobial resistance. World health report on infectious diseases 2000. Online. Available: www.who.int/infectious-disease-report/2000/index-rpt2000_text.html

Wormser G P, Nadelman R B, Dattwyler R J et al 2000 Practice guidelines for the treatment of Lyme disease. Clinics in Infectious Diseases 31(suppl 1):S1–S14

Yeung S, Davies E Gm 2001 Infection in the fetus and neonate. Medicine 29:78–83

GASTROENTEROLOGY

Ahmad T, Armuzzi A, Bunce M et al 2002 The molecular classification of the clinical manifestations of Crohn's disease. Gastroenterology 122:854–866

Barrett S, Goh J, Coughlan B et al 2001 The natural course of hepatitis C virus infection after 22 years in a unique homogenous cohort: spontaneous viral clearance and chronic HCV infection. Gut 49:423–430

Booth J C, O'Grady J, Neuberger J et al 2001 Clinical guidelines on the management of hepatitis C. Gut 49(suppl 1):i1–i21

Cole T R, Sleightholme H V 2000 ABC of colorectal cancer. The role of clinical genetics in management. British Medical Journal 321:943–946

Day C P 2002 Non-alcoholic steatohepatitis (NASH): where are we now and where are we going? Gut 50:585–588

Efthimiou E, Crnogorac-Jurcevic T, Lemoine N R, Brentnall T A 2001 Inherited predisposition to pancreatic cancer. Gut 48:143–147

El-Omar E M 2001 The importance of interleukin 1 beta in *Helicobacter pylori* associated disease. Gut 48:743–747

Elson C O 2002 Genes, microbes, and T cells – new therapeutic targets in Crohn's disease. New England Journal of Medicine 346:614–616

Goel A, Arnold C N, Boland C R 2001 Multistep progression of colorectal cancer in the setting of microsatellite instability: new details and novel insights. Gastroenterology 1497–1502

Goodwin C S, Mendall M M, Northfield T C 2002 *Helicobacter pylori* infection. Lancet 349:265–269

Hanauer S B, Feagan B G, Lichtenstein G R et al 2002 Maintenance infliximab for Crohn's disease: the ACCENT 1 randomised trial. Lancet 359:1541–1549

Houlston R, Crabtree M, Phillips R et al 2001 Explaining differences in the severity of familial adenomatous polyposis and the search for modifier genes. Gut 48:1–5

Medical Research Council Oesophageal Cancer Working Party 2002 Surgical resection with or without preoperative chemotherapy in oesophageal cancer: a randomised controlled trial. Lancet 359:1727–1733

Parkes M, Jewell D 2001 Ulcerative colitis and Crohn's disease: molecular genetics and clinical implications. Expert Reviews in Molecular Medicine 19: 1–18. Online. Available: www.ermm.cbcu.cam.ac.uk/010039Ixh.htm

Present D H, Rutgeerts P, Targan S et al 1999 Infliximab for the treatment of fistulas in patients with Crohn's disease. New England Journal of Medicine 340:1398–1405

Ransohoff D F, Sandler R S 2002 Screening for colorectal cancer. New England Journal of Medicine 346:40–44

Reid A E 2001 Nonalcoholic steatohepatitis. Gastroenterology 121:710–723

Rhodes J M 2000 Colorectal cancer screening in the UK: joint position statement by the British Society of Gastroenterology, the Royal College of Physicians, and the Association of Coloproctology of Great Britain and Ireland. Gut 46:746–748

UK Flexible Sigmoidoscopy Screening Trial Investigators 2002 Single flexible sigmoidoscopy screening to prevent colorectal cancer: baseline findings of a UK multicentre randomised trial. Lancet 359:1291–1300

Wheeler J M D, Mortensen N J McC 2000 DNA mismatch repair genes and colorectal cancer. Gut 47:148–153

NEPHROLOGY

Andrews P A 2002 Renal transplantation. British Medical Journal 324:530–534

Bhil G, Meyers A 2001 Recurrent renal stone disease – advances in pathogenesis and management. Lancet 358:651–656

Borghi L, Schianchi T, Meschi T et al 2002 Comparison of two diets for the prevention of recurrent stones in idiopathic hypercalciuria. New England Journal of Medicine 346:77–84

Cahalan M D 2002 The ins and outs of polycystin-2 as a calcium release channel. Nature Cell Biology 4:E56–E57

Casadevall N, Nataf J, Viron B et al 2002 Pure red cell aplasia and anti-erythropoietin antibodies in patients treated with recombinant EPO. New England Journal of Medicine 346:469–475

Cattran D C 2001 Idiopathic membranous glomerulonephritis. Kidney International 59:1983–1994

Cooper M E 1998 Pathogenesis, prevention and treatment of diabetic nephropathy. Lancet 352:213–219

Ducloux D, Bresson-Vautrin C, Chalopin J 2001 Use of pentoxifylline in membranous nephropathy. Lancet 357:1672–1673

Flanigan R C, Salmon S E, Blumenstein B A et al 2001 Nephrectomy followed by interferon alfa2b compared with interferon alone for metastatic renal cell cancer. New England Journal of Medicine 345:1655–1659

Foggensteiner L, Mulroy S, Firth J 2001 Management of diabetic nephropathy. Journal of the Royal Society of Medicine 94:210–217

Halloran P F, Melk A, Barth C 1999 Rethinking chronic allograft nephropathy. Journal of the American Society of Nephrology 10:167–181

Harris P C 2002 Molecular basis of polycystic kidney disease. Current Opinion in Nephrology and Hypertension 11:309–314

Karumanchi S A, Merchan J, Sukhatme V P 2002 Renal cancer: molecular mechanisms and newer therapeutic options. Current Opinion in Nephrology and Hypertension 11(1):37–42

Kugler A, Stuhler G, Walden P et al 2000 Regression of human metastatic renal cell carcinoma after vaccination with tumour cell-endritic cell hybrids. Nature Medicine 6:332–336

Levy J 2001 New aspects in the management of ANCA-positive vasculitis. Nephrology, Dialysis, Transplantation 16:1314–1317

Macdougall I C, Cooper A 2002 The inflammatory response and EPO sensitivity. Nephrology, Dialysis, Transplantation 17(S1):48–52

Margreiter R 2002 Efficacy and safety of tacrolimus compared with ciclosporin microemulsion in renal transplantation: a randomised multicentre study. Lancet 359:741–746

Morton A R, Iliescu E A, Wilson J W 2002 Investigation and treatment of recurrent kidney stones. Canadian Medical Association Journal 166:213–218

Parving H H, Lehnert H, Brochner-Mortensen J et al 2001 The effect of irbesartan on the development of diabetic nephropathy in patients with type 2 diabetes. New England Journal of Medicine 345:870–878

Pascual M, Theruvath T, Kawai T et al 2002 Strategies to improve long-term outcomes after renal transplantation. New England Journal of Medicine 346:580–590

Peters D J, Breuning M H 2001 Autosomal dominant polycystic kidney disease: modification of disease progression. Lancet 354:1439–1444

Ponticelli C, Passerini P 2001 Treatment of membranous nephropathy. Nephrology, Dialysis, Transplantation 16(S5):8–10

Proceedings of the 10th International Vasculitis and ANCA workshop 2002 Cleveland Clinic Journal of Medicine 69(suppl 2)

Saunders R N, Metcalfe M S, Nicholson M L 2001 Rapamycin in renal transplantation: a review of the evidence. Kidney International 59:3–16

Savage C O S 2001 ANCA-associated renal vasculitis. Kidney International 60:1614–1627

Torres A, Dominguez-Gil B, Carreno C et al 2002 Conservative versus immunosuppressive treatment of patients with idiopathic membranous nephropathy. Kidney International 61:219–227

Update on all European vasculitis trials run by EUVAS, including CYCLOPS and MEPEX. Online. Available: www.vasculitis.org

Valderrabano F 2002 Anaemia management in chronic kidney disease patients: an overview of current practice. Nephrology, Dialysis, Transplantation 17(S1):13–18

Waugh N R, Robertson A M 2000 Protein restriction for diabetic renal disease. Cochrane Database System Review 2:CD002181

GENETICS

Aitman T J 2001 DNA microarrays in medical practice. British Medical Journal 323:611–615

Banks R E, Dunn M J, Hochstrasser D F et al 2000 Proteomics: new perspectives, new biomedical opportunities. Lancet 356:1749–1756

Brugarolas J, Haynes B F, Nevins J R 2001 Towards a genomic-based diagnosis. Lancet 357:249–250

Sampath D, Plunkett W 2001 Design of new anticancer therapies targeting cell cycle checkpoint pathways. Current Opinons in Oncology 13(6):484–490

IMMUNOLOGY

Armstrong A, Eaton D, Ewing J C 2001 Cellular immunotherapy for cancer. British Medical Journal 323:1289–1293

Bell S, Kamm M A 2000 Antibodies to TNFα as treatment for Crohn's disease. Lancet 355:858–860

Bolland S, Ravetch J V 2000 Spontaneous autoimmune disease in FcgRIIB-deficient mice results in strain-specific epistasis. Immunity 13:277–285

Breedveld F C 2000 Therapeutic monoclonal antibodies. Lancet 355:735–740

Cobleigh M A, Vogel C L, Tripathy D et al 1999 Multinational study of efficacy and safety of humanised anti-HER2 monoclonal antibody in women who have HER-2 overexpressing metastatic breast cancer that has progressed after chemotherapy. Journal of Clinical Oncology 17:2639–2648

Davidson A, Diamond B 2001 Autoimmune disease. New England Journal of Medicine 345(5):340–350

Drewe E, Powell R J 2002 Clinically useful monoclonal antibodies in treatment. Journal of Clinical Pathology 55:81–85

Jager E, Jager D, Knuth A 2002 Clinical cancer vaccine trials. Current Opinion in Immunology 14:178–182

Jayne D R, Chapel H, Adu D et al 2000 Intravenous immunoglobulin for ANCA-associated systemic vasculitis with persistant disease activity. Quarterly Journal of Medicine 93:433–439

Kamradt T, Mitchison N A 2001 Tolerance and autoimmunity. New England Journal of Medicine 334:655–664

Kazatchkine M D, Kaveri S V 2001 Immunomodulation of autoimmune and inflammatory diseases with intravenous immune globulin. New England Journal of Medicine 345:747–755

O'Shea J J, Ma A, Lipsky P 2002 Cytokines and autoimmunity. Nature Reviews. Immunology 2:37–45

Pardoll D M 2002 Spinning molecular immunology into successful immunotherapy. Nature Reviews, Immunology 2:227–238

Pisetsky D S, St Clair E W 2001 Progress in the treatment of rheumatoid arthritis. Journal of the American Medical Association 286:2787–2790

Poland G P, Murray D, Bonilla-Guerrero R 2002 New vaccine development. British Medical Journal 324:1315–1319

Sakaguchi S 2001 Regulatory T cells: key controllers of immunologic self tolerance. Cell 101:455–458

Samuelsson A, Towers T L, Ravetch J V 2001 Anti-inflammatory activity of IVIG mediated through the inhibitory Fc receptor. Science 291:484–486

Shevach E M 2002 CD4+ CD25+ suppressor T cells: more questions than answers. Nature Reviews, Immunology 2:389–400

CARDIOLOGY

Abraham W T, Fisher W G, Smith A L et al 2002 Cardiac resynchronization in chronic heart failure. New England Journal of Medicine 346:1845–1853

Cazeau S, Leclercq C, Lavergne T et al 2001 Effects of multisite biventricular pacing in patients with heart failure and intraventricular conduction delay. New England Journal of Medicine 344:873–880

Clopidogrel and acute coronary syndrome. Drug and Therapeutics Bulletin 2002 40:41–42

Connolly S J, Hallstrom A P, Cappato R et al 2000 Meta-analysis of the implantable cardioverter defibrillator secondary prevention trials. AVID, CASH and CIDS studies. Antiarrhythmics vs implantable defibrillator study. Cardiac Arrest Study Hamburg. Canadian Implantable Defibrillator Study. European Heart Journal 21:2071–2078

DVLA 2001 At-a-glance guide to the current medical standards of fitness to drive. DVLA, Swansea

Heart Outcomes Prevention Evaluation (HOPE) Study Investigators 2000 Effects of ramipril on cardiovascular and microvascular outcomes in people with diabetes mellitus: results of the HOPE study and MICRO-HOPE substudy. Lancet 355:253–259

Huikuri H V, Castellanos A, Myerburg R J 2001 Sudden death due to cardiac arrhythmias. New England Journal of Medicine 345:1473–1482

Lloyd-Williams F, Mair F S, Leitner M 2002 Exercise training and heart failure: a systematic review of current evidence. British Journal of General Practice 52:47–55

Morice M C, Serruys P W, Sousa J E et al 2002 A randomized comparison of a sirolimus-eluting stent with a standard stent for coronary revascularization. New England Journal of Medicine 346:1773–1780

MRC/BHF 2002 Heart protection study of cholesterol lowering with simvastatin in 20,536 high-risk individuals: a randomised placebo-controlled trial. Lancet 360:7–22

Pitt B, Zannad F, Remme W J et al (Randomized Aldactone Evaluation Study Investigators) 1999 The effect of spironolactone on morbidity and mortality in patients with severe heart failure. New England Journal of Medicine 341:709–717

Recommendations for exercise training in chronic heart failure patients. European Heart Journal 2001 22:125–135

Recommendations on the management of the asymptomatic patient with valvular heart disease. European Heart Journal 2002 23:1253–1266

Towbin J A, Bowles N S 2001 Molecular genetics of left ventricular dysfunction. Current Molecular Medicine 1:81–90

Yusuf S, Zhao F, Mehta S R 2001 Effects of clopidogrel in addition to aspirin in patients with acute coronary syndromes without ST-segment elevation. New England Journal of Medicine 345:494–502

RHEUMATOLOGY

Bohan A, Peter J B 2000 Polymyositis and dermatomyositis. New England Journal of Medicine 292:344–347, 403–407

Bombardier C, Laine L, Reicin A et al 2000 Comparison of upper gastrointestinal toxicity of rofecoxib and naproxen in patients with rheumatoid arthritis. New England Journal of Medicine 343:1520–1528

Calin A 1998 Ankylosing spondylitis. In: Maddison P J, Isenberg D A, Woo P, Glass D N (eds) Oxford textbook of rheumatology (vol 2). Oxford University Press, Oxford p 681–690

Callen J P 2000 Dermatomyositis. Lancet 355:53–57

Dalakas M C, Illa I, Dambrosia J M et al 1993 A controlled trial of high-dose intravenous immune globulin infusions as treatment for dermatomyositis. New England Journal of Medicine 329:1993–2000

Del Rincon I, Williams K, Stern M et al 2001 High incidence of cardiovascular events in rheumatoid arthritis cohort not explained by traditional cardiac risk factors. Arthritis and Rheumatism 44:2737–2745

Egland A G 2000 Temporal arteritis. eMedicine Journal 2(10). Online. Available: www.emedicine.com

Etanercept and infliximab for rheumatoid arthritis. Drug and Therapeutics Bulletin 39:49–52

Hall F, Walport M 1998 Systemic lupus erythematosis. Medicine 26:5–11

Kirwin J, Edwards A, Huitfeldt B et al 1993 The course of established ankylosing spondylitis and the effects of sulphasalazine over 3 years. British Journal of Rheumatology 32:729–733

Klippel J H 2000 Biological therapy for rheumatoid arthritis. New England Journal of Medicine 343:1640–1641

Manzi S, Meilhn E N, Rairie J E et al 1997 Age specific incidence rates of myocardial infarction and angina in women with SLE: comparison with the Framingham study. American Journal of Epidemiology 145:408–415

Miller M L Pyogenic arthritis in adults. In: Maddison P J, Isenberg D A, Woo P, Glass D N (eds) Oxford textbook of rheumatology (vol 2). Oxford University Press, Oxford p 529–538

NICE 2001 Guidance on COX II inhibitors for osteoarthritis and rheumatoid arthritis (press release 025). Issued 26 July 2001

NSAIDs and COX-2 inhibitors. Internet On-line Medical Monograph Series 1999 9(3). Online. Available: webcampus.med.mcphu.edu/cme/medicine/med_study.html

Nuki G 1998 Gout. Medicine 26:54

Nuki G Crystal arthropathies: calcium pyrophosphate dihydrate (CPPD) deposition. In: Maddison P J, Isenberg D A, Woo P, Glass D N (eds) Oxford textbook of rheumatology (vol 2). Oxford University Press, Oxford p 997–1001

Rahman P, Gladman D D, Urowitz M B et al 1999 The cholesterol lowering effect of antimalarial drugs is enhanced in patients with lupus taking corticosteroid drugs. Journal of Rheumatology 26(2):325–330

Reginster J Y, Deroisy R, Rovati L et al 2001 Long-term effects of glucosamine sulphate on osteoarthritis progression: a randomised, placebo-controlled clinical trial. Lancet 357:251–256

Siguregeirsson B, Lindelöf B, Edhag O, Allander E 1992 Risk of cancer in patients with dermatomyositis or polymyositis. New England Journal of Medicine 325:363–367

Silversteine F, Faich G, Goldsteine J et al 2000 Gastrointestinal toxicity with celecoxib vs non-steroidal anti-inflammatory drugs for osteoarthritis and rheumatoid arthritis: The CLASS study. Journal of the American Medical Association 284:1247–1255

Snaith M L 1995 ABC of rheumatology: gout, hyperuricaemia, and crystal arthritis. British Medical Journal 310:521–524

Sturrock R D 2000 Gout, easy to misdiagnose. British Medical Journal 320:132–133

Svenungsson B 1994 Reactive arthritis. British Medical Journal 308:671–672

Van Doornum S, McColl G, Wicks I P 2002 Accelerated atherosclerosis: an extra-articular feature of rheumatoid arthritis? Arthritis and Rheumatism 46:862–873

EPIDEMIOLOGY

Christen W G, Ajani U A, Glynn R J et al 2000 Blood levels of homocysteine and increased risk of cardiovascular disease: causal or casual? Archives of Internal Medicine 160:422–434

Cleophas T J, Hornstra N, van Hoogstraten B et al 2000 Homocysteine, a risk factor for coronary artery disease or not? A meta-analysis. American Journal of Cardiology 86:1005–1009

Ford E S, Smith S J, Stroup D F et al 2002 Homocysteine and cardiovascular disease: a systematic review of the evidence with special emphasis on case-control studies and nested case-control studies. International Journal of Epidemiology 31:59–70

Hennekens C H, Buring J E, Mayrent S L 1987 Epidemiology in medicine, 1st edn. Little Brown, Boston

Last J M 1995 A dictionary of epidemiology, 3rd edn. Oxford University Press, New York

NEUROLOGY

Ad hoc Subcommittee of the American Academy of Neurology AIDS Task Force 1991 Research criteria for diagnosis of chronic inflammatory demyelinating polyneuropathy (CIDP). Neurology 41:617–618

Association of British Neurologists 2001 Guidelines for the use of beta interferon and glatiramer acetate in multiple sclerosis. January 2001

Berger P, Young P, Suter U 2002 Molecular cell biology of Charcot–Marie–Tooth disease. Neurogenetics 4:1–15

Canger R, Battino D, Canevini M P et al 1999 Malformations in offspring of women with epilepsy: a prospective study. Epilepsia 40:1231–1236

Clarke C 2000 Medical management of Parkinson's disease. Journal of Neurology, Neurosurgery and Psychiatry 72(suppl 1):122–127

Collinge J 1999 Variant Creutzfeldt–Jakob disease. Lancet 354:317–323

Dalmau J O, Posner J B 1999 Paraneoplastic syndromes. Archives of Neurology 56:405–408

Galton C, Hodges J 1999 The spectrum of dementia and its treatment. Journal of the Royal College of Physicians, London 33:234–239

Hebb A, Cusimano M 2001 Idiopathic normal pressure hydrocephalus: a systemic review of diagnosis and outcome. Neurosurgery 49:1166–1184

IFNB Multiple Sclerosis Study Group 1993 Interferon beta-1b is effective in relapsing-remitting multiple sclerosis. Neurology 43:655–661

Jacobs L D, Cookfair D L, Rudick R A et al 1996 Intramuscular interferon beta-1a for disease progression in relapsing multiple sclerosis. Annals of Neurology 39:285–294

Lindblad K, Schalling M 1999 Expanded repeat sequences and disease. Seminars in Neurology 19(3):289–299

Moore A 2000 What to refer to a neurosurgeon. Medicine 28:82–84

Nobile-Orazio E, Carpo M 2001 Neuropathy and monoclonal gammopathy. Current Opinion in Neurology 14:615–620

Parkinson Study Group 2000 Pramipexole verus levodopa as initial treatment for Parkinson's disease. Journal of the Americal Medical Association 284:1931–1938

Plasma Exchange/Sandoglobulin Guillain–Barré Syndrome Trial Group 1997 A randomised trial of plasma exchange, intravenous immunoglobulin, and combined treatments in Guillain–Barré syndrome. Lancet 349:225–230

PRISMS Study Group 1998 Randomised double-blind placebo controlled study of interferon-1a in relapsing/remitting multiple sclerosis. Lancet 352:1498–1504

Rascol O, Brooks D, Korczyn A et al 2000 A five year study of the incidence of dyskinesia in patients with early Parkinson's disease who were treated with ropinirole or levodopa. New England Journal of Medicine 342:1484–1491

Reiff-Eldridge R, Heffner C R, Ephross S A et al 2000 Monitoring pregnancy outcomes after prenatal drug exposure through prospective pregnancy registries: a pharmaceutical company commitment. American Journal of Obstetrics and Gynecology 182:159–163

Spencer M D, Knight R S, Will R G 2002 First hundred cases of variant Creutzfeldt–Jakob disease: retrospective case note review of early psychiatric and neurological features. British Medical Journal 324:1479–1482

Van der Meche F G, Schmitz P I for the Dutch Guillain–Barré Study Group 1992 A randomised trial comparing intravenous immune globulin and plasma exchange in Guillain–Barré syndrome. New England Journal of Medicine 326:1123–1129

Van Gijn J, Rinhel G J 2001 Subarachnoid haemorrhage: diagnosis, causes and management. Brain 124:249–278

Vincent A, Palace J, Hilton-Jones D 2001 Myasthenia gravis. Lancet 357:2122–2128

Will R G, Zeidler M, Stewart G E et al 2000 Diagnosis of new variant Creutzfeldt–Jakob disease. Annals of Neurology 47:575–582

HAEMATOLOGY

Eikelboom J W, Quinlan D J, Douketis J D 2001 Extended-duration prophylaxis against venous thrombosis after total hip or knee replacement: a meta-analysis of the randomised trials. Lancet 358:9–15

Giardina P J, Grady R W 2001 Chelation therapy in beta-thalassaemia: an optimistic update. Seminars in Hematology 38:360–366

Hankey G J 2000 Clopidogrel and thrombotic thrombocytopenic purpura. Lancet 356:269–270

Kemmeren J M, Algra A, Grobbee D E 2001 Third generation oral contraceptives and risk of venous thrombosis: meta-analysis. British Medical Journal 323:1–9

Lennard A L, Jackson G H 2000 Stem cell transplantation. British Medical Journal 321:433–437

Merson L, Olivier N 2002 Orally active iron chelators. Blood Reviews 16:127–134

Nachbaur D, Bonatti H, Oberaigner W et al 2001 Survival after bone marrow transplantation from cytomegalovirus seropositive sibling donors. Lancet 358:1157–1159

Porte R J, Molenaar I Q, Begliomini B et al 2000 Aprotinin and transfusion requirements in orthotopic liver transplantation: a multicentre randomised double-blind study. Lancet 355:1303–1309

Powles R, Mehta J, Kulkani S et al 2000 Allogeneic blood and bone-marrow stem-cell transplantation in haematological malignant diseases: a randomised trial. Lancet 355:1231–1237

Regan F, Taylor C 2002 Recent developments: blood transfusion medicine. British Medical Journal 325:143–147

Scurr J H, Machin S J, Bailey-King S et al 2001 Frequency and prevention of symptomless deep-vein thrombosis in long-haul flights: a randomised trial. Lancet 357:1485–1489

Taylor C M 2001 Complement factor H and the haemolytic uraemic syndrome. Lancet 358:1200–1202

Todd W T A 2001 Prospects for the prevention of haemolytic-uraemic syndrome. Lancet 359:1636–1638

Weatherall D J, Provan A B 2000 Red cells I: inherited anaemias. Lancet 355:1169–1175

Zornberg G L, Jick H 2000 Antipsychotic drug use and risk of first-time idiopathic venous thromboembolism: a case-control study. Lancet 356:1219–1223

MOLECULAR BIOLOGY

Chaudhari N, Landin A M, Roper S D 2000 A metabotropic glutamate receptor variant functions as a taste receptor. Nature Neuroscience 3:113–119

Donnelly R, Yeung J M 2002 Therapeutic angiogenesis: a step forward in intermittent claudication. Lancet 359:2048–2050

Ebrahim I O, Howard R S, Kopelman M D et al 2002 The hypocretin/orexin system. Journal of the Royal Society of Medicine 95:227–230

Eichhorst S T, Kramner P H 2001 Derangement of apoptosis in cancer. Lancet 358:345–346

Haslett C, Savill J 2001 Why is apoptosis important? British Medical Journal 322:1499–1500

Henry T D 1999 Therapeutic angiogenesis. British Medical Journal 318:1536–1539

Lederman R J, Mendelsohn F O, Anderson R D et al 2002 Therapeutic angiogenesis with recombinant fibroblast growth factor-2 for intermittent claudication (the TRAFFIC study): a randomised trial. Lancet 359:2053–2058

Leonard J V, Schapira A H V 2000a Mitochondrial respiratory chain disorders I: mitochondrial DNA defects. Lancet 355:299–304

Leonard J V, Schapira A H V 2000b Mitochondrial respiratory chain disorders II: neurodegenerative disorders and nuclear gene defects. Lancet 355:389–394

Marban E 2002 Cardiac channelopathies. Nature 415:213–218

Maxwell P H 2002 Oxygen homeostasis and cancer: insights from a rare disease. Clinical Medicine 2:356–362

McKemy D, Neuhausser W M, Julius D 2002 Identification of a cold receptor reveals a general role for TRP channels in thermosensation. Nature 416:52–58

Morris K 2000 Candidate receptor turns on human pheromone debate. Lancet 356:835

Rayman M P 2000 The importance of selenium to human health. Lancet 356:233–241

Renehan A G, Booth C, Potten C S 2001 What is apoptosis, and why is it important? British Medical Journal 322:1536–1538

Rose M R 1998 Neurological channelopathies. British Medical Journal 316:1104–1105

Schuld A, Hebebrand J, Geller F, Pollmacher T 2000 Increased body-mass index in patients with narcolepsy. Lancet 355:1274–1275

Seeman E 2002 Pathogenesis of bone fragility in women and men. Lancet 359:1841–1850

Sjostrom J, Bergh J 2001 How apoptosis is regulated, and what goes wrong in cancer. British Medical Journal 322:1538–1539

Stewart P S, Costerton J W 2001 Antibiotic resistance of bacteria in biofilms. Lancet 358:135–138

Taheri S, Zeitzer J M, Mignot E 2002 The role of hypocretins (orexins) in sleep regulation and narcolepsy. Annual Review of Neuroscience 25:283–313

Waxman S G 2001 Acquired channelopathies in nerve injury and MS. Neurology 56:1621–1627

Zasloff M 2002 Antimicrobial peptides of multicellular organisms. Nature 415:389–395

ONCOLOGY

Baas P 2002 Inductive and adjuvant treatment strategies for localzed nonsmall cell lung cancer in operable and inoperable patients. Current Opinion in Oncology 14:180–184

Batchelor T 2000 Temozolomide for malignant brain tumours. Lancet 355:1115–1116

Body J J 2000 Current and future directions in medical therapy – hypercalcaemia. Cancer 88:3054–3058

Clemons M, Goss P 2001 Estrogen and the risk of breast cancer. New England Journal of Medicine 344:276–285

Diel I J, Solomayer E F, Bastert G 2000 Bisphosphonates and the prevention of metastasis. Cancer 88:3080–3088

Dong C, Hemminki K 2001 Second primary neoplasms among 53,159 haematolymphoproliferative malignancy patients in Sweden, 1958–1996: a search for common mechanisms. British Journal of Cancer 85:997–1005

Glioma Meta-analysis (GMT) Group 2002 Chemotherapy in adult high-grade glioma: a systematic review and meta-analysis of individual patient data from 12 randomised trials. Lancet 359:1011–1018

Hoffman P C, Mauer A M, Vokes E E 2000 Lung cancer. Lancet 355:479–485

Klein M, Heimans J J, Aaronson N K et al 2002 Effect of radiotherapy and other treatment-related factors on mid-term to long-term cognitive sequelae in low-grade gliomas: a comparative study. Lancet 360:1361–1368

Lonning P E 2001 Aromatase inhibitors and inactivators in breast cancer. British Medical Journal 323:880–881

Mundy G R 2002 Metastasis to bone: causes, consequence and therapeutic opportunities. Nature Reviews. Cancer 2:584–593

Ng A K, Bernardo P, Weller E et al 2002 Second malignancy after Hodgkin disease treated with radiation therapy with or without chemotherapy: long-term risks and risk factors. Blood 100:1989–1996

Relling M V, Rubnitz J E, Rivera G K et al 1999 High incidence of secondary brain tumours after radiotherapy and antimetabolites. Lancet 354:34–39

Robison L L 1996 Second primary cancers after childhood cancers. British Medical Journal 312:861–862

Van Klaveren J D, Pedersen J H, de Koning H J et al 2001 Lung cancer screening by low-dose spiral computed tomography. European Respiratory Journal 18:857–866

Writing group for the Women's Health Initiative (WHI) investigators 2002 Risks and benefits of estrogen plus progestin in health postmenopausal women. Journal of the American Medical Association 288:321–333

Abbreviations

ACE	angiotensin converting enzyme
ACTH	adrenocorticotrophic hormone
ADH	antidiuretic hormone
ADP	adenosine diphosphate
ALT	alanine transaminase
ANCA	antineutrophil cytoplasmic antibodies
APS-1	autoimmune polyendocrinopathy syndrome type 1
ATP	adenosine triphosphate
AV	atrioventricular
BCG	bacille Calmette-Guérin
BMI	body mass index
BP	blood pressure
bpm	beats per minute
CI	confidence interval
CK	creatine kinase
CMR1	cold and menthol receptor
CMV	cytomegalovirus
CNS	central nervous system
COPD	chronic obstructive pulmonary disease
COX	cyclo-oxygenase
CPAP	continuous positive airway pressure
CPEO	chronic progressive external ophthalmoplegia
CPK	creatine phosphokinase
CRP	C-reactive protein
CSF	cerebrospinal fluid
CT	computerised tomography
CVA	cerebrovascular accident
DNA	deoxyribonucleic acid
EBV	Epstein–Barr virus
ECG	electrocardiograph
EEG	electroencephalograph
ELISA	enzyme-linked immunosorbent assay
EMG	electromyography
ERCP	endoscopic retrograde cholangiopancreatography
ESR	erythrocyte sedimentation rate
ET	endothelin
FAP	familial adenomatous polyposis
FEV_1	forced expiratory volume in 1 second
FGF	fibroblast growth factor
FVC	forced vital capacity
GABA	gamma-aminobutyric acid
GAD	glutamic acid decarboxylase
GCS	Glasgow coma score

GM-CSF	granulocyte–macrophage colony stimulating factor
HbA1c	glycosylated haemoglobin
hCG	human chorionic gonadotrophin
HDL	high density lipoprotein
HHV	human herpesvirus
HIV	human immunodeficiency virus
HLA	human leucocyte antigen
HMSN	hereditary motor sensory neuropathy
HUS	haemolytic–uraemic syndrome
IAA	islet-associated antigens
IBD	inflammatory bowel disease
ICD-10	International classification of disease, version 10
IFN	interferon
IgA	immunoglobulin A
IgE	immunoglobulin E
IGF	insulin-like growth factor
IgG	immunoglobulin G
IgM	immunoglobulin M
IU	international unit
LDH	lactate dehydrogenase
LDL	low density lipoprotein
LVH	left ventricular hypertrophy
MELAS	myoclonus, epilepsy, lactic acidosis and stroke-like episodes
MEN	multiple endocrine neoplasia
MERRF	myoclonic epilepsy with ragged red fibres
MHC	major histocompatibility complex
MRI	magnetic resonance imaging
MRSA	methycillin-resistant *Stapylococcus aureus*
NF-κB	nuclear factor-κB
NICE	National Institute for Clinical Excellence
NMDA	N-methyl-d-aspartate
NSAIDs	non-steroidal anti-inflammatory drugs
NYHA	New York Heart Association
PCR	polymerase chain reaction
PET	positron emission tomography
PGE_2	prostaglandin E_2
PGI_2	prostaglandin I_2
PMP	peripheral myelin protein
POEMS	polyneuropathy, organomegaly, endocrinopathy, monoclonal band, skin changes
PPAR-γ	peroxisome proliferator-activated receptor gamma
PTH	parathyroid hormone
PTHrP	parathyroid hormone-related peptide
PUVA	psoralen + ultraviolet A
RANK	receptor activator of nuclear factor-κB
RCC	renal cell carcinoma
RNA	ribonucleic acid
rtPA	recombinant tissue plasminogen activator
SLE	systemic lupus erythematosus
SSRI	serotonin reuptake inhibitor
TGF	transforming growth factor

Th1 cells	type 1 helper T cells
Th2 cells	type 2 helper T cells
TIA	transient ischaemic attack
TNF	tumour necrosis factor
TRAIL	TNF-related apoptosis-inducing ligand
TSH	thyroid stimulating hormone
TTP	thrombotic thrombocytopenic purpura
UKPDS	UK prospective diabetes study
UV	ultraviolet
UVA	ultraviolet wavelength A
UVB	ultraviolet wavelength B
vCJD	variant Creutzfeldt–Jakob disease
VQ scan	ventilation perfusion isotope scan
VVI pacing	fixed rate ventricular pacing
VZV	varicella zoster virus
WCC	white cell count
WHO	World Health Organization

Index

Page numbers in italic indicate tables